The Geriatric Admission

A Handbook for Hospitalists

Other World Scientific Titles by the Editor

M(odified) E(ssay) Q(uestions) for Medicine Finals
With Solutions and Tips
Volume 3
ISBN: 978-981-122-855-1
ISBN: 978-981-123-009-7 (pbk)

M(odified) E(ssay) Q(uestions) for Medicine Finals
With Solutions and Tips
Volume 2
ISBN: 978-981-3109-54-4
ISBN: 978-981-3109-55-1 (pbk)

M(odified) E(ssay) Q(uestions) for Medicine Finals
With Solutions and Tips
ISBN: 978-981-4412-28-5 (pbk)

The Geriatric Admission

A Handbook for Hospitalists

Derrick Chen Wee Aw
Sengkang General Hospital, Singapore

Anupama Roy Chowdhury
Singapore General Hospital, Singapore

World Scientific

NEW JERSEY • LONDON • SINGAPORE • BEIJING • SHANGHAI • HONG KONG • TAIPEI • CHENNAI • TOKYO

Published by

World Scientific Publishing Co. Pte. Ltd.
5 Toh Tuck Link, Singapore 596224
USA office: 27 Warren Street, Suite 401-402, Hackensack, NJ 07601
UK office: 57 Shelton Street, Covent Garden, London WC2H 9HE

British Library Cataloguing-in-Publication Data
A catalogue record for this book is available from the British Library.

THE GERIATRIC ADMISSION
A Handbook for Hospitalists

ISBN 978-981-127-069-7 (hardcover)
ISBN 978-981-127-130-4 (paperback)
ISBN 978-981-127-070-3 (ebook for institutions)
ISBN 978-981-127-071-0 (ebook for individuals)

For any available supplementary material, please visit
https://www.worldscientific.com/worldscibooks/10.1142/13260#t=suppl

Contents

List of Contributors (in Alphabetical Order)

Angkodjojo, Stanley (Rheumatology)
Aw, Chen Wee, Derrick (Dermatology)
Cai, Jiashen (Renal Medicine)
Chawla, Mayank (Renal Medicine)
Chen, Weizhen, Jessica (Geriatric Medicine)
Cheong, Li Anne (Internal Medicine)
Chowdhury, Anupama Roy (Geriatric Medicine)
Chua, Peng Wei, Melvin (Geriatric Medicine)
Chuah, Tyng Yu (Rheumatology)
Foo, Swee Sen (Geriatric Medicine)
Goh, Kai Heng, Raymond (Geriatric Medicine)
Goh, Teow Koon, Jonathan (Gastroenterology)
Guo, Weiwen (Renal Medicine)
Hanif, Muhammad Ibrahim (Internal Medicine)
Ho, Huimin, Kayleigh (Internal Medicine)
Koh, Chien Hsiang, Cedric (Internal Medicine)
Koh, Hsien Hui, Kenneth (Respiratory Medicine)
Kwan, Kah Wai, Clarence (Gastroenterology)
Lee, Pei Shan (Renal Medicine)
Lee, Wai Ching, Deanna (Internal Medicine)
Lim, Kai Xiong (Internal Medicine)
Lim, Shao Jiao, Dorcas (Internal Medicine)
Lingegowda, Pushpalatha Bangalore (Infectious Disease)
Mahesh, Lalmalani Roshan (Geriatric Medicine)
Moy, Wai Lun (Internal Medicine)
Naing, Chaw Su (Internal Medicine)
Narasimhalu, Kaavya (Neurology)
Ng, Kwan Geok (Rehabilitation Medicine)
Peh, Wee Ming (Internal Medicine)
Phoon, Yee Wei (Dermatology)
Roslan, Nur Emillia (Rheumatology)
Sachdeva, Pooja (Internal Medicine)

See, Kee Yon, Lionel (Internal Medicine)
Sivagame, Maniya (D/O) (Advance Specialty Care Nursing)
Soh, Xiao Jue, Jade (Infectious Disease)
Suantio, Astrid Melani (Geriatric Medicine)
Tan, Boon Hian (Geriatric Medicine)
Tan, Wee Beng, Alvin (Geriatric Medicine)
Tan, Yan, Denise (Haematology)
Tay, Sok Boon (Respiratory Medicine)
Teh, Swee Ping (Renal Medicine)
Teo, Qiao Qi (Rehabilitation Medicine)
Tey, Tze Tong (Gastroenterology)
Than, Zaw Oo (Internal Medicine)
Wong, Hwei May, Victoria (Palliative Medicine)
Wong, Shan Li, Shandy (Geriatric Medicine)
Yeoh, Lee Ying (Renal Medicine)
Yiu, Cheung, Richard (Haematology)
Zheng, Shuwei (Infectious Disease)

Foreword by Pang Weng Sun

Issues related to care of the elderly in Singapore were highlighted in the Ministry of Health's Report by the Committee on the Problems of the Aged in 1984. This led to the setting up of the first Geriatric Medicine Department in Tan Tock Seng Hospital in 1988 and by 2000, hospital departments and community services were established nationwide.

In 1996, the Gerontological Society published the first local textbook *Geriatric Medicine for Singapore* and in 1997, the Ministry of Health released a second book, *Caring for the Elderly: a Guide for Family Physicians. Medicine and Surgery in the Older Person* was co-written by colleagues from both Hong Kong and Singapore and was published in 2000. It is indeed timely now for a new and updated local publication on the subject.

In this latest book, the authors have adopted a very practical, problem-based approach to clinical challenges in the elderly. Each chapter deals with a common presenting problem, with typical symptoms and complaints that clinicians regularly encounter in practice. Thought-provoking questions lead the reader on a journey of clinical reasoning to arrive at not just a diagnosis but also the issues faced by the patient. Treatment options are offered and discussed. Key messages summarise the issues in each case and references are provided for further reading. This pedagogical approach certainly makes the book an interesting read and an excellent resource for teaching.

I have no doubt that clinicians both in hospitals and primary care practices will find this book useful. Residents will appreciate the problem-oriented approach. These case studies can also be used for tutorials on the topics.

My congratulations to the team on this excellent piece of work. Care of the elderly in Singapore has progressed considerably over the years and it is great to see our colleagues continuing this journey of improvement.

Professor Pang Weng Sun
Dean, Healthcare Leadership College, MOHH
Vice Dean, Clinical Affairs, Lee Kong Chian School of Medicine
Senior Consultant, Geriatric Medicine, Khoo Teck Puat Hospital

Foreword by
Teo Eng Kiong

I have always believed that the practice of holistic medicine is the way to deliver excellent care to the patient. I read this book with enthusiasm and nostalgia. Enthusiasm as every case reflects the daily clinical challenges faced by our clinicians in our acute wards; nostalgia as it brings back memories of the teachings from my mentors who were both astute diagnosticians and experts in therapeutics in their field of specialty.

A typical patient in our acute wards, regardless of whether the patient was admitted for orthopaedic, surgical, or medical issues, is likely to be in the geriatric age group and has multiple comorbidities that increase the complexity of care. The collection of cases in this book reflects the daily challenges faced by the authors of the chapters and how they have assessed the patients to make an accurate diagnosis and deliver the care that matters to the patient. From physical challenges like falls to psychological, physiological, and end-of-life matters, this book takes a holistic approach with questions that nudge the reader to think critically. The answers serve as a guide rather than a prescription to stimulate the reader to think even further on how they can combine the science of the subject with the art of medicine to cater to the specific needs of their own patients.

I will certainly recommend this book to any person who practises in the clinical realm — doctors, nurses, pharmacists, and other allied health professionals. As you read through the chapters, think about our past patients as they were our best teachers. With the knowledge shared by the authors, consider how you can improve your care delivery to your future patients.

Enjoy.

Professor Teo Eng Kiong
Deputy Group Chairman Medical Board (Regional Hospital Network), Singhealth
Chief Executive Officer, Sengkang General Hospital
Senior Consultant, Internal Medicine and Gastroenterology
Singapore

Preface by Anupama Roy Chowdhury

As a geriatrician practising geriatric medicine as well as looking after general medicine patients in a busy regional hospital, what has struck me over the years is the increasing proportion of older patients and their increasing multimorbidity and complexity as they live longer. Age-related changes and their heterogeneity can make diagnosis and management challenging, leaving the clinician overwhelmed as he or she tries to make sense of atypical presentations with non-specific symptoms to come up with a working diagnosis and holistic management plan. Looking after the older person doesn't end with sorting out medical issues and almost always requires attention to function and social needs as well.

Given the rapidly ageing population, all doctors regardless of specialty (with the exception of paediatrics and neonatology) will need to have some basic knowledge of medicine for the older individual and a practical approach to the elderly patient. I am grateful to my colleague, Dr Derrick Aw, for spearheading this book and inviting me to join him in this endeavour.

I am grateful to all the contributors for making the time and effort despite their busy schedules to write their chapters and review them. Without their precious contributions and support, this book wouldn't exist.

We hope this makes for an enjoyable read and at the same time provides the reader with useful and practical tips that can be used in daily practice.

Dr Anupama Roy Chowdhury
Head and Senior consultant, Department of Geriatric Medicine,
Singapore General Hospital

Preface by Derrick Aw

As specialists in a regional hospital, my colleagues and I contribute significantly to general medicine inpatient work and in the course of doing so, encounter a considerable number of elderly patients in the wards. We do have a strong geriatric team, but they would no doubt be overwhelmed if every single geriatric case gets referred to them. As such, I conceived of this guide which would benefit not just ourselves but our medical officers, medical students, advanced practice nurses, family medicine physicians, and so on — essentially the non-geriatricians — so that we can all manage our patients more capably, appropriately, and holistically.

This guide is the product of a close collaboration between the general medicine and geriatric faculties in our department. Anupama and I began by brainstorming the commonest clinical situations in the general medicine setting, and then we invited contributors from the department. Specialists were tagged with geriatricians for the various chapters. I am deeply appreciative of their dedication and immensely thankful for their patience with the multiple rounds of vets and edits. I am grateful to my colleague and friend, Associate Professor Melvin Chua Peng Wei, Chair of Division of Medicine, for his steadfast support for the writing of this book. I also wish to thank Benjamin Ng for his secretarial assistance.

This is not a textbook. Basic medical knowledge is presumed, but certain background information will be highlighted where we deem it helpful to aid understanding. Some thematic concepts may appear repetitive, but as I always tell my students and younger educators, repetition is always good for reinforcement!

I hope you will enjoy reading and learning from the fruits of our efforts as much as I have delighted in writing and editing this book. More importantly, I hope we can all chip in to adequately and more confidently handle the silver tsunami which is looming upon us as you are reading this.

A/Prof Derrick Aw Chen Wee
Campus Education Director, Sengkang General Hospital
Senior consultant, Dermatology, Singapore

Introduction

Congratulations on purchasing this extraordinary book! Whether you are a general practitioner, polyclinic doctor, resident in a general medicine ward, advanced practice nurse, or even a medical student, you will find this guide useful in bringing greater awareness, diagnostic insight, and therapeutic reasoning to the breadth of medical problems commonly encountered in the elderly.

You probably have already seen the content page — each chapter is a clinical presentation of an elderly patient. However, there is another content page at the back of the book! It is what you may refer to *after* you have completed this book — each chapter is the same clinical presentation but with corresponding thematic highlights. The index may be helpful if you need to perform rapid searches.

The premise for each chapter is based on a realistic clinical scenario. Do attempt the questions littered throughout the chapters — as you read the subsequent text, you will be able to reflect upon your initial thoughts and answers. You will find the recommended solutions at the end of each chapter which, together with the key messages, will help fortify your learning of the topic. Each chapter is bursting with practical pointers and geriatric pearls that you can immediately use when you encounter your next geriatric patient! Where there are alternative drugs suitable for a condition, we have included the latest estimated costings to give you an additional perspective in your decision-making process. Chapters are self-contained and can probably be read in any order, though we recommend reading from front to back.

Now it's time to enjoy the book.

1 Falls I (Blood Pressure Changes)

Moy Wai Lun, Astrid Melani Suantio

A 65-year-old man, resident of a psychiatric institution, was admitted to the acute hospital for two episodes of fall preceded by dizziness. He has a past medical history of Parkinson disease with dementia, cervical spondylosis, lumbar stenosis which was surgically decompressed, and major depressive disorder.

Question 1: Based on this short provision of the patient's condition, what are some of the predisposing factors for fall in this patient?

Multiple factors often predispose and/or precipitate the fall in an elderly patient. Most of the times, a thorough physical examination and history taking can elucidate the risk factors for the fall. A detailed fall risk assessment includes:

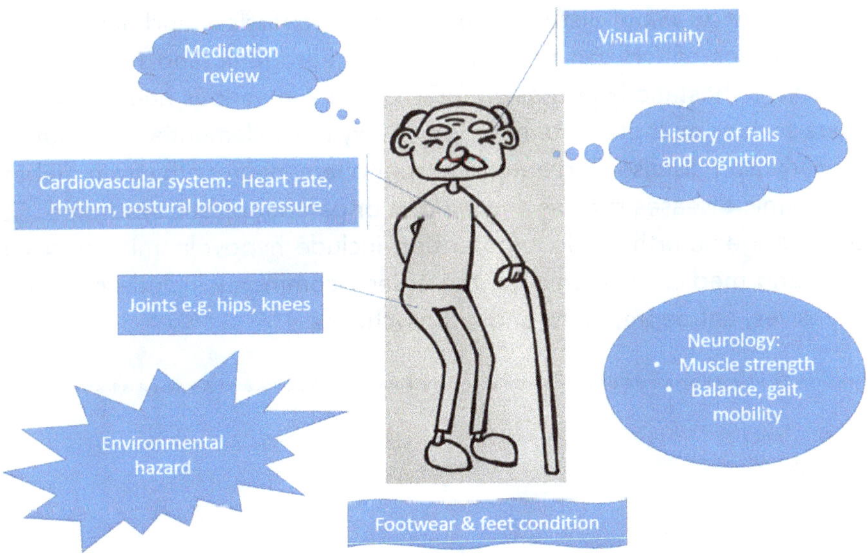

Illustrating elements of a detailed fall assessment. (Graphic by Ms Tan Wanjun.)

If you are unsure about the risk of falls after your initial assessment, you can always ask your friendly geriatrician to further elucidate the risk factors in your patient.

****

The team reviewing the patient noticed that his lying, sitting, and standing blood pressures (BP) were very different:

BP while lying down was 131/78 mmHg
BP while sitting was 103/69 mmHg
BP while standing was 88/61 mmHg

The patient felt very giddy and could not stand for another 3 minutes. He requested to sit down. His mucous membranes were dry and he had reduced skin turgor.

Question 2: What are the most likely contributing causes for the changes in BP in this patient?

This patient has orthostatic hypotension (OH). By consensus definition, OH is a sustained ***decrease in systolic blood pressure (SBP) of ≥20*** **mmHg** or a decrease in diastolic blood pressure (DBP) of **≥10** ***mmHg within 3 minutes of standing***. Occasionally, delayed orthostatic hypotension may occur after 3 minutes of standing.

Patients with significant OH commonly present with postural dizziness, presyncope, and falls. It is also important to recognise other less common symptoms such as visual disturbances, fatigue, confusion, and nausea.

The causes of OH can be divided into neurogenic and non-neurogenic. Neurogenic orthostatic hypotension (nOH) occurs in various neurodegenerative disorders such as multiple system atrophy, Lewy body dementia, pure autonomic failure, Parkinson disease, and autonomic peripheral neuropathy from diabetes or other systemic diseases such as amyloidosis or paraneoplastic syndrome. Causes of non-neurogenic orthostatic hypotension include hypovolaemia, poor cardiac function, and medications which in the elderly commonly include multiple anti-hypertensives, antidepressants, and antipsychotics.

****

The team performed a medication reconciliation and found that the patient was taking the following medications:

Aripiprazole 7.5 mg BD
Captopril 6.25 mg ON
Escitalopram 5 mg ON
Lorazepam 0.5 mg TDS
Madopar (levodopa 100 mg, benserazide 25 mg) 5 am, 9 am, 1 pm, 5 pm, and 9 pm

Question 3: Which medication(s) would you stop/adjust at this point?

Captopril was stopped as the patient's BP was generally low on the day of admission. As aripiprazole may contribute to postural hypotension possibly due to its α-1 adrenergic receptor antagonism, a psychiatrist was consulted. The dose of aripiprazole was cut down to once a day as the patient was not overtly agitated. His escitalopram was kept in view of his depression, but his lorazepam dose was changed to PRN dosing. His Madopar regimen was kept, even though it can contribute to postural hypotension, as it was necessary to minimise his rigidity.

****

After the medication adjustments, the following BP trend was observed:

	Day 1		Day 2					
Time	16:26	21:39	2:11	5:06	10:13	13:46	15:55	17:29
BP (mmHg)	181/109	185/118	161/80	123/88	95/61	170/120	103/69	166/110
Position	Supine	Supine	N/A	N/A	Sitting	Supine	N/A	Supine

Question 4: What is the most appropriate management?

a. Drink half a litre of water at bedtime

b. Enforce rest in bed in the daytime

c. Start nifedipine long-acting 30 mg ON

d. Start hydralazine 25 mg OM

e. Start midodrine 2.5 mg BD (in the morning and afternoon) and elevate the head of the bed when in supine position

This patient has orthostatic hypotension with supine hypertension. By consensus criteria, supine hypertension is defined as a SBP of ≥140 mmHg and/or a DBP of ≥90 mmHg after at least 5 minutes of supine rest.

The management of orthostatic hypotension can be broadly divided into non-pharmacologic and pharmacologic interventions:

A. Non-pharmacologic interventions should be implemented first to manage the symptoms associated with orthostatic hypotension. These interventions include but are not limited to:
   - Increasing oral intake of salt and fluid if there are no contraindications such as heart failure or chronic kidney disease
   - Counter-pressure manoeuvres such as crossing legs and clenching the legs and buttocks muscles while standing
   - Waist-high compression stockings or abdominal binder
   - Lower body strengthening exercises

B. If the symptoms of orthostatic hypotension are not well controlled despite non-pharmacological interventions, pharmacologic treatments to augment the BP may be instituted.

Medication	Midodrine	Fludrocortisone	Pyridostigmine
Pharmacologic class	α-1 agonist	Synthetic mineralocorticoid	Acetylcholinesterase inhibitor
Mechanism of action	Peripheral vasoconstriction	Increases plasma volume (off label use)	Amplifies ganglionic neurotransmission in the sympathetic baroreflex pathway
Dose	2.5 to 10 mg BD-TDS during daytime	0.05 to 0.20 mg daily	30 to 60 mg BD-TDS
Remarks and precautions	– Raises both supine and standing BPs (duration of action 2–3 hours) – ***Should not be administered <4 hours before bedtime*** to minimise further exacerbation of supine hypertension	– Contraindicated in patients with congestive cardiac failure and chronic kidney disease – ***Hypokalaemia*** is common, so oral potassium supplement is often necessary	– Useful in mild to moderate OH only – Can be used as an ***adjunct*** to midodrine and fludrocortisone – Does not worsen supine hypertension

Droxidopa is a synthetic noradrenaline precursor that is approved by the US FDA for the treatment of symptomatic nOH in adults. At the time of writing, droxidopa is not available in Singapore.

Uncontrolled supine hypertension occurs in up to half of patients with neurogenic hypotension. It may lead to pressure natriuresis causing nocturia, disturbed sleep, volume depletion overnight, and exacerbation of nOH in the morning.

The management of supine hypertension can also be broadly divided into non-pharmacological and pharmacological interventions:

A. Non-pharmacologic management of supine hypertension include:
   - Avoiding lying down flat during daytime, especially after taking medications that treat orthostatic hypotension
   - Raising the head of bed by at least 30° when resting or sleeping
   - Avoiding evening dose of vasopressor medication such as midodrine and droxidopa
   - Avoiding fludrocortisone in patients with supine hypertension in view of its long duration of action
   - Limiting water intake to 60 to 90 minutes before bedtime
   - Eating carbohydrate-rich snacks before bedtime

B. If non-pharmacologic treatment fails to control supine hypertension, short-acting antihypertensive medication may be administered just before bedtime.

Medication	Losartan	Captopril	Nitro-glycerine patch	Hydralazine
Starting dose	25 mg at bedtime	6.25 mg at bedtime	0.1 mg/hour (apply at bedtime, remove in the morning)	10 mg at bedtime
Onset	Up to 6 hours	≤15 minutes	30 minutes	1 hour
Duration of action	Up to 24 hours*	6–12 hours	The effect should wear off soon after the patch is removed	3–8 hours

*Losartan is effective in lowering night-time supine blood pressure, reducing night-time natriuresis, and may have a neutral effect on orthostatic hypotension even though the duration of action is long.

Should the above therapies fail, other potential second-line options may include nebivolol, eplerenone, clonidine, and short-acting nifedipine, all of which can be considered subject to the individual patient profile and availability in your institution.

Key messages

1. The main goals of the management are to improve symptoms, reduce falls and risk of injury, increase mobility, and maximise independence in performing daily activities.
2. ***Normalisation of standing BP is neither necessary nor feasible in most cases.*** The treatments that elevate orthostatic BP may very often also increase supine BP. Likewise, any treatment of supine hypertension may potentially worsen orthostatic hypotension. Treatment must be individualised to the patient.
3. Patient and caregiver education on the topic and blood pressure recording is necessary since both orthostatic hypotension and supine hypertension pose risks to patient safety.
4. Treatment should be based on the patient's comorbidities, concomitant medications, prognosis, and expectations. As it may be very challenging to manage this condition, it is pertinent for the treating physician to manage the patient's and caregiver's expectations accordingly.
5. In elderly patients, remember to ***start LOW, go SLOW, and only start one agent at a time***. Regular follow-up is needed to monitor the patient's response to the medications and any adverse effects.

Answer key

1. Cervical spondylosis and lumbar stenosis which may have affected the patient's ambulation, gait, and balance; autonomic dysfunction from Parkinson disease; effects from medications; poor safety awareness from dementia.
2. Dehydration; Parkinson disease; and the medications to treat Parkinson disease, dementia and depression.
3. Captopril, aripiprazole, lorazepam.
4. E.

References

American Geriatric Society and British Geriatrics Society (2010) Clinical Practice Guideline for the Prevention of Falls in Older Persons. New York: American Geriatric Society; www.medcats.com/FALLS/frameset.htm.

Cutsworth-Gregory JK, Low PA (2019) Neurogenic Orthostatic Hypotension in Parkinson Disease: A Primer. *Neurol Ther* **8**(2): 307–324.

Fanciulli A, Jordan J, Biaggioni I, *et al.* (2018) Consensus statement on the definition of neurogenic supine hypertension in cardiovascular autonomic failure by the American Autonomic Society (AAS) and the European Federation of Autonomic Societies (EFAS). *Clin Auton Res* **28**: 355–362.

Figueroa JJ, Basford JR, Low PA (2010) Preventing and treating orthostatic hypotension: As easy as A, B, C. *Cleve Clin J Med* **77**(5): 298–306.

Jodan J, Fanciulli A, Tank J, *et al.* (2019) Management of supine hypertension in patients with neurogenic orthostatic hypotension: scientific statement of the American Autonomic Society, European Federation of Autonomic Societies, and the European Society of Hypertension. *J Hypertens* **37**(8): 1541–1546.

2 Falls II (Movement Disorder)

Tan Boon Hian, Melvin Chua Peng Wei

This chapter is a compilation of four clinical scenarios of falls due to an undiagnosed movement disorder which prominently features Parkinsonism.

<u>*CASE 1*</u>

Mr A is a 70-year-old Chinese male who presented to the hospital with a fall. This is his first fall this year. While walking to a nearby coffee-shop for breakfast, the children playing nearby bumped into him causing him to lose balance. He fell and hit his head but did not complain of any loss of consciousness or physical injuries.

Mr A has been complaining of gradually increasing slowness and stiffness for more than a year. He noted tremors on his right arm, which have now progressed to both arms and worsen when he is watching television over the last 5 years. He ignored the tremors as he thought it was part of "growing old". He did not experience any giddiness, chest pain, dyspnoea, palpitations, or numbness.

He is independent in his instrumental activities of daily living and had visited the general practitioner by himself for a routine check-up last month. He has a significant history of diverticular disease, haemorrhoids, and long-standing constipation despite high doses of laxatives; his most recent visit to the gastroenterologist was unremarkable with colonoscopy not showing any significant abnormality. The gastroenterologist had been careful to avoid the use of prokinetics such as metoclopramide.

He also has had visits to the psychiatrist for depressive symptoms relating to his decreasing ability to walk which have been managed without medication. He has a history of talking in his sleep for many years in the past which has responded to melatonin.

Physical examination reveals a man who doesn't blink much but who is otherwise alert and speaking slowly albeit clearly. There is no dysphonia. At rest, a pill-rolling tremor is observed. Lead-pipe rigidity and bradykinesia are demonstrated in all *limbs with full power. There are no cerebellar signs or upgoing plantar reflexes. The extra-ocular movements are full. Seborrheic dermatitis is noted over his scalp. His blood pressure is 140/90 mmHg with no postural drop. His gait speed is <0.8 m/s and he exhibited festinating gait with decreased right arm swing. Pull test is positive. Visual acuity is 6/6 bilaterally and no cataract is seen. There is no significant crepitus in the knees and the rest of the examination is unremarkable.*

Screening laboratory investigations are normal. CT brain shows no cerebral atrophy or old vascular injury. ECG shows normal sinus rhythm.

Question 1: What is the most likely underlying cause of Parkinsonism in this patient?

A clinical diagnosis of Parkinsonism is established given the hallmark features of bradykinesia, rigidity, and tremors. This is the first and often the most difficult step as the diagnosis is a clinical one requiring an index of suspicion and confirmation with clinical examination of these findings.

Idiopathic Parkinson Disease (iPD) is a neurodegenerative disease, often with prodromal ("pre-disease") symptoms of constipation, anxiety and depressive illness, and rapid eye movement sleep behaviour disorder (RBD). Other prodromal symptoms absent in Mr A include anosmia and early daytime somnolence. These prodromal symptoms can occur ten years prior to the onset of motor symptoms. Note, however, that these prodromal symptoms (especially RBD) can also be exhibited in other α-synucleinopathies (e.g., multiple system atrophy, dementia with Lewy bodies).

Important clinical clues to iPD include:

a. asymmetrical, upper limb-first presentation of the disease
b. slow and insidious progression of disease — remember that the disease is as "slow" as the patient!
c. relatively intact cognition — in this patient the motor symptoms had been present for more than a year with intact cognition (in contrast to Lewy body dementia in which there is often concurrent manifestations of motor symptoms and cognitive decline)
d. the eventual development of non-motor symptoms, which is best presented in the Movement Disorder Society-Sponsored Revision of the Unified Parkinson's Disease Rating Scale (MDS-UPDRS)

While Mr A's tremors and slowness have been present for years, he only started falling recently. It should be emphasised that patients with early-stage Parkinson disease often have symptoms limited to the upper limbs and do not manifest as frequent falls (Table 2.1); frequent falls early in the disease presentation suggest Parkinson plus syndromes.

Table 2.1. Hoehn and Yahr Scale for Parkinson disease (Mr A is in Stage III). Note that the scale is non-linear: patient does not remain at each stage for the same number of years, and a stage does not represent a given amount of pathology in the brain.

Stage	Symptom	Diagnostic implication	Therapeutic implication
I	Unilateral involvement	This stage is often missed entirely but its history may be elicited in retrospect when patient presents at a more advanced stage.	One can function almost normally with adequate therapy. The goals of therapy are to (a) treat symptoms (b) restore function Dopamine agonists, monoamine oxidase-B (MOAB) inhibitors, or levodopa can be started at this stage as all treatments are not disease- modifying.
II	Bilateral involvement	"Midline" or "axial" signs become apparent (e.g., facial masking, decreased blinking, monotony of speech, truncal rigidity). This stage may be mistaken for "advanced age" if patient only presents with slowness and lack of spontaneous movement.	
III	Mild-to-moderate bilateral involvement with some postural instability but ADL-independent	***Loss of balance*** with inability to make rapid automatic movements to protect against falling is key to the diagnosis of this stage.	Higher treatment doses are needed to resolve symptoms of rigidity, tremors, and bradykinesia, but at the risk of developing dyskinesia at optimal doses.
IV	Severe disability but still able to stand and walk independently	Non-motor symptoms such as cognitive impairment and hallucinations start presenting. The patient is unable to lead an independent life.	One will have residual symptoms despite the most optimised treatment.
V	Wheelchair-bound or bedridden unless assisted	This stage is similar to the end stages of other neurodegenerative diseases (e.g., Alzheimer's disease). Patient's needs are completely dependent on caregivers. Complications of immobility and dysphagia will start occurring with increasing frequency.	The aims of treatment are to (a) allow ease of nursing and transfers by continuing dopaminergic therapy (b) minimise psychiatric, orthostatic, and gastrointestinal side-effects of dopaminergic therapy (c) palliate with support from the relevant services It is also important to prevent complications of immobility and dysphagia.

Question 2: What pharmacological and non-pharmacological treatments would you initiate for Mr A to address his physical function?

iPD is a neurodegenerative disease and at present there are no disease-modifying therapies. The medications used for the motor symptoms of Parkinson disease are for symptomatic relief. The goal of treatment is amelioration of lost function and preservation of function and quality of life.

There has been, in the past, a concern that starting dopaminergic agents early would lead to rapid progression of disease, but this has been addressed with the recent clinical trials. The observation of progression of motor symptoms is a manifestation of the natural history of a neurodegenerative disease, rather than because of initiation of dopaminergic agents.

There are important non-pharmacological managements for the motor symptoms of Parkinson disease. The management of Parkinson disease is interdisciplinary and interprofessional. Exercise, particularly involving balance, resistance, and strength training in a gradual and increasing fashion, helps build intrinsic capacity and maintenance of function in all elderly, Parkinson disease or otherwise. Optimising nutrition is important to prevent complications of malnutrition such as frailty and sarcopenia which would lead to functional decline. For the non-motor symptoms, they each have their own non-pharmacological management strategies.

Dopaminergic medications bind to proteins in the stomach which leads to their absorption being affected. A practical tip to optimise absorption would be to obtain the usual meal timings of the patient and time the dosing of dopaminergic agents one hour pre- or two hours post-meal. To aid titration of medications, instruct the patient to note how long the medication takes to reach a desirable effect, how long the effect lasts, and if there is any dyskinesia with treatment.

Many patients with iPD have dyspepsia and constipation as part of the disease spectrum. Metoclopramide should be avoided as it can penetrate the blood-brain barrier leading to drug-induced Parkinsonism. Domperidone could be considered as it does not cross the blood-brain barrier.

Question 3: What key aspects should the doctor look out for when reviewing Mr A in the clinic after discharge?

Remember that the diagnosis of iPD is a clinical one; other differential diagnoses include multiple system atrophy-Parkinsonian type (MSA-P), progressive supranuclear palsy (PSP), dementia with Lewy bodies (DLB) and vascular Parkinsonism.

One should look out for

(a) rapid progression of disease or lack of response to treatment as iPD is very responsive to dopaminergic replacement

(b) worsening cognition especially in the first year of diagnosis, which is suggestive of a revision of diagnosis to DLB (in ambiguous cases, some use the label "Lewy body disease")

(c) profound orthostatic hypotension or involvement of speech or swallowing early in disease — this is suggestive of an alternative diagnosis
(d) recurrent falls early in the disease as such a presentation in the early stages of iPD is atypical

Orthostatic hypotension should be managed by (a) addressing any underlying medical causes such as dehydration or bleeding, (b) ensuring that the titration of Madopar is indeed gradual and necessary, (c) reducing high doses of other blood pressure medications (e.g., calcium channel blockers), or (d) instituting non-pharmacological measures for treatment [refer to Chapter 1 on Falls I (Blood Pressure Changes)]. One should bear in mind that up to 50% of patients with iPD have neurogenic orthostatic hypotension due to the disease itself, and the patients may need medications such as midodrine or fludrocortisone as part of management.

Dyskinesia is divided into peak-dose dyskinesia, wearing-off/off-dose dyskinesia, and diphasic dyskinesia. Peak-dose dyskinesia is treated by fractionating the total dose of levodopa (e.g., 125 mg TDS into 62.5 mg QDS), increasing the dosing interval, or combining therapy with a dopaminergic agent, amantadine, or MAOB inhibitor with a consequent lower total dose of levodopa. Wearing off/off-dose dyskinesia is suggestive of progression of disease requiring increased frequency of dosing (e.g., 125 mg Q4H from Q6H), use of entacapone (catechol-O-methyltransferase inhibitor which inhibits the metabolism of levodopa), or long-acting formulations such as HBS or combination therapy. Diphasic dyskinesia is also seen in advanced iPD which may require reducing the peak dose but prolonging the duration of treatment following the principles above. As the disease advances, there is a higher likelihood of dyskinesia and it may not be completely treatable. In intractable cases, apomorphine (a short-acting dopaminergic drug) infusions or deep brain stimulation in appropriate patients in consultation with neurologists can be considered.

In the older patient, a levodopa formulation is generally better tolerated than the other agents including dopamine agonists and MAO-B inhibitors due to their side-effect profile (including but not limited to gastrointestinal side-effects and postural hypotension). Hence, in the elderly you will often see Madopar or Sinemet being used as first-line treatment.

Freezing of gait (FOG) is more commonly seen in advanced iPD of Hoehn and Yahr 3 onwards. It is managed with up-titration of therapy, addressing psychological causes such as fear of falling, and rehabilitation. Unfortunately, FOG is often refractory to therapy.

Key messages

1. iPD is a clinical diagnosis with prodromes and it follows a slow and predictable trajectory of progression over many years.
2. It is important to elicit and address both motor and non-motor symptoms in a patient with iPD as they affect the patient's function and quality of life.
3. Apart from titrating medications to these symptoms, clinical assessment early in the disease diagnosis also involves looking out for the development of Parkinson disease plus syndromes.

Answer key

1. Idiopathic Parkinson disease.
2. A reasonable starting dose is Madopar 62.5 mg (L-dopa 50 mg + benserazide 12.5 mg) TDS pre-meal, referral to physiotherapy and occupational therapy to address balance, gait, and strength, and optimising function and assessing the home environment.

   NB. While Madopar HBS is available in the formulary, we do not recommend routinely starting patients on it. The initiation of Madopar helps us to assess responsiveness to therapy, and a slow release agent can complicate the assessment. Secondly, HBS formulations start out as 125 mg which is a high dose for early iPD and more strongly predisposes to dyskinesia.
3. As Mr A is a patient with recently diagnosed iPD, one would want to look out for Parkinson plus symptoms. Side-effects to therapy need to be checked and dosage adjustments made accordingly.

References

de Bie RMA, Clarke CE, Espay AJ, Fox SH, Lang AE (2020) Initiation of pharmacological therapy in Parkinson's disease: when, why, and how. *Lancet Neurol* **19**(5): 452–461.

Goetz CG, Fahn S, Martinez-Martin P, *et al.* (2007) Movement Disorder Society-sponsored revision of the Unified Parkinson's Disease Rating Scale (MDS-UPDRS): Process, format, and clinimetric testing plan. *Mov Disord* **22**(1): 41–47.

Hoehn MM, Yahr MD (1967) Parkinsonism: onset, progression and mortality. *Neurology* **17**(5): 427–442.

Postuma RB, Berg D, Stern M, *et al.* (2015) *MDS* clinical diagnostic criteria for Parkinson's disease. *Mov Disord* **30**(12): 1591–1601.

<u>*CASE 2*</u>

Mdm B is a 65-year-old female who presented to the hospital for a fall. She was pacing about in the Institute of Mental Health long-stay ward when she tripped against a chair, lost her balance, and fell. She hit her head but did not lose consciousness. There was no antecedent trigger prior to the fall such as cardiac symptoms, weakness, giddiness, or inter-current illness.

Her background history is significant for paranoid schizophrenia which has been well controlled on chlorpromazine 25 mg TDS for the past 30 years. Prior to the fall, which is her first, she was bADL-independent and was engaged in an in-hospital job programme where she had been performing well for the past 30 years. Her annual cMMSE is 25/28. She has no other medical problems. Her sleep prior to these two weeks was normal with no verbalisations and her bowel habits were normal.

Unfortunately, Mdm B's psychosis worsened in the past two weeks after a new inmate became aggressive towards her. She developed paranoia towards oral medications, requiring a switch to colourless risperidone syrup 1 mg twice daily. Despite this dose of risperidone, she remained alert. She was also found to be increasingly slow and stiff since a few days ago. She seemed to have developed a nascent inner sense of restlessness requiring her to move from one place to another, and the fall occurred during an episode of her pacing about. Her vitals are stable and there is no fever or no orthostatic hypotension.

On examination, she has paucity of facial expression, symmetrical rigidity of all four limbs, and bradykinesia. There is no tremor noted, though there are choreiform movements of the tongue. Her right upper limb was in an involuntarily persistent state of internal rotation. She looked restless in her chair. There were no myoclonic jerks or action myoclonus. The rest of the neurological and cardiac examination was unremarkable. CT brain did not show any acute deficit; in particular, there were no notable lesions in the basal ganglia or the midbrain.

Question 1: What is the most likely underlying cause of Parkinsonism in this patient?

From history, there is a temporal relationship between the initiation of a higher equivalent dose of an antipsychotic and the development of the symptoms of slowness and akathisia (inner sense of restlessness). This occurred in the setting of a patient who works in a job programme (thus having relatively preserved cognition),

The patient is likely to have developed drug-induced Parkinsonism (DIP) or otherwise known as the extra-pyramidal side-effects (EPSE) of her new, high-dose risperidone. This is usually the top differential diagnosis in a patient who is on high-dose or long-term antipsychotic medications.

The onset of DIP may be days to weeks after starting the offending antipsychotic. However, on occasion it may also occur after several months of use. DIP may be seen in up to 80% of patients on antipsychotics. Symptoms and signs are often symmetrical with rigidity and bradykinesia; tremors are infrequently seen. Other EPSE symptoms seen to co-exist with DIP — and which are hardly seen in iPD — include dystonia, akathisia, and tardive dyskinesia. Symptoms resolve in 50–90% of patients within weeks to months after cessation or down-tapering of the offending medication.

As unmasking of pre-clinical iPD remains a possibility, three other clinical outcomes are possible:

(1) persistent symptoms with no progression
(2) persistence with progression
(3) cessation of symptoms with recurrence of symptoms in the absence of drugs years later

The progression of Parkinsonism in the last two scenarios would suggest the presence of underlying iPD.

Question 2: What is an appropriate management plan?

Clinical observation over time will reveal and affirm the underlying cause of the Parkinsonism. The antipsychotic should be stopped, tapered, or switched in consultation with the primary psychiatrist. It may be worthwhile to note that antipsychotics such as quetiapine and clozapine have 3–4% incidence of DIP compared to 6–14% with olanzapine, haloperidol, aripiprazole, and risperidone.

If the Parkinsonism is debilitating, a short course of antimuscarinic agents such as benztropine (can start at 1 mg ON) or dopaminergic agents such as levodopa, amantadine, or dopamine agonists may be considered (it is reasonable to start levodopa 62.5 mg BD-TDS to see the response), taking into consideration the potential for worsening of psychosis (by stimulating D2 receptors while the patient is already being treated with antipsychotics). To avoid labelling patients with DIP as Parkinson disease, one should follow up closely and monitor the treatment response, document clearly the reasons for starting these medications, and stop these medications once DIP no longer exists upon cessation of the culprit drugs.

Non-pharmacological methods include rehabilitation and treatment with aims to avoid contractures, improve gait and mobility, and address the underlying triggers for the psychosis.

As DIP is not a neurodegenerative disease, it is not expected to progress nor recur, assuming no new offending medications are taken. Should the symptoms of Parkinsonism recur or persist, a trial of Madopar and assessing its effectiveness may help to resolve this diagnostic dilemma. Nevertheless, the gold standard for diagnostic confirmation is to monitor the patient longitudinally.

Should there be a need to obtain further objective evidence to support the diagnosis of DIP, specific brain scans are available locally:

a. Dopamine transport (DAT) scan — a single-photon emission computed tomography (SPECT) scan which tags dopamine transporters in the brain. We are looking for loss of dopamine transporters in the substantia nigra.
b. Nigrosome scan — T2-weighted MRI which detects for presence of clusters of dopaminergic cells within the substantia nigra. A reduction of nigrosomes is observed in Parkinson disease.
c. MIBG cardiac (cardiac [123I]metaiodobenzylguanidine scintigraphy) scan — reflects postganglionic cardiac autonomic denervation. Of all the α-synucleinopathies, MSA is mostly "preganglionic" while Parkinson disease, pure autonomic failure, and DLB are mostly "postganglionic". In MSA, the MIBG is normal and lights up compared to iPD and other postganglionic α-synucleinopathies.

Key messages

1. DIP is usually a static disease with a clear temporal relationship with the precipitating medication.
2. DIP has atypical extrapyramidal signs which are not typically seen in iPD.
3. Stopping the medication will usually lead to resolution of physical signs.

Answer key

1. Extra-pyramidal side-effects of high-dose risperidone.
2. The risperidone should be stopped, tapered, or switched (to an alternative drug; e.g., quetiapine) in consultation with the primary psychiatrist. Physical therapy should also be initiated.

References

de Germay S, Montastruc F, Carvajal A, Lapeyre-Mestre M, Montastruc JL (2020) Drug-induced Parkinsonism: Revisiting the epidemiology using the WHO pharmacovigilance database. *Parkinsonism Relat Disord* **70**: 55–59.

D'Souza RS, Hooten WM (2021) Extrapyramidal Symptoms. 2021 Aug 3. In: StatPearls [Internet]. Treasure Island (FL): StatPearls Publishing; PMID: 30475568.

Wisidagama S, Selladurai A, Wu P, Isetta M, Serra-Mestres J (2021) Recognition and Management of Antipsychotic-Induced Parkinsonism in Older Adults: A Narrative Review. *Medicines (Basel)* **8**(6): 24.

CASE 3

Mdm C is a 65-year-old lady who was admitted to the hospital for a fall. She was found having had a fall at home as a result of hallucinations of children prompting her to chase them. While running, she felt giddy, lost her balance, and fell. She had no inter-current illness.

Mdm C's hallucinations have been occurring regularly in the past year. They initially occurred in the late evening and subsequently started manifesting even during the day. She has had intermittent episodes of confusion and disorientation to time, place, and person over the past year in the early morning upon awakening, and recently in the evening as well. She feels that the hallucinations are real and can describe the hallucinations in fine detail, indicating that her memory is relatively preserved. There are no complaints with her mood as she was seen laughing with the illusory children at times and still enjoys watching television.

She used to work as a cleaner but stopped due to getting lost in her cleaning site multiple times over the past year. She also used to jog but her family discovered her getting lost while outside and frequently talking to herself. Her movements significantly slowed in the past six months. Due to her hallucinations and her recurrent progressive episodes of confusion, she was no longer able to handle her finances or go out into the community unaccompanied. She saw a private psychiatrist three months ago who diagnosed her with adjustment disorder. She was not on any regular medications.

On examination during morning ward rounds, she is inattentive and not orientated to time, place, and person. She sees children of various ethnicities in the ward talking to her. She appears distressed and unkempt with evidence of poor self-care. While her vital signs are stable, she has a systolic drop in blood pressure of 40 mmHg on standing without reflex tachycardia and feels giddy. Neurological examination reveals bradykinesia and symmetrical rigidity in all limbs. There is generalised hyperreflexia with downgoing plantars and no myoclonus. Her neck is supple and there is no orofacial dyskinesia. Her gait is slow but not festinating. There are no tremors noted. There is no ideomotor apraxia, cerebellar signs, nystagmus, or ophthalmoplegia. She is constipated with impacted stool in the rectum. The rest of the neurological, cardiac, ophthalmic, and general examination is normal. Her cMMSE is 15/28 with loss of 6 points in orientation, 0/5 for serial 7s, 0/1 construction, and 2/3 for 3-step commands. Her screening geriatric depression scale is 1/15.

Blood tests for general health and for reversible causes of cognitive impairment (e.g., thyroid function, vitamin B12, folate, calcium) are normal. Neuroimaging showed generalised atrophy with preference for the parieto-occipital regions with no evidence of previous strokes. Her hippocampal volumes are preserved.

Electroencephalogram and lumbar puncture were unremarkable. While in the ward, she continues to be intermittently confused and there are episodes of her shouting in the middle of the night while asleep and kicking in her bed, which the family shared has been worsening for the past ten years.

Question 1: What are the top two differential diagnoses of Parkinsonism in this patient?

The likely underlying diagnosis is dementia with Lewy bodies (DLB). There is a subacute-to-chronic progressive and clear deterioration of function due to cognitive decline. Despite the preservation of memory, she has prominent fluctuations in orientation with inattention and loss of executive function. Important diagnostic clues also include classic visual hallucinations, manifested rapid eye movement sleep behaviour disorder (RBD) and Parkinsonism. Autonomic dysfunction (severe neurogenic orthostatic hypotension and constipation) are additional suggestive features of DLB.

The crucial differential to rule out in this patient is delirium as it is often due to potentially life-threatening causes, which when addressed often lead to resolution of the altered mental state and back to the patient's premorbid cognition. Delirium can last up to 6 months in some cases! Subacute delirium is either recurrent delirium due to similar unaddressed causes, subacute causes (e.g., autoimmune encephalitis, tuberculous meningitis, carcinomatous meningitis, neurosyphilis/HIV encephalopathy, psychiatric, or toxic causes), or the unmasking of a dementing process.

In this patient, other differential diagnoses to consider after excluding delirium are:

a. Parkinson disease dementia (PDD) — from the history, PDD is unlikely due to the Parkinsonism occurring within one year of the cognitive symptoms, also known as the "1-year rule". (Parkinsonism and cognitive decline occurring within a year of each other suggest an alternative diagnosis to iPD. In iPD patients who develop dementia, this usually occurs on a background of established Parkinson disease for a few years.)
b. Other Parkinson's plus syndromes — for example, multiple system atrophy (MSA) which often presents with recurrent falls, treatment-resistant and rapidly progressing Parkinsonism, or symptoms pertaining to dysautonomia rather than cognitive/psychiatric complaint as the first and most prominent symptom.

If the patient did <u>not</u> have Parkinsonism, additional differential diagnoses to consider are:

a. Late-onset psychosis, which is usually static for years as opposed to the rapid progression seen in this patient with DLB.
b. Psychotic depression — there will be an obvious depressive illness during assessment; this patient's hallucinations are also not depressive (i.e., not "mood congruent") in nature.
c. Autoimmune encephalitis — characterised by subacute onset, behavioural manifestation, and fluctuations of the clinical course. Various encephalitides such as viral, bacterial, carcinomatous, and tuberculous meningitis may also mimic it.

Question 2: How can the hallucinations be addressed in this patient?

For the hallucinations, one has to first review if a new condition (e.g., depression or delirium) has occurred. In the absence of a new condition, if hallucinations are not bothersome, non-pharmacological methods of distraction and engagement of the patient is first line. A trained professional could teach the caregivers to engage the patient with activities that the patient previously enjoyed and to normalise the hallucinations to make them less distressing to the patient. Cognitive enhancers with acetylcholinesterase inhibitors such as rivastigmine (oral formulation: start at 1.5 mg BD and titrate up gradually to max 12 mg/day; patch formulation: start at 4.6 mg/day and increase to 9.5 mg/day) or donepezil (starting dose 2.5–5 mg once daily; may be increased to 10 mg daily) may help manage the hallucinations in DLB and PDD. These acetylcholinesterase inhibitors are unlikely to cause EPSE.

Patients with DLB often have RBD, which is best treated non-pharmacologically by ensuring safety of the patient using bedrails and moving dangerous items (e.g., electrical wires, fragile or sharp items) away from the bed. The patient may be left alone if the risk of falling off the bed is addressed and if the vocalisations by the patient are tolerable. If the RBD disturbs the patient, affects others, or puts the patient at risk of falls, melatonin (start at 2 mg ON) which is safe and relatively free of side-effects can be considered. A suitable second-line therapy is clonazepam (start at 0.25 mg ON) — take note of the risks of sedation and falls.

The other non-motor symptoms such as urinary retention and constipation should be addressed. It is important to avoid anti-cholinergic medications; these patients are also sensitive to neuroleptics. As the prognosis is generally three to four years after diagnosis with continued decline to be expected, advance care planning and close care with allied health, community, and palliative services should be initiated and coordinated.

Key messages

1. Dementia with Lewy bodies (DLB is a challenging diagnosis which requires detailed history documenting of the type of Parkinsonism, the type of memory deficit, and the temporal sequence of one with the other whilst ruling out other treatable causes.
2. Delirium needs to assessed and treated prior to making the diagnosis of DLB.
3. Acetylcholinesterase inhibitors in these patients may be used for the management of hallucinations.

Answer key

1. Dementia with Lewy bodies and subacute delirium.
2. After excluding depression and delirium, non-pharmacological treatments should be started first. A trained professional can work with the caregivers to distract and engage the patient. Pharmacological treatment with rivastigmine or donepezil is considered if the hallucinations pose a danger to the patient or caregiver. In suicidal cases or at high risk of harm, commence pharmacological treatment right away in tandem with non-pharmacological measures.

References

Armstrong MJ, McFarland N (2019) Recognizing and treating atypical Parkinson disorders. *Handb Clin Neurol* **167**: 301–320.

McKeith IG, Boeve BF, Dickson DW, *et al.* (2017) Diagnosis and management of dementia with Lewy bodies: Fourth consensus report of the DLB Consortium. *Neurology* **89**(1): 88–100.

<u>*CASE 4*</u>

Mr D is a 65-year-old Chinese gentleman who presented to the hospital for a fall. He was outside the house when his neighbours' dog ran past him, causing him to lose balance. He fell and hit his head. There were no pre-fall symptoms, slurring of speech, or visual disturbance. He does not feel stiff nor does he feel slow. You notice the patient's hands shaking and he shared with you that he has been having these tremors for forty years; his father and his uncles all share similar tremors. There is no history of dementia, early death, or liver disease in the family. He shared that usually his hands start to shake when he stretches out to reach for something or when he is bringing something from the kitchen to the dining table in the living room. He has not sought any medical attention for these tremors because he is not troubled by it. Over the years, he finds that his head occasionally shakes when he tries to take a drink, and that over the years he would lose his balance inside the bus when it comes to a sudden standstill.

This is his first hospitalisation and fall this year. He has a history of hypertension and hyperlipidaemia for which he is taking atenolol and simvastatin. His yearly thyroid panel by the polyclinic is normal. He has worked for years in a desk-bound job. There is no history of use of traditional medicines or exposure to unusual chemicals or metals.

On physical examination, there is a 4–8 Hz bilateral tremor over both hands which is precipitated by sustaining a posture or reaching out for a cup; it does not occur at rest. There is no rigidity and bradykinesia. There is no focal weakness, dystonia, myoclonus, dysmetria, nystagmus, or dysdiadochokinaesia. An ophthalmic examination did not reveal any sun-flower cataracts or Kayser–Fleischer rings. Tandem gait is mildly impaired; Romberg's test is negative. There is absence of stigmata of chronic liver disease and uraemic fetor. There is no orthostatic hypotension. cMMSE is 27/28.

MRI brain showed neither infarcts nor cerebral or cerebellar atrophy. His liver, thyroid, and renal panels are within normal limits. Serum caeruloplasmin is within normal limits.

Question 1: What is the most likely underlying cause of falls in this patient?

Essential tremor (ET) and Parkinsonism are similar-presenting movement disorders. ET is increasingly seen as a syndromic, slow neurodegenerative disorder which may have additional clinical features as the disease progresses.

The tremors of ET are often 4–8 Hz and are precipitated by maintaining posture or during action but as the disease persists, tremors under different situations such as at rest, on intention, or over unusual regions (e.g., neck, head, upper airway, jaw) may manifest. Other features of ET (which prompt a label of "ET-plus") include dystonia, bradykinesia, rigidity, gait ataxia, and in advanced cases, possibly cognitive impairment. In summary, the disease transforms from an initial single-symptom mild disease with minimal impact on function to that of multiple symptoms with greater effect on function as the disease progresses.

Diagnostic clues include the prominent tremor in the absence of clear neurological signs of any other disorder, the long history of disease without progression (the latest international consensus statement recommends a minimum of three years of symptom duration highlighting the chronicity of this disorder), and autosomal dominant familial history of a similar disorder. It is important to rule out a stroke in cases that come in with new symptoms or falls in the setting of ataxia.

As per idiopathic Parkinson disease, clinical observation in unclear cases would reveal the true diagnosis over time.

Question 2: What is an appropriate management plan?

The prognosis of this condition is usually good. Most cases of ET are benign and the progression of disease is recognised as slow if at all, and it is currently a topic under investigation. As with most neurological diseases, non-pharmacological measures include inter-professional and inter-disciplinary management such as physiotherapy with regards to gait and balance training, occupational therapy for coping strategies for tremors, orthoses, and aids for walking and stabilisation. Pharmacological treatments include propranolol 10 mg TDS and primidone (please refer to a neurologist). Primidone is a phenobarbitone derivative, and sedation and malaise occur in 1/3 of patients compared to 8% in propranolol. Consultation with a neurologist for long-term follow-up is recommended.

Key messages

1. Patients with purely essential tremor (ET) do not exhibit bradykinesia and rigidity.
2. ET is also a neurodegenerative disease that progresses with time.

Answer key

1. Gait ataxia due to essential tremor.
2. As Mr D is at risk of falls from ambulating and taking the bus, long-term suppressive therapy is recommended. His atenolol can be switched to propranolol as it can simultaneously control his tremor and hypertension. Atenolol (β-1 selective adrenergic antagonist) is inferior to propranolol (non-selective β-adrenergic

antagonist, so it can block the peripheral β-2 receptors located in the muscle spindles) for controlling essential tremor as its action is cardioselective. The usual dose is 10 mg TDS. Referrals to physiotherapy and occupational therapy would also be helpful. Upon discharge, it would be good to refer to neurology for long-term follow-up.

References

Bhatia KP, Bain P, Bajaj N, *et al.* (2018) Consensus Statement on the classification of tremors: from the task force on tremor of the International Parkinson and Movement Disorder Society. *Mov Disord* **33**: 75–87.

Espay AJ, Lang AE, Erro R, Merola A, Fasano A, Berardelli A, Bhatia KP (2017) Essential pitfalls in "essential" tremor. *Mov Disord.* **32**(3): 325–331.

Haubenberger D, Hallett M (2018) Essential Tremor. *N Engl J Med.* **378**(19): 1802–1810.

Louis ED, Bares M, Benito-Leon J, Fahn S, Frucht SJ, Jankovic J, Ondo WG, Pal PK, Tan EK (2020) Essential tremor-plus: a controversial new concept. *Lancet Neurol.* **19**(3): 266–270.

Louis ED (2021) The Essential Tremors: Evolving Concepts of a Family of Diseases. *Front Neurol.* **12**: 650601.

3 Falls III (Bone Problem)

Stanley Angkodjojo, Raymond Goh Kai Heng

Mdm L is a 75-year-old Chinese lady who was admitted after a fall. She was mopping the floor at home when she accidentally slipped and sat down on the floor. She did not report any giddiness before the fall and was well prior to it. She was able to get up on her own and reported some soreness on the back.

Mdm L reported three near falls in the past one year, which she described as mostly accidental when she was trying to reach for items in her kitchen wall cabinets or on a wet floor in the kitchen.

Her past medical history was significant for hypertension and diabetes mellitus. Her chronic medications were losartan and metformin. Mdm L does not smoke or drink.

Physical examination was largely unremarkable. She weighed 70 kg and her height was 1.65 m.

A thoracolumbar (TL) X-ray did not show any vertebral fractures.

Mdm L and her family were concerned about her risks for osteoporosis and fractures.

Question 1: What clinical tools can be used to assess her risks for osteoporosis and fractures?

The Agency for Care Effectiveness (ACE) has published a comprehensive and easy-to-follow guide on Osteoporosis — identification and management in primary care, on 7 November 2018. If you have not read it, please read it now via this QR code:

The guide will teach you how to use the Osteoporosis Self-Assessment Tool for Asians (OSTA) to estimate a woman's osteoporosis risk and, depending on the risk level, the decision to proceed with bone mineral density (BMD) assessment.

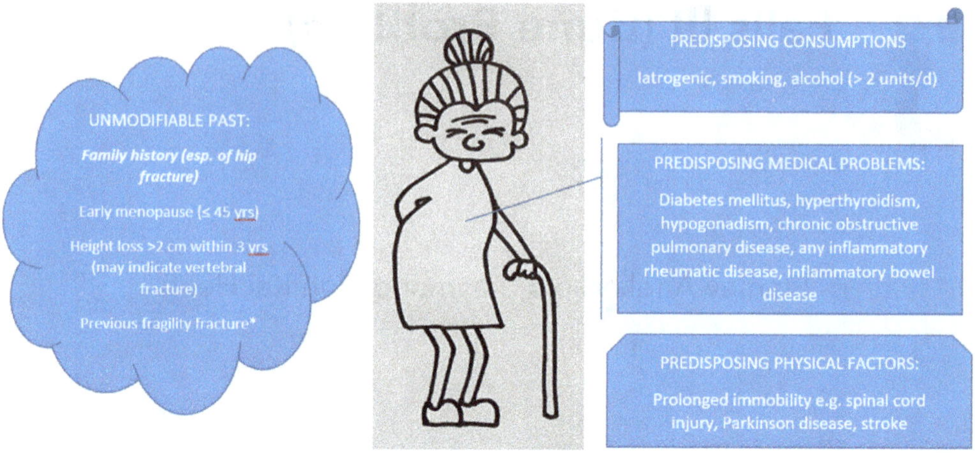

Fig. 3.1. Figure illustrating risk factors associated with osteoporosis and fragility fractures. (Graphic by Ms Tan Wanjun.)
*Fragility fracture (esp. of hip, wrist, spine) is one that occurs as a result of minimal trauma (e.g., fall from standing height or less) or no identifiable trauma.

Aside from age and low body weight which are osteoporosis risk factors already factored in the OSTA, it is imperative to conduct a clinical risk assessment for other factors known to be associated with osteoporosis and fragility fractures (Fig. 3.1).

Iatrogenic consumptions predisposing to osteoporosis

- *Immune suppressants esp. >5 mg/d prednisolone or its equivalent for >3 months, calcineurin inhibitors*
- *Very common drugs, e.g., proton pump inhibitors, anticoagulants (heparin and warfarin)*
- *CNS drugs, e.g., selective serotonin reuptake inhibitors, anticonvulsants*
- *Hormones, e.g., medroxyprogesterone acetate, aromatase inhibitors, androgen deprivation therapy*
- *Thiazolidinediones*

BMD assessment using dual energy X-ray absorptiometry (DXA) is the definitive investigation to assess osteoporosis. With its result, you may estimate fracture risk using the Fracture Risk Assessment Tool FRAX®, whose link is also found in the ACE guide.

Question 2: Aside from clinical risk assessment for osteoporosis risks, what other component of evaluation is important in the assessment of Mdm L's future fracture risk?

3 out of 10 people aged above 65 years and 5 out of 10 people aged above 80 years have a rate of falling at least once a year. A history of falls is a major risk factor for fracture. A multifactorial assessment should thus be performed in older people reporting a fall or who are at risk of falling — you may refer to the Fig. 1.1.

In particular, the impact of hazards in and around the home cannot be underestimated! Patients and their caregivers should review their home environment using a home safety checklist. That and other practical information can be found in Your Bone Health Handbook by the Asia Pacific Fragility Fracture Alliance (APFFA):

****

Mdm L was subsequently discharged from the hospital and was given a follow-up appointment with the geriatrician in the falls clinic. Her BMD revealed a T-score of −1.2 at the lumbar spine and −1.7 at her femoral neck. Her daughter was concerned as she had read on the internet that post-menopausal women are at increased risk of fragility fractures. She enquired whether there are ways she can help her mother optimise her bone health. She also wondered whether her mother needs to be started on specific medications for osteoporosis.

Question 3: What is your interpretation of the BMD result?

Question 4: The following are useful lifestyle advice which you can give Mdm L *except* for which statement?

a. Advise on smoking cessation and appropriate alcohol intake

b. Educate on falls prevention, home safety, and footwear choices

c. Optimise calcium and vitamin D intake, e.g., milk, oily fish, sunshine

d. Optimise phosphate intake, e.g., beans, nuts, lentils

e. Take up exercises such as walking, elastic band exercises, Tai Chi

The diagnosis of osteoporosis is universally defined by either the presence of a fragility fracture OR hip and/or spine DXA BMD T-score ≤ –2.5. T-score ≥ –1 is normal and T-score > –2.5 to < –1 denotes osteopenia.

Healthy lifestyle choices can reduce osteoporosis-associated risks:

Optimise bone nutrition • Appropriate calcium intake (800 mg/d for 19 to 50 years, 1,000 mg/d elemental calcium for ≥51 years). (*Source: Singapore Health Promotion Board*) • Optimise vitamin D intake (600 IU/d for 51 to 70 years, 800 IU/d for >70 years). (*Source: Institute of Medicine*)	**Lifestyle advice: ↑ Exercise** Details on appropriate weight-bearing, muscle-strengthening, and balance exercises are found in the APFFA guide. Importantly, the exercise should ▪ be ongoing for continued benefits ▪ be undertaken for ≥3 hours/week ▪ minimise the risk of harm (including falls)
Provide education • about osteoporosis, fragility fractures, and their implications • review home environment for hazards in and around the home: ➢ Poor lighting, e.g., around stairs ➢ Trip hazards, e.g., cords ➢ Slip hazards, e.g., bathroom ➢ Structural hazards, e.g., uneven walkway • fall risk and footwear	**Lifestyle advice: ↓ Vices** ➢ smoking cessation ➢ appropriate alcohol intake

Question 5: The FRAX® risk assessment tool is used to determine whether Mdm L needs to be started on osteoporosis-specific medication. Estimate her ten-year probability of a major osteoporotic fracture using the information provided so far.

The decision to start a patient on any osteoporosis-specific medication involves making a clinical judgement weighing the overall risks and benefits of different management options in individual patient circumstances and discussing them with the patient (including treatment duration).

Initiation of osteoporosis-specific medication can be considered in the following groups:

- Patients presenting with a fragility fracture.
- Patients without a fragility fracture, but with DXA BMD T-score ≤ –2.5.
- Patients with osteopenia (DXA BMD T-score > –2.5 but < –1) without a fragility fracture, but with high or very high fracture risk.

Mdm L has no fragility fracture and her DXA BMD showed that she has osteopenia. The FRAX® risk assessment tool can be used to assess her 10-year probability of a hip fracture or a major osteoporotic fracture (clinical spine, hip, forearm, or humerus fracture) and thereby categorise her fracture risk as low, high, or very high. Although other fracture risk calculators are available (e.g., Garvan fracture risk calculator, QFracture), FRAX® is recommended given its multi-country validation and the availability of a Singapore model. FRAX® thresholds for treatment should be country-specific. USA guidelines use a fixed threshold of ≥20% for major osteoporotic fractures based on cost-effectiveness criteria. Singapore-specific thresholds are under development and will be made available at ace-hta.gov.sg once validated.

****

Mdm L subsequently was started on calcium carbonate 1,250 mg OM and cholecalciferol 1,000 IU OM. After discussion with both herself and her daughter, the decision was to monitor her bone health condition with annual DXA-BMD. On her third year DXA-BMD, a diagnosis of osteoporosis was made:

T-score –1.0 (lumbar spine)
T-score –2.5 (femoral neck)

Question 6: What could have accounted for the increase in her T-score in the lumbar spine as compared to three years ago?

Before starting osteoporosis-specific treatment, some laboratory investigations are useful.

Laboratory investigation	Rationale
Serum creatinine	This helps to determine the baseline renal function and inform treatment options. It may also indicate the presence of chronic kidney disease and hence its related mineral and bone disorder.
Serum calcium and albumin	This helps to calculate the corrected serum calcium levels. Increased serum calcium levels might indicate the presence of diseases such as primary hyperparathyroidism, malignancy, or granulomatous infections (e.g., tuberculosis). Decreased serum calcium levels might indicate the presence of malabsorption or vitamin D deficiency. Correct hypocalcaemia before starting bisphosphonate, anti-RANKL monoclonal antibody, or sclerostin inhibitor treatments.

(Continued)

(*Continued*)

Laboratory investigation	Rationale
25-hydroxy (OH) vitamin D level	It is important to obtain a baseline level for vitamin D. Aim for **>20 mg/mL** for optimal bone and muscle strength.
Full blood count	This helps to identify a range of disorders such as the presence of malignancy and malabsorption.
Other tests if secondary causes are suspected:	
Erythrocyte Sedimentation Rate (ESR)	High ESR levels might indicate the presence of rheumatological or haematological diseases such as multiple myeloma (in the appropriate clinical context).
Thyroid-stimulating hormone	Thyrotoxicosis is an important cause of osteoporosis.
Serum alkaline phosphatase (ALP)	Increased serum ALP levels might indicate liver disease, Paget's disease, recent fracture, or other bone pathology.
Serum phosphate	Abnormal levels might indicate vitamin D deficiency or renal phosphate wasting.
Spot urine calcium/creatinine ratio	Elevated levels might indicate idiopathic hypercalciuria. Urinary calcium (mmol/l)/creatinine (mmol/l) level >0.6 suggests the need to check 24-hour urine calcium levels.
Serum total testosterone	Consider checking in men <70 years of age with osteoporosis or in those with hypogonadal symptoms. Decreased serum testosterone levels might indicate hypogonadism.

Table 3.1 provides a succinct overview of the osteoporosis treatments currently available in Singapore.

Table 3.1. Overview of osteoporosis treatments in Singapore. The main mechanisms of action together with the clinical evidence of efficacy are reported.

Drug		Bone targets and mechanism of action	Dose in osteoporosis treatment	Effects on fracture risk reduction demonstrated in clinical trials			Adverse events, contraindications, and warnings
				Vertebral	Non-vertebral (excluding hip)	Hip	
Bisphosphonates	**Alendronate**	**Inhibitors of bone resorption:** inhibit osteoclasts activity and induce osteoclast apoptosis.	70 mg/wk (oral)	+	+	+	**Adverse events:** **Common:** Oral drugs: Upper gastrointestinal adverse reactions. IV drugs: Acute phase reaction (fever, flu-like symptoms, myalgia, arthralgia, headache). **Uncommon:** Bone, joint, and muscle pain. **Rare:** Eye inflammation. Femoral shaft or subtrochanteric fractures with atypical radiographic features with long-term use. ***Osteonecrosis of the jaw (ONJ).*** **Contraindications:** Hypersensitivity. Hypocalcemia. Oral drugs: Oesophageal abnormalities that delay emptying. ***Inability to remain upright.*** IV drugs: Renal impairment with creatinine clearance ***<35 ml/min***. **Warning:** People with severe renal impairment should use oral drugs with caution.
	Risedronate		35 mg/wk (oral)	+	+	+	
	Zoledronate		5 mg/yr (IV) (S$541.18 per 5 mg dose)	+	+	+	

(Continued)

Table 3.1. (*Continued*)

Drug		Bone targets and mechanism of action	Dose in osteoporosis treatment	Effects on fracture risk reduction demonstrated in clinical trials			Adverse events, contraindications, and warnings
				Vertebral	Non-vertebral (excluding hip)	Hip	
Anti-RANKL monoclonal antibodies	**Denosumab**	**Inhibitors of bone resorption:** humanised monoclonal antibodies binding selectively and with high affinity to RANKL. Prevent the effect of RANKL on osteoclast differentiation, activation, and survival.	60 mg/6 months (SC)($237.50 per 60 mg dose)	+	+	+	**Adverse events:** **Uncommon:** Rash. **Rare:** Cellulitis. Femoral shaft or subtrochanteric fractures with atypical radiographic features. ***ONJ***. **Contraindications:** Hypersensitivity. ***Hypocalcemia***. Pregnancy and in women trying to get pregnant. **Warning:** Multiple vertebral fractures have occurred when denosumab is discontinued.

Parathyroid hormone receptor agonist	**Teriparatide**	**Activators of bone formation:** intermittent administration of PTH increases the number and activity of osteoblasts.	20 μg/day (SC) (S$719.59 per 600 μg/2.4 ml vial)	+	+	–	**Adverse events:** **Common:** Muscle cramps. Increase serum/urine calcium or serum uric acid. Mild/transient injection site reactions. **Uncommon:** Orthostatic hypotension. Hypercalcemia. Myalgia. Arthralgia. **Contraindications:** Hypersensitivity. Paget's disease of the bone. **Warning:** Should not be used in children or adolescents with open epiphyses or patients with Paget's disease of the bone, previous external beam or implant radiation involving the skeleton, bone metastases, history of skeletal malignancies, other metabolic bone diseases, or hypercalcaemic disorders. Maximum duration of therapy over a patient's lifetime is 24 months.

(*Continued*)

Table 3.1. *(Continued)*

Drug		Bone targets and mechanism of action	Dose in osteoporosis treatment	Effects on fracture risk reduction demonstrated in clinical trials			Adverse events, contraindications, and warnings
				Vertebral	Non-vertebral (excluding hip)	Hip	
Sclerostin inhibitor	**Romosozumab**	Activators of bone formation: Inhibits sclerostin, a regulatory factor in bone metabolism that inhibits the Wnt/Beta-catenin signaling pathway regulating bone growth; romosozumab increases bone formation and, to a lesser extent, decreases bone resorption.	210 mg/month (SC) for up to 12 months. (~S$780 per 210 mg dose)	+	+	+	**Adverse events:** **Very common:** Viral upper respiratory tract infection. Arthralgia. **Common:** Rash, dermatitis. Headache, neck pain, muscle spasms. Cough. Peripheral oedema. Injection site reactions. **Uncommon:** Hypocalcemia. Urticaria. **Rare:** Angioedema. Erythema multiforme. **Contraindications:** Uncorrected ***hypocalcemia***. Hypersensitivity. **Warning:** Should not be initiated in patients who have had a myocardial infarction or stroke within the preceding year.

SERMs	**Raloxifene**	**Inhibitors of bone resorption:** non-steroidal agents that bind to the oestrogen receptor and act as oestrogen agonists on bone.	60 mg/day (oral)	+	Post hoc	–	**Adverse events:** **Common:** Vasomotor symptoms. Muscle cramps. **Uncommon:** Venous thrombosis. **Contraindications:** ***Venous thromboembolism***. Pregnancy. **Warning:** Discontinue in the event of a condition or illness leading to a prolonged period of immobilisation.

IV: intravenous. RANKL: receptor activator of nuclear factor kappa B ligand. SC: subcutaneous. SERMs: selective oestrogen-receptor modulators. +: effect on fracture demonstrated. –: effect on fracture not demonstrated.

Some practical considerations when deciding which drug to use in the older patient would include their ability to sit upright, follow instructions, and cooperate with administration. Many elderly patients have poor dentition and it would be prudent to refer to a dentist to optimise dentition prior to commencement of therapy. ONJ albeit rare can be chronic and troublesome, hence measures to reduce its risk such as stabilising oral disease prior to initiation of antiresorptives and maintaining good oral hygiene are important. Antibiotics may be used when tooth extraction is required and wounds must be closed if possible.

Patients with dementia, chronic pain, or disabilities may not be able to cooperate with sitting upright after ingestion of the oral medications. In addition, those in the advanced stage of the disease may pocket their medications in their mouth instead of swallowing them. Given that many older patients have multiple comorbidities and polypharmacy, this must also be taken into account when deciding on the best pharmacological option for the patient once a decision to commence treatment has been made.

Key messages

1. Early identification of patients at risk for osteoporosis is key to fracture prevention.
2. A careful assessment of the patient's risk profile is needed to identify the need for bone mineral density assessment (BMD) using dual energy X-ray absorptiometry (DXA).
3. Diagnose osteoporosis in patients with a fragility fracture or DXA BMDT-score ≤ -2.5.
4. The FRAX® risk assessment tool is available on the web for calculating the 10-year fracture risk in women and men.
5. Treat patients diagnosed with osteoporosis or patients with osteopenia and high fracture risk.
6. Any pharmacological intervention for postmenopausal osteoporosis and osteoporosis of the elderly should be preceded and accompanied by the elimination of risk factors.

Answer key

1. The OSTA combined with clinical risk assessment for other risk factors known to be associated with osteoporosis and fragility fractures.
2. Falls risk assessment.

3. Osteopenia.
4. D.
5. 12%.
6. Degenerative spine conditions and lumbar spondylosis can artificially elevate spinal BMD and T-score. Other DXA artifacts that can affect and artificially inflate spinal BMD values include the presence of calcification in organs and vessels (such as atherosclerosis involving the aorta) and the presence of compression vertebral fractures.

References

ACE Agency for Care Effectiveness (2018) Osteoporosis — Identification and management in primary care. https://www.ace-hta.gov.sg.

Compston JE, *et al.* (2019) Osteoporosis. *Lancet* **393**: 364–376.

Implementing the minimum clinical standards of the Asia Pacific Consortium on Osteoporosis (APCO) Framework; (2021). https://apfracturealliance.org/.

Kanis JA, *et al.* (2020) Algorithm for the management of patients at low, high and very high risk of osteoporotic fractures. *Osteoporos Int* **31**: 1–12.

4 Falls IV (Joint Problem)

Nur Emillia Binte Roslan, Chuah Tyng Yu,
Raymond Goh Kai Heng

Mrs G is a 75-year-old woman who was evaluated for a swollen right knee that developed the day before. Two days prior she had had a fall. Regarding the fall, she gave a history of trying to cross a kerb while going home from the market when she felt sudden pain in her right knee causing her to lose balance and fall over. She did not report any giddiness before the fall and was well prior to it. She was able to get up after the fall with the help of some passers-by and did not report any broken skin, bruise, or other injuries apart from the sore right knee. She has no fever.

Mrs G also reported a three-year history of pain in both hands, wrists and knees that worsens with activity. There was no redness or swelling of these joints but she experienced morning stiffness lasting half to one hour. There is no personal or family history of psoriasis.

Her past medical history is significant for hypertension and diabetes mellitus. Her chronic medications are losartan-hydrochlorothiazide combination and metformin, as well as frusemide 40 mg OM/PRN prescribed recently for leg swelling. She is scheduled for a cataract surgery in two months.

On physical examination, vital signs including postural blood pressure are normal. BMI is 30 kg/m^2. There is a large right knee effusion. The knee is erythematous, warm, and tender. Examination of the hands revealed mildly tender bony hypertrophy of the proximal and distal interphalangeal joints. There are no rashes or nail changes. Neurological and cardiovascular examination was unremarkable.

Question 1: What is the precipitating factor for her fall?

a. **Obesity**

b. **Poor eyesight**

c. **Poor safety awareness**

d. **Recent change in medications**

e. **Right knee pain**

A precipitating factor refers to the specific event or trigger that resulted in the fall, whereas predisposing factors are those that put the patient at risk of a fall. The causes of falls in the elderly are often multifactorial, thus a careful history and appropriate physical examination are necessary.

A comprehensive falls history would encompass when the patient first started falling, the number of falls, the frequency of falls, and details surrounding each fall including preceding symptoms, location of the fall, time of day, injuries, hospitalisations, and whether the person was able to get up on his or her own. The patient's past medical history including cognitive history and social circumstances also gives us important information with regards to predisposing factors and safety respectively. An older person living alone or left at home alone for several hours who is unable to get up after a fall without assistance is at risk of a long lie and complications of rhabdomyolysis, dehydration, kidney injury, and pressure injuries.

A detailed drug history is also essential in view of possible polypharmacy and drug–drug interactions in an older adult. Given the history of knee pain in this case, the change in medication is likely to be more of a predisposing factor of her fall rather than the exact precipitating factor.

A detailed physical examination from head to toe is essential. This would include checking the patient's vision, visual fields, and eye movements. Persons with limitation in vertical gaze have difficulty negotiating steps and uneven ground. Abnormalities of tone in the limbs (e.g., Parkinsonism, cervical myelopathy) as well as proprioceptive loss in the lower limbs increase risk of falls. Painful, deformed, or unstable joints especially in the lower limbs also predispose the older person to falls.

****

In the Emergency Department, X-ray of the right knee was done and she was given paracetamol and colchicine. Diagnostic knee tap was planned to be performed upon admission.

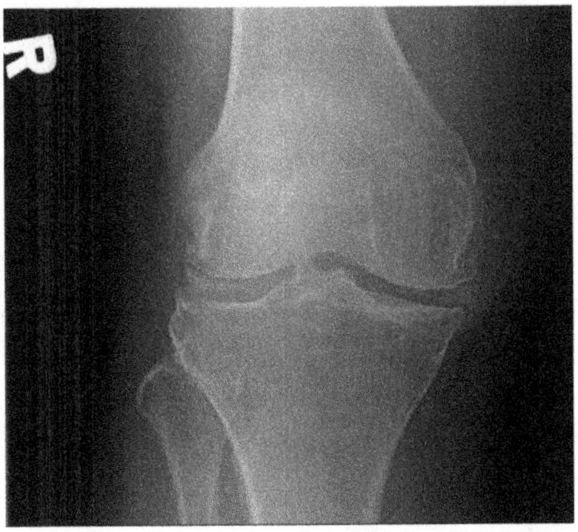

Question 2: What does this radiograph of her right knee show? Choose all that apply.

a. **Fracture**
b. **Chondrocalcinosis**
c. **Osteomyelitis**
d. **Osteophytes**
e. **Subchondral cyst**

Question 3: Which of the following synovial fluid tests is most helpful in establishing a diagnosis?

A. **Acid-fast bacilli smear and culture**
B. **Alizarin red stain on light microscopy**
C. **Crystal analysis, gram stain, and culture**
D. **Glucose and protein measurement**
E. **Leucocyte count**

Question 4: What other pertinent investigations would you perform?

In this elderly lady with a history of a fall, it is prudent to exclude a fracture as a cause of her painful right knee swelling. Plain radiography will help to identify fractures of the knee, which may involve the patella, femur, tibia, and fibula.

Joint infection is also an urgent consideration in acute to subacute-onset monoarthritis. Elevated inflammatory markers may suggest infectious arthritis but cannot confirm or exclude other inflammatory causes. Ultimately, synovial fluid aspiration will give helpful information that is not otherwise available from any blood test or imaging.

In the first instance, gross observation of the aspirated fluid will allow recognition of hemorrhagic or turbid synovial fluid, which would suggest haemarthrosis or septic arthritis, respectively. Laboratory analysis of the synovial fluid provides information that helps to distinguish between inflammatory and non-inflammatory disease, and to diagnose infection versus crystal-related disease.

Synovial fluid leucocyte counts greater than 2,000/μL are consistent with inflammatory fluid — the higher the count, the more inflammatory the fluid and the greater the suspicion for crystal-related or infectious disease, but it does not differentiate between them! A positive gram stain and culture confirms septic arthritis. If there is a high suspicion for septic arthritis, it is prudent to start empirical antibiotics first while awaiting further confirmation from the synovial fluid investigations.

Glucose and protein from synovial analysis do not add any useful information and do not distinguish between infectious and non-infectious synovial fluid.

Basic calcium phosphate (BCP) deposition is a common cause of cartilage calcification and may be radiologically indistinguishable from calcium pyrophosphate (CPP) deposition. Unlike CPP, BCP crystals commonly deposit in the periarticular tendons, bursae, and other soft tissues. Patients are more often asymptomatic although BCP crystals can also stimulate inflammation via pathways similar to that of monosodium urate (gout) and CPP (pseudogout) crystals. Diagnosis of BCP deposition is made clinically or by joint aspiration with visualisation of non-birefringent clumps that stain with alizarin red.

Inflammatory arthritis is suspected when an individual has chronic joint pain that persists for more than 6 weeks. Morning stiffness of the joints is considered significant if it lasts more than 30 minutes. The joint pain and stiffness of inflammatory arthritis improve with movement, and worsen with rest or immobility. This is in contrast to mechanical joint pains, which commonly occur from degenerative musculoskeletal conditions like osteoarthritis. The chronic pains are also in contrast to the recurrent episodic acute pains of crystal arthropathy.

It is prudent to check the rheumatoid factor in this elderly lady with chronic pain affecting her hands, wrists, and knees symmetrically. More than a third of cases of rheumatoid arthritis are diagnosed in populations that are older than 60 years old. The elderly patient with newly diagnosed rheumatoid arthritis may present slightly differently from the younger age group by having a more abrupt onset, more prominent morning stiffness, severe constitutional symptoms, and higher disability.

The bony hypertrophy of the proximal and distal interphalangeal joints in this lady are Bouchard's and Heberden's nodes, respectively. These are features of osteoarthritis of the hands — a common incidental finding in many elderly patients, the majority of whom remain fairly asymptomatic.

****

Her serum uric acid (SUA) level is raised at 425 µmol/L. The right knee synovial fluid aspirate demonstrated needle-shaped crystals. While most of these crystals were strongly negatively birefringent on polarised microscopy, there was also co-existing weakly positive birefringent crystals. Gram stain and culture were negative.

Question 5: What further history do you want to obtain from the patient and family?

Early gout flares are typically monoarticular (90%), begin abruptly, and reach maximal intensity within hours. Periarticular erythema and swelling of a gout flare may progress to resemble cellulitis and can often be confused with an infectious process. Gout flares can also occur in periarticular sites (e.g., the Achilles tendon) or in various bursae (e.g., olecranon, prepatellar).

The demonstration of monosodium urate (MSU) crystals in aspirates of synovial fluid or tophi remains the gold standard for the diagnosis of gout. Intracellular or extracellular MSU crystals are needle-shaped, approximately the size of a white blood cell, and are strongly negatively birefringent on polarised microscopy. MSU crystals can also be identified in joint aspirates during inter-critical periods, i.e., when the joints are quiescent in between gout flares.

The presence of crystals does not exclude septic arthritis. It must be noted that synovial fluid during a flare of crystal arthropathy (gout and/or pseudogout) is typically very inflammatory with a leukocyte count of 20,000–100,000/µL and neutrophil-predominant, making it indistinguishable from septic arthritis. Adding to this challenge is the fact that septic synovial fluids may also contain MSU crystals. Thus, it is important to obtain a gram stain and culture for the purpose of ruling out concomitant septic arthritis.

The weakly positive birefringent crystals in this lady's synovial fluid aspirates suggest the co-existence of calcium pyrophosphate deposition disease or pseudogout. Concomitant gout and pseudogout are not uncommon.

****

Mrs G was treated with oral colchicine 500 mcg TDS, and topical ice compression was applied over the right knee. The next day, her symptoms improved by 50% and she could ambulate independently. Further history from family revealed that there were four other similar episodes in the past year that were triggered by intake of rich broth with internal organ meat.

Question 6: What is the MOST effective next course of action?

A. Cessation of frusemide

B. Discharge with regular colchicine

C. Initiation of allopurinol with anti-inflammatory prophylaxis

D. Intra-articular hyaluronic acid injection

E. Referral for physiotherapy

This lady has concomitant gout and pseudogout.

Treatment of gout requires lifelong urate lowering therapy (ULT). This is indicated in the following situations:

- frequent flares — defined as ≥2 episodes over a period of 1 year
- nephrolithiasis (urate or calcium)
- tophaceous gout (clinical or radiographical)
- moderate-to-severe chronic kidney disease (CKD)

Anti-inflammatory prophylaxis is recommended to reduce the risk of gout flares precipitated by the initiation of ULT and should be initiated concomitantly with ULT. Agents most commonly used in prophylaxis include low-dose non-steroidal anti-inflammatory drugs (NSAIDs) and oral colchicine. In elderly patients or those with a GFR of 30–50 mL/min, colchicine doses may need to be reduced (500 mcg per day or every other day) or avoided altogether with more advanced CKD. NSAIDs are best avoided in the older patient, but should they be deemed necessary then they must be used for the shortest duration possible and with close monitoring for side-effects including peptic ulcer disease, worsening of kidney function, and fluid retention. Low dose glucocorticoid treatment can be used for prophylaxis in those contraindicated for NSAIDs/colchicine. Prophylaxis should be continued for the initial 3–6 months of ULT or longer in patients suffering from frequent gout flares. It is important to note that ULT should neither be reduced nor stopped in a patient who is admitted with a gout flare.

Allopurinol is the commonest urate-lowering therapy used in patients with gout. Specific dose titration schedule is left to the physician and patient to individualise, based on the patient's comorbidities and preferences, and should be carried out over a reasonable time frame (e.g., weeks to months, not years).

Acute treatment for gout flares are similar to those used in pseudogout flares, i.e., colchicine and/or NSAIDs or prednisolone. The choice of medication depends

Tips for prescribing allopurinol (adapted from 2020 American College of Rheumatology Guideline for the Management of Gout as well as various randomized controlled trials):

- *Consider HLA-B5801 testing in patients with high risk for allopurinol-induced severe cutaneous adverse reactions, particularly those with renal impairment and older age.*
- *Aim to achieve and maintain SUA level of <360 μmol/L and <300 μmol/L for non-tophaceous and tophaceous gout respectively.*
- *Common starting dose is 100 mg once daily, titrate upwards in 100 mg increments every 3–4 weeks according to SUA level (max 800 mg once daily).*
- *In patients with chronic kidney disease, start at lower doses e.g., ≤50 mg once daily and titrate in a similar fashion.*

on the patient's drug allergies, age, and comorbidities. For example, NSAIDs are best avoided in patients with renal impairment, cardiovascular risks, and those at higher risk of peptic ulcer disease. Colchicine is used with caution and at lower doses in patients with renal impairment. In those with renal impairment, oral prednisolone 0.5 mg/kg/day or 30 mg/day for 5–10 days can be considered, but the doctor must be mindful to weigh the benefits against the risks which include hyperglycaemia and infection.

Cessation of frusemide (and the hydrochlorothiazide) does not treat the aetiology and by itself will not prevent future gout flares. The diuresis may be continued as clinically indicated.

Intra-articular hyaluronic acid is a viscosupplementation approved to treat osteoarthritis. It is a naturally occurring synovial fluid component that allows for smooth gliding of bones upon each other. When conventional drugs fail for calcium pyrophosphate deposition disease, this chondroprotective option may be considered to increase joint mobility and improve joint function. However, this does not treat the aetiology for the concomitant gout.

Key messages

1. In an elderly person with a single painful, swollen joint, the more urgent diagnoses to exclude are septic arthritis and fracture in the right clinical context.
2. The leukocyte count in the synovial fluid is remarkably raised (typically 20,000–100,000 leukocytes/μL) in both septic arthritis and crystal arthropathy flare.
3. Synovial fluid gram stain and culture are essential to confirm or exclude septic arthritis.
4. The presence of MSU crystals in synovial fluid, or tophi, is the gold standard for the diagnosis of gout.

5. Further careful history from the patient and family is needed to elicit details of joint pain that may resemble chronic inflammatory arthritis, recurrent episodic acute arthritis, or mechanical joint pain.

Answer key

1. E.
2. B (chondrocalcinosis, blue arrows) and D (osteophytes, red arrows).

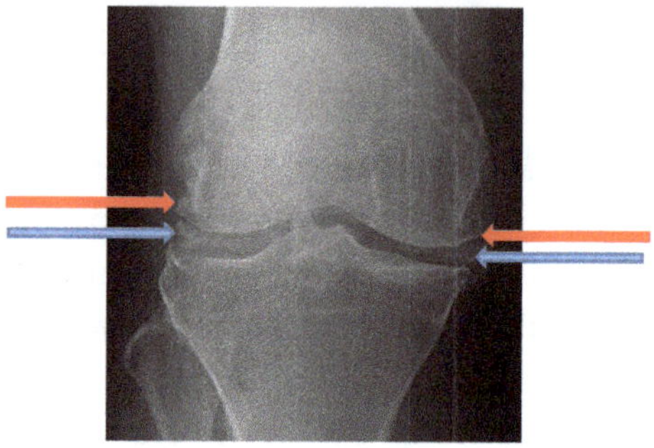

3. C.
4. Full blood count, erythrocyte sedimentation rate, rheumatoid factor, serum uric acid, radiographs of the hands and wrists.
5. Obtain a detailed history from the patient and her family about recurrent severely painful swelling of the joints and identify any dietary trigger.
6. C.

References

ACE Agency for Care Effectiveness (2019) Gout: Achieving the management goal; https://www.ace-hta.gov.sg.

FitzGerald JD, Dalbeth N, Mikuls T, *et al.* (2020) 2020 American College of Rheumatology Guideline for the management of gout. *Arthritis Care Res* **72**(6): 744–760.

Lahaye C, Tatar Z, Dubost JJ, Tournadre A, Soubrier M (2019) Management of inflammatory rheumatic conditions in the elderly. *Rheumatology* **58**(5): 748–764.

5 Functional Decline I (Electrolyte Disturbances)

Naing Chaw Su, Mayank Chawla, Anupama Roy Chowdhury

Mdm S is an 82-year-old female who presented to the Emergency Department after a fall at home. She complained of lethargy, loss of appetite for one week, and a near syncopal episode. On the day before, she was walking from the living room to the kitchen when her legs suddenly gave way, resulting in the fall. She did not have chest pain or palpitations. Her medical history is significant for hypertension and hypercholesterolemia. Her medications include hydrochlorothiazide (HCTZ) 25 mg OM, amlodipine 5 mg OM, and atorvastatin 20 mg ON. She neither drinks alcohol nor smokes.

Clinical examination revealed mild volume depletion. She was fully oriented to time, place, and person. Her blood pressure was 120/76 mmHg without any postural drop. Jugular venous pressure was not elevated, heart sounds are normal, and there is no peripheral oedema. Other examinations were unremarkable. There was no focal neurological deficit. Her body weight was 60 kg.

Initial laboratory investigations were as follows:

	Hospital Day
	On admission
Serum urea, mmol/L	*3.5*
Serum sodium, mmol/L*	*114*
Serum potassium, mmol/L	*4.0*
Serum chloride, mmol/L	*80*
Serum bicarbonate, mmol/L	*23.4*
Serum glucose, mmol/L	*7.4*
Serum creatinine, µmol/L	*63*
Serum osmolality, mOsm/kg	*270*
Urine sodium, mmol/L	*73*
Urine osmolality, mOsm/kg	*560*

**Previous serum sodium one year ago was 136 mmol/L.*

Thyroid function test and short Synacthen test were normal. CT brain showed no significant findings.

Question 1: What are the likely causes of hyponatraemia in this patient?

Question 2: Which of the following is the most appropriate sodium target for treating hyponatraemia at this point of time?

a. **aim for serum Na^+ level to be 118–120 mmol/L over the first 24 hours with daily monitoring of Na^+**
b. **aim for serum Na^+ level to be 122–124 mmol/L over the first 24 hours with daily monitoring of Na^+**
c. **aim for serum Na^+ level to be 118–120 mmol/L over the first 24 hours with monitoring of Na^+ 6 hourly**
d. **aim for serum Na^+ level to be 118–120 mmol/L over the first 24 hours with monitoring of Na^+ 2-4 hourly and urine output hourly**
e. **aim for serum Na^+ level to be 122–124 mmol/L over the first 24 hours with monitoring of Na^+ 2-4 hourly and urine output hourly**

This patient's symptoms of lethargy, gait disturbance, and fall are mostly due to symptomatic hyponatraemia. There are many causes of falls in the elderly, but the very low sodium level of 114 mmol/L in this patient is an adequate explanation. The cause of hyponatraemia is contributed by HCTZ which can occur by several mechanisms including volume depletion. Typically, HCTZ-induced hyponatraemia has laboratory values similar to the syndrome of inappropriate antidiuretic hormone secretion (SIADH) as suggested by the inappropriately high urine osmolality. Thus, the differentiation from concomitant underlying SIADH is the main diagnostic question especially in an euvolaemic patient. A CNS event (e.g., stroke, subdural haemorrhage) was excluded through lack of focal neurology and CT brain findings.

Diuretic-induced hyponatraemia is usually chronic and should be carefully managed. The most important first step is discontinuation of the offending agent, which is HCTZ in this patient.

In the case of symptomatic severe hypotonic hyponatremia, volume replacement with 0.9% saline to euvolaemia generally suffices to correct the low sodium level. Restoring this volume can be done with intravenous infusion of 0.9% saline at 0.5 mL/kg/hr. However, beware that volume repletion will result in increased urine output as the ADH activity is suddenly suppressed, resulting in rapid rise of sodium above the target value.

Measurement of urine electrolytes and calculation of ***urine/plasma electrolyte ratio [(urine Na^+ + urine K^+)/serum Na^+]*** are helpful during correction. A urine/serum electrolyte ratio <0.5 is indicative of increased water excretion, which is associated with potentially over-correction of hyponatraemia. However, the usual time lag of the result limits its practical value at the initial management.

Importantly, frequent measurement of serum electrolytes every few hours (e.g., 2–4 hourly) and monitoring of hourly urine output are mandatory for the safe and effective correction of hyponatraemia during active correction. This is because the increase in urine output and decrease in urine osmolality will usually precede any increase in sodium concentration.

****

0.9% sodium chloride solution 1 L was infused over the first two hours. Electrolyte panel was repeated four hours after:

	Hospital Day	
	On admission	*4 hours*
Serum urea, mmol/L	*3.5*	*2.5*
Serum sodium, mmol/L	*114*	*122*
Serum potassium, mmol/L	*4.0*	*3.8*
Serum chloride, mmol/L	*80*	*88*
Serum bicarbonate, mmol/L	*23.4*	*24.0*
Serum glucose, mmol/L	*7.4*	
Serum creatinine, mmol/L	*63*	*59*
Serum osmolality, mOsm/kg	*270*	
Urine sodium, mmol/L	*73*	
Urine osmolality, mOsm/kg	*560*	
Intervention	*1 L N/S*	
Daily intake, mL	*NA*	
Daily output, mL		*920*

Question 3: Outline your management plan at this stage.

Unexpected water diuresis from volume repletion resulting in a rapid rise in sodium concentration can potentially cause osmotic demyelinating syndrome (ODS). A more conservative goal of correcting hyponatraemia ***no more than 6 mmol/L in the first 24 hours*** is appropriate for this patient to avoid the complication of ODS as the duration of hyponatraemia is unknown and chronic hyponatraemia has an inherent risk of developing ODS. Sudden increase in urine output to >100 mL/h signals increased risk of rapid rise in serum sodium concentration.

In this patient, the trajectory of the rise of sodium is expected to exceed the daily maximal limit as suggested by water diuresis resulting in rapid raise of serum sodium (by 8 mmol/L in 4 hours). Hence, to avoid overcorrection, ***therapeutic re-lowering of sodium level*** should be undertaken at this point in time. It is appropriate to start an infusion of electrolyte-free water (e.g., D5W) at 10 mL/kg/hr. Subsequent D5W infusion should be adjusted based on serum sodium level after each infusion and careful evaluation of urine output until it has returned to below target levels. Furthermore, subsequent administration of desmopressin 2 µg every 8 hours is recommended to prevent further water losses. At this point, consulting an expert is strongly recommended.

****

Mdm S was given 5% dextrose solution initially at 10 mL/kg/hr and the amount was adjusted based on subsequent sodium trend and urine output. She recovered well and her sodium level prior to discharge was 135 mmol/L.

Question 4: What would be the most appropriate action concerning Mdm S's usual diuretic medication?

a. Just stop HCTZ

b. Resume HCTZ at an attenuated dose of 12.5 mg OM

c. Resume HCTZ at usual dose of 25 mg OM

d. Switch HCTZ to frusemide 40 mg OM

e. Switch HCTZ to angiotensin-converting enzyme inhibitor

The first step in prevention of thiazide-induced hyponatraemia is the awareness that thiazide diuretics are amongst the most common causes of drug-induced hyponatraemia, particularly in the elderly, females, or those with low body mass. That risk is further augmented in the elderly with comorbidities like heart failure, liver disease, or malignancy, as well as those on polypharmacy (especially medications like non-steroidal anti-inflammatory drugs and selective serotonin-reuptake inhibitors). Serum sodium should be monitored in the first one or two days after initiation of the diuretic. However, thiazide-induced hyponatraemia can appear after many months of uncomplicated thiazide therapy especially when the steady balance is upset by concurrent illness. Patients should be educated about this expected side-effect and advised to temporarily stop the diuretic if there is any intercurrent illness resulting in poor oral intake or gastro-intestinal loss such as diarrhea or vomiting. It is also recommended that serum electrolytes are rechecked within 4–6 weeks and thereafter every 6–12 months.

Thiazide diuretics should be discontinued in this patient and replaced with an alternative antihypertensive not associated with hyponatraemia.

****

Mdm S presented to the Emergency Department six months later with a two-day history of a painful vesicular rash over her right back (Fig 5.1). She characterised the pain as intense, constant, stabbing, and unresponsive to paracetamol. These symptoms were accompanied by lethargy, fatigue, and loss of appetite.

Clinical examination revealed a lethargic woman who was alert and orientated. Vital signs were temperature 36.0°C, pulse rate 89/min, and blood pressure 140/90 mmHg. She was clinically euvolaemic.

Question 5: What is the most appropriate management?

a. **Betamethasone valerate 0.1% et clioquinol cream BD**
b. **Cephalexin 500 mg TDS**
c. **Mupirocin 2% cream BD**
d. **Valacyclovir 1 g TDS**
e. **Warm compresses BD**

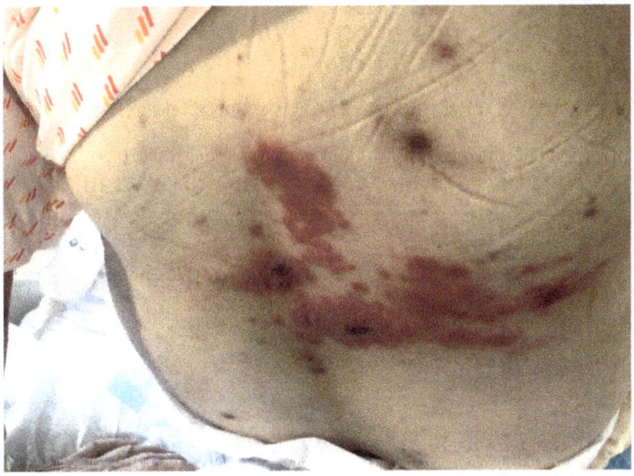

Fig. 5.1. Photograph courtesy of Dr Astrid Melani Suantio.

The rash consists of clusters of hemorrhagic vesicles on an erythematous base over the right T8/9 dermatomes suggesting acute herpes zoster infection. Zoster is a clinical diagnosis and treatment (acyclovir 800 mg 5x/d for 7 days or valacyclovir 1,000 mg 3x/d for 7 days) should be started within 72 hours for the best outcome. Dose adjustment is required for creatinine clearance <50 mL/min. Note that acyclovir may reduce INR in patients taking warfarin.

****

These are her laboratory investigations:

	Hospital Day
	On admission
Serum urea, mmol/L	*2.2*
Serum sodium, mmol/L	*115*
Serum potassium, mmol/L	*3.8*
Serum chloride, mmol/L	*81*
Serum bicarbonate, mmol/L	*21.3*
Serum glucose, mmol/L	*6.0*
Serum creatinine, mmol/L	*64*
Serum osmolality, mOsm/kg	*240*
Urine sodium, mmol/L	*104*
Urine osmolality, mOsm/kg	*387*

Liver function and thyroid function tests were normal and 8 am cortisol level was robust. Chest X-ray revealed no remarkable findings.

Question 6: What is your diagnosis at this point of time?

Question 7: What parameters need to be monitored in the management for her hyponatraemia?

Diagnostic workup should include history of drug intake and physical examination with specific attention to possible causes as well as symptoms from hyponatraemia. Given the clinical and initial laboratory investigations of inappropriately high urine osmolality in the presence of hypo-osmolality, hyponatraemia, and euvolaemia, Mdm S most likely has SIADH. The cause of SIADH is likely due to localised herpes zoster infection causing pain as a non-osmotic stimulus of ADH secretion.

Euvolaemic hyponatraemia has many causes, the commonest being SIADH. SIADH remains a ***diagnosis of exclusion.*** The Schwartz diagnostic criteria for SIADH is a composite of:

(1) Hyponatraemia
(2) Plasma osmolality <275 mOsm/kg
(3) Urine osmolality >100 mOsm/kg
(4) Urinary sodium excretion (UNa >30 mmol/L) with normal dietary salt and water intake
(5) Normal thyroid and adrenal function
(6) No recent use of diuretic medication

It should be kept in mind that diuretics can alter urine sodium concentration and confuse the work up of hyponatraemia.

Hyponatraemia in SIADH is usually chronic and hence slow correction is needed. However, in severe symptomatic or acute cases 3% NaCl should be considered at an initial infusion rate of ***1 mL/kg/hr with an estimation to raise the serum Na^+ by 1 mmol/L/h*** within the first 4 hours.

Fluid restriction (<1 L/day) is the initial treatment for chronic hyponatraemia in SIADH with the aim to increase free water excretion more than intake. Again, measurement of ***urine/plasma electrolyte ratio [(urine Na^+ + urine K^+)/serum Na^+]*** is useful to guide the extent of fluid restriction.

- Ratio <0.5 (indicating high urine electrolyte-free water) → fluid restriction is adequate.
- Ratio >1 (indicating concentrated urine) → <500 mL/day of fluid restriction is recommended.

Generally, fluid intake should be at least 500 mL below the patient's urine output; thus, usually 1 L or less.

If fluid restriction is not effective, salt tablets can be considered. Normally, ADH regulates urine volume in response to change in fluid intake. In patients with SIADH, where ADH is produced inappropriately in excess, urine osmolality is relatively fixed and urine volume varies with changes in solute excretion in the urine. Hence, increasing solute excretion by administering salt tablets (or urea tablets — presently not available locally) will increase urine volume and raise the serum sodium.

The desired increase in serum sodium in chronic hyponatremia should be 4–8 mmol/L in the first 24 hours (4–6 mmol/L per day in high risk for ODS) and <18 mmol/L over 48 hours. The rate of correction should be slower in conditions with higher risk of osmotic demyelination such as severe malnutrition, alcoholism, advanced liver disease, initial $Na^+ \leq 105$ mmol/L, and hypokalaemia.

****

Mdm S was managed with fluid restriction of 500 mL per 24 hours with addition of 3 sodium chloride tablets TDS:

	Hospital Day (hr)							
	On admission	*6 hr*	*12*	*18*	*24*	*30*	*36*	*48*
Serum urea, mmol/L	*2.2*	*2.2*			*2.7*			*3.9*
Serum sodium, mmol/L	*112*	*114*	*118*	*119*	*120*	*122*	*126*	*127*
Serum potassium, mmol/L	*3.8*	*4.0*			*4.0*			*3.7*
Serum chloride, mmol/L	*81*	*79*			*78*			*89*
Serum bicarbonate, mmol/L	*21.3*	*22.9*			*19.2*			*25.6*
Serum glucose, mmol/L	*6.0*				*7.4*			*7.7*
Serum creatinine, mmol/L	*43*	*48*			*47*			*65*
Serum osmolality, mOsm/kg	*240*							
Urine sodium, mmol/L	*104*							
Urine osmolality, mOsm/kg	*387*							
Intervention	*Fluid restricted to 500 mL/day, NaCl tablets 3 TDS*							
Daily intake, mL					*500*			*500*
Daily output, mL					*2,100*			*1,850*

Key messages

1. Elderly females are at higher risk than others for hyponatraemia from thiazide diuretics. The clinical picture along with blood and urine investigations of hyponatraemia are often complicated by some element of volume depletion from thiazide use. It may result in normal or elevated urine sodium even though there is underlying volume depletion. The main treatment is to stop the thiazide diuretic and at times fluid replacement is required.
2. It is usually not an emergency to treat chronic hyponatremia, which is asymptomatic and not associated with cerebral or cardiac signs and symptoms. If symptoms are severe, rapid controlled correction is necessary in the first few hours to reduce the risk of cerebral oedema.
3. Close monitoring of serum sodium concentration and fluid balance is crucial during the correction of hyponatraemia.
4. The fundamental concepts behind increasing serum sodium concentration in SIADH are that (i) the free water excretion should be more than intake and (ii) intake of solute should be more than its excretion.

Answer key

1. Thiazide diuretic, underlying SIADH, recent loss of appetite (possibly poor solute intake), recent dehydration.
2. D.
3. Consider re-lowering of Na^+ level with 5% dextrose water; monitor urine output hourly and monitor serum sodium level after each infusion; refer to nephrologist/endocrinologist regarding intranasal desmopressin.
4. E.
5. D.
6. Severe hyponatraemia likely secondary to SIADH.
7. Volume status and neurological status; weigh daily; serum Na^+, K^+ (4 to 12 hourly); serum osmolality daily; urine Na^+, K^+, osmolality daily; strict monitoring of input and output.

References

Spasovski G, Vanholder R, Allolio B, *et al.* (2014) Hyponatraemia Guideline Development Group: Clinical practice guideline on diagnosis and treatment of hyponatraemia. *Nephrol Dial Transplant* **29**(Suppl 2): i1–i39.

Verbalis JG, Goldsmith SR, Greenberg A, *et al.* (2013) Diagnosis, evaluation, and treatment of hyponatremia: expert panel recommendations. *Am J Med* **126**(10 Suppl 1): S1–S42.
Wang CC, Shiang JC, *et al.* (2011) Syndrome of inappropriate secretion of antidiuretic hormone associated with localized herpes zoster ophthalmicus. *J Gen Intern Med* **26**(2): 216–220.

6 Functional Decline II (Joint Problem)

Ng Kuan Geok, Teo Qiao Qi, Anupama Roy Chowdhury

Mr M is a 70-year-old Malay taxi driver who was admitted to the hospital due to a fall after his knees gave way. In the past year, he has experienced four to five falls, all due to knee pain and knees giving way. He has a long-standing history of bilateral knee pain, left worse than right, with worsening of pain with physical activity including walking — this has greatly affected his daily activities and social life. He has been taking two tablets of paracetamol three times a day, with which he has had minimal relief of pain. He has previously tried to reduce his weight through exercises with no yield as his knee pain has limited his physical ability. He used to be able to walk two to three blocks to nearby markets and coffee shops to meet his friends, but has been largely homebound this year. He reports no other joint pain and is otherwise well with no fever and systemic symptoms. He used to play soccer in college and he does not recall any history of sports injury. His medical history is notable for diabetes, hypertension, hyperlipidaemia, chronic kidney disease stage 4, and ischaemic heart disease with ischaemic cardiomyopathy.

Clinical examination revealed an obese man (BMI 30) with varus knee deformities. Both knees were warm to palpation, with suprapatellar effusions and medial joint line tenderness. Knee extensions were reduced by about 10° with crepitus on range of movement testing. Neurological examination of the lower limbs was unremarkable except for slight weakness in extension of both knees.

Question 1: What is your impression for Mr M, and what is the most likely differential diagnosis?

This patient is likely to have osteoarthritis (OA) of the knees. The typical joints affected by OA are the knees, hips, distal and proximal interphalangeal joints, first carpometacarpal and metatarsophalangeal joints, and the facet joints of the spine. It is characterised by joint line tenderness, reduced range of movement, crepitus, joint effusions, and valgus or varus deformity. Heberden and Bouchard nodules (swellings over the distal and proximal interphalangeal joints, respectively) may be present.

Pain is usually the most prominent symptom, which tends to come in two forms: a constant background aching pain and intermittent intense pain. Early in the course, the pain is predictable and caused by specific and often high impact activities. Over time, pain and other joint symptoms become less predictable and more constant, intense, and severe which result in patients avoiding certain activities. When activities of daily living become impaired, patients start to experience loss of independence and an impaired quality of life with a negative impact on mental health.

The OA is likely primary in Mr M. In other patients, secondary OA can occur in the setting of chondrocalcinosis, a history of joint trauma, metabolic bone disorders, hypermobility syndromes, and neuropathic diseases.

It is important to consider the differential diagnosis of a crystal arthropathy. Unlike classical gout in middle-aged men, gout in the elderly has a more equal gender distribution, frequent polyarticular presentation with involvement of finger joints, a more indolent chronic clinical course with fewer acute gouty episodes, and an increased incidence of tophi. Moreover, long-term diuretic use in patients with renal insufficiency and prophylactic low-dose aspirin are factors particularly associated with hyperuricaemia and gout in the elderly. Check this patient's drug history carefully as he has chronic renal disease and ischaemic heart disease!

Pseudogout in the elderly patient can be acute or chronic and can have a variety of clinical presentations. Although pseudogout most commonly affects the knee, it should still be considered in the evaluation of any patient with OA occurring in an atypical distribution. Other joints commonly involved are the wrists and second and third metacarpophalangeal joints.

The other differential diagnoses viz. haemarthrosis, inflammatory arthritis (rheumatoid arthritis, psoriatic arthritis, ankylosing spondylitis), septic arthritis, and ligamentous and meniscus injuries appear to be less likely in this scenario.

****

X-rays of both knees were performed. The right knee X-ray is shown below:

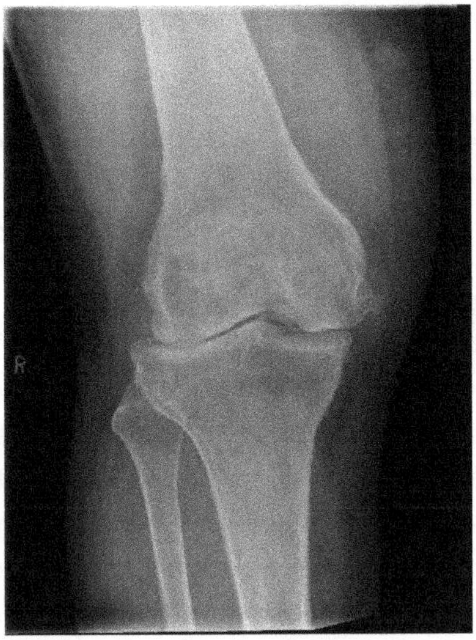

Question 2: What is the grade of OA according to the Kellgren–Lawrence classification system?

Although OA is primarily a clinical diagnosis, plain radiographs (weight-bearing views recommended) can be helpful to confirm it (at least grade 2 of the Kellgren–Lawrence radiographic classification) and rule out other pathologies. Note that the severity of radiographic changes does *not* correlate with the knee pain, but that the degree of discordance diminishes as the severity and persistence of knee pain increases.

Kellgren–Lawrence classification system *(radiographic severity of OA)*

Grade 0 (none): no joint space narrowing or reactive changes.
Grade 1 (questionable): doubtful joint space narrowing, possible osteophytic lipping.
Grade 2 (mild): ***definitive osteophytes****, possible joint space narrowing.*
Grade 3 (moderate): moderate osteophytes, ***definite joint space narrowing****, and possible bone end deformity.*
Grade 4 (severe): large osteophytes, marked joint space narrowing, ***severe sclerosis, definite bone end deformity****.*

Ultrasound offers many advantages, including low cost, no radiation, ability to image structure dynamically, and can be used to guide interventional procedures. MRI, rarely needed, can provide information on the structural integrity of cartilage and identify predisposing factors for OA such as meniscal damage and anterior cruciate ligament injury.

****

Question 3: Suggest an appropriate management plan for Mr M's knee problem.

Holistic management of OA requires consideration of the patient's premorbid functional status, lifestyle, comorbidities, severity of symptoms, and even personal preference.

Modifiable risk factors should be managed as far as possible. Muscle weakness should be addressed with physiotherapy. Rehabilitation usually comprises of a combination of supervised exercises and home programmes, and it includes strengthening, low impact aerobic exercise, aquatic exercise, tai chi, and balance training. Modalities like knee brace (tibiofemoral and patellofemoral braces), walking cane, kinesiotaping, and thermal intervention may also be employed. If the patient is still working and the job involves repetitive knee bending for instance, it would be prudent to discuss about revocationalising. Patients with metabolic syndrome or high BMI (especially if ≥25; high BMI is a strong risk factor for developing hand OA!) should be recommended weight loss programmes for dietary control and low-impact exercises.

Concurrent pharmacologic treatment for pain control is recommended. Regular acetaminophen may be used first line due to it being one of the safer analgesics when used at prescribed doses. A topical NSAID such as ketoprofen plaster may be added onto the affected joint. In the event that an oral NSAID is considered, the patient's comorbidities such as renal impairment, peptic ulcer disease or gastritis, and underlying heart disease must be taken into account. Using an oral NSAID in Mr M puts him at risk of worsening renal function, heart failure, and gastrointestinal bleeding if he is on an antiplatelet agent. Hence, it would not be a wise choice to start Mr M on an oral NSAID with other alternatives available.

Should regular acetaminophen and topical NSAID not be adequate in controlling the pain, a low dose of tramadol can be added with gradual titration upwards monitoring for adverse effects such as confusion, nausea and constipation. In a robust older patient with no obvious contraindications, should an oral NSAID be considered for use, it must be prescribed for the shortest duration possible with close monitoring for side-effects such as worsening renal function.

Duloxetine (start at 30 mg/day, $3.17 each, to mitigate nausea and gradually titrate to a maximum of 120 mg/day) may be added for patients with partial response to the aforesaid analgesics to improve pain control and physical functioning.

Glucosamine, chondroitin, and vitamin D may be helpful in patients with mild to moderate knee OA; the evidence, however, is inconsistent and limited.

For patients who cannot tolerate or respond only partially to oral analgesia, decline surgery, or prefer complementary and alternative medicine, referral to a acupuncture service can be offered. It has been shown to significantly reduce pain intensity and improve functional mobility and quality of life in OA.

Intra-articular corticosteroid injections can achieve short-term pain relief. The clinical effects decrease over time and usually last no longer than six months. Its benefit may be less predictable in obese patients and patients with advanced OA. Other intra-articular therapies such as hyaluronic acid (viscosupplementation), platelet-rich plasma, botulinum toxin, and hyperosmolar dextrose (prolotherapy) are presently not recommended for routine use.

Total knee replacement is the definitive treatment for advanced knee OA after failing conservative treatments. Genicular nerve radiofrequency ablation is generally reserved for patients with symptomatic knee OA who have failed conservative treatment or have failed or are poor candidates for total knee replacement surgery. It has been shown to consistently provide short-term (3- to 6-month) and sometimes longer pain relief and can be safely re-administered as necessary.

****

Mr M was started on tramadol for pain control but he was unable to tolerate higher doses due to constipation, nausea, vomiting, and drowsiness. Physiotherapy and occupational therapy services were engaged. He did not obtain adequate pain relief with knee brace and ice packs, which impaired his ability to participate in daily therapy sessions. Intra-articular corticosteroid injection was thus performed to improve his functional status. His knee pain significantly improved and he was discharged with outpatient orthopaedic surgical appointment for consideration of total knee replacement.

In view of significant cardiac history with impaired cardiac function, he was deemed to have high surgical risk for total knee replacement. In any case, Mr M was not keen for surgery. He was then referred for genicular nerve blocks to better manage his knee pain.

Key messages

1. OA is a clinical diagnosis. X-rays are useful for assessing severity, especially in the later stages.

2. It is important to consider other differential diagnoses or concomitant pathologies (in particular, crystal arthropathies) as treatment options and outcomes can be very different.
3. In those who opt for conservative management or are deemed unsuitable surgical candidates, there is a multitude of physical modalities and therapeutic interventions that can be explored to help improve quality of life of these patients.

Answer key

1. Bilateral knee primary OA with functional decline. An important differential diagnosis is crystal arthropathy (i.e., gout or pseudogout).
2. Grade 4.
3. Pain control with tramadol added on (since paracetamol alone was not effective and NSAIDs are contraindicated due to Stage 4 chronic kidney disease); referral for physiotherapy and occupational therapy; referral to weight loss management clinic; referral to orthopaedic service for consideration of surgical intervention.

References

Abramoff B, Caldera FE (2020) Osteoarthritis: Pathology, Diagnosis, and Treatment Options. *Med Clin North Am* **104**(2): 293–311.

Kohn MD, Sassoon AA, Fernando ND (2016) Classifications in Brief: Kellgren-Lawrence Classification of Osteoarthritis. *Clin Orthop Relat Res* **474**(8): 1886–1893.

Kolasinski SL, *et al.* (2020) 2019 American College of Rheumatology/Arthritis Foundation Guideline for the Management of Osteoarthritis of the Hand, Hip, and Knee. *Arthritis Care Res* **72**(2): 149–162.

7 Delirium I (Infection)

Pooja Sachdeva, Alvin Tan Wee Beng

Mr Z is an 85-year-old Chinese male who is independent in his activities of daily living and community ambulant with a walking stick. His medical history consists of hyperlipidemia, hypertension, ischaemic heart disease, degenerative disc disease with T12 compression fracture, gout, and asthma/COPD overlap. His medications include gabapentin 300 mg ON, amlodipine 2.5 mg OM, aspirin 100 mg OM, and atorvastatin 20 mg ON. He is also using a salbutamol inhaler, 2 puffs QDS/PRN. He has no known allergies.

Prior to the current admission, he complained of left wrist pain and swelling which had developed insidiously and progressed over five days. This was associated with fever, highest temperature recorded at home being 38°C, which responded to paracetamol. The family also noted that his speech was irrelevant and that his answers to their questions were inappropriate. There were no other systemic complaints like chest pain, orthopnea, or paroxysmal nocturnal dyspnoea. Mr Z had long-standing exertional dyspnoea but no change in effort tolerance recently.

Systemic review for infective screen was negative; in particular, he did not have nocturia, polyuria, frothy urine, jaundice, or abdominal swelling. He has occasional constipation which improves with drinking water and walking. Mr Z is not observing any fluid restriction; however, he is compliant to medications.

Question 1: The above history is obtained from the Emergency Department. What other relevant aspects of history would you want to probe further at initial assessment?

Mr Z experienced gouty attacks at least 4–5 times in a year that usually involved the hands, fingers, and wrists. He is not taking any preventive medication. The current attack, however, was preceded by fever. He has not sought any consultation for the above nor has he taken any medication for it apart from paracetamol.

Functionally, Mr Z can shower, dress, and feed himself. He uses a walking stick to ambulate in the community. He goes for evening walks to meet his friends daily. There had been no decline in his cognition noted by family. He was able to recognise family, manage money, and buy his own food. There had been no prior incidents of him losing his way or wandering about. The episode of talking irrelevantly prior to this admission was new and the first of such an occurrence.

Socially, the patient is a widower and stays with his son, daughter-in-law, and three grandchildren. There is a helper in the family but is not designated for his care. His medical appointments are managed by his son and medications are served by a helper. He does not need home care support or community support.

Clinical examination revealed a hydrated and comfortable patient. However, he was not orientated to time, place, and person. Vitals signs were temperature 38.3°C, blood pressure 126/66 mmHg, heart rate 78/min, and SpO_2 96% in room air. He was agitated, talking loudly, giving unrelated responses to questions asked, and was trying to climb out of bed.

His left wrist joint was warm and swollen with overlying erythema and tenderness extending to the dorsum of his hand. Active and passive range of motion of the left wrist joint was limited due to the pain and swelling. Active synovitis of the left 1st and 2nd metacarpophalangeal joints (MCPJs) and proximal interphalangeal joints (PIPJs) of the middle finger were also noted. A gouty tophus was noted over the left 3rd finger PIPJ.

Heart sounds were dual with no murmurs, breath sounds were vesicular, and abdominal examination did not reveal organomegaly or ascites. Neurological examination was limited by disorientation, but he was moving all four limbs spontaneously.

Question 2: The 4AT is a brief tool that we can use to screen for delirium. You can access it by downloading the free app "SIGN decision support". Calculate the 4AT score for Mr Z.

The domains to calculate the 4AT score for acute delirium are:

(1) Alertness (drowsy/somnolent/hyperactive)
(2) Attention (count backwards months in a year)
(3) AMT4 (age, date of birth, place, year)
(4) Acute onset (less than 2 weeks) and/or fluctuating course (symptoms present in the last 24 hours)

A score ≥4 suggests delirium. It is a *screening* test, not a diagnostic test and it has less specificity. A detailed cognition history should be taken to further delineate the timeline of cognitive decline, if any, and the nature of the acute change in mental status observed. Alternatively, you can use the Confusion Assessment Method which has >90% sensitivity for diagnosing delirium [covered in Chapter 8 on Delirium II (Medication)].

Question 3: What are some bedside tests that can be done to look out for other common precipitating factors for delirium in an elderly person?

Mr Z has acute hyperactive delirium from fever with polyarthritis. The many possible causes include crystal arthropathy, septic arthritis, and inflammatory arthritis such as rheumatoid arthritis, psoriasis, reactive arthritis, or traumatic arthritis with superimposed infection. With a previous history of gout, crystal arthropathy would often be considered as the first differential; however, considering the patient's age, fever, and the presence of delirium, septic arthritis must be excluded. Note that fever may be absent in elderly patients with septic arthritis due to the atypical presentations of illness in this age group! Hence, a high index of suspicion is needed to diagnose this potentially life threatening condition. Hydroxyapatite crystal deposition in the hands and joints may also cause acute inflammatory syndromes that mimic septic arthritis.

****

Laboratory investigations showed:

WBC count	*10.26 x 10^9/L*	*(4–10)*
Haemoglobin	*13.0 g/dL*	*(12–16)*
Platelet count	*126 x 10^9/L*	*(140–440)*
Blood urea	*10.3 mmol/L*	*(2.7–6.9)*
Sodium	*139 mmol/L*	*(136–146)*
Potassium	*4.4 mmol/L*	*(3.5–5.1)*
Serum creatinine	*118 µmol/L*	*(45–84)*
C-reactive protein	*95 mg/L*	*(0.2–9.1)*
Serum procalcitonin	*1.14 mcg/L*	*(<0.49)*
Creatine kinase	*72 U/L*	*(56–336)*
CKMB	*1.2 µg/L*	*(1–5)*
Trop-T	*59 ng/L*	*(<29)*
ProBNP	*2,796 pg/ml*	*(<149)*

Chest X-ray: no congestion or opacities.

Blood and urine cultures were taken.

X-rays of left hand and wrist: There is soft tissue swelling involving the left middle finger and index finger. Bony erosions are seen in the proximal third metacarpal. There is no fracture. Significant joint space narrowing, marginal spurring, and articular/peri-articular erosive changes are noted at the left middle finger PIPJ.

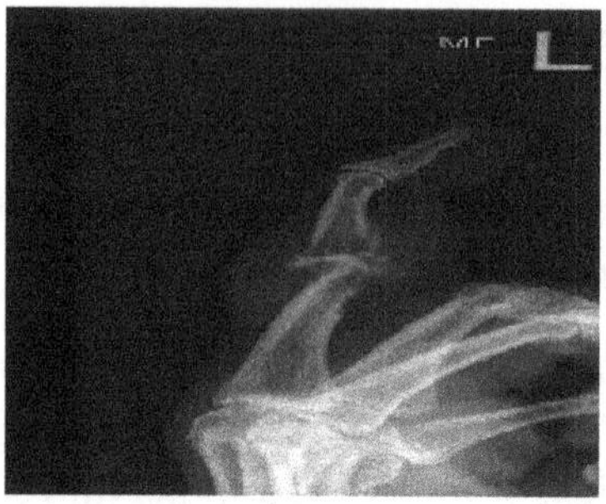

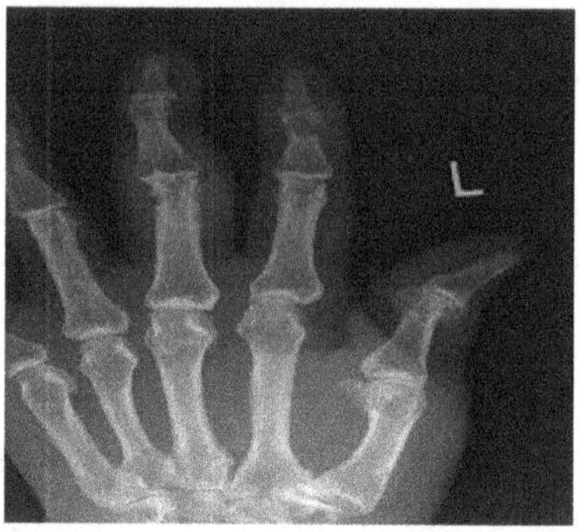

Question 4: Which of the following is the next *most* appropriate investigation?

a. **Imaging (e.g., CT, MRI)**
b. **Joint aspiration and analysis**
c. **Rheumatoid factor**
d. **Serum uric acid level**
e. **Synovial biopsy**

The radiographic findings of an effusion/arthritis may include soft tissue swelling, displacement of muscle surrounding the joint, widening of the joint space, increased opacity within the joint, distension of the joint capsule, subluxation, erosion or disappearance of the epiphysis or metaphysis, or erosion of subchondral bone.

The diagnosis of septic arthritis requires joint aspiration and fluid analysis with culture. For smaller joints such as MCPJs and PIPJs that may not be aspirated, a diagnosis can be made on MRI or ultrasonography (USG). For the bigger joints such as hip and sacro-iliac joints, imaging can help in the diagnosis of an effusion. Both MRI and USG have high sensitivity for effusion. Imaging also helps in the diagnosis of concomitant osteomyelitis and trauma.

Synovial biopsy is not a routine procedure. Indications for synovial biopsy include refractory mono-arthritis, a high degree of suspicion for atypical infectious agents (mycobacterium, fungal infections), or evaluation for intra-articular tumors.

Serum uric acid level is ***NOT*** useful in the setting of acute gout.

****

Although acute gouty arthritis was the working diagnosis, left wrist septic arthritis with overlying cellulitis could not be excluded. MRI was ordered for the left wrist joint to exclude septic arthritis; however, it could not be performed as Mr Z was unable to keep his hand and wrist in the required position for the duration of the scan despite analgesia with subcutaneous fentanyl. Empirical intravenous cefazolin and oral colchicine were commenced.

His mental state gradually improved. On day three of admission, he was orientated to time, place, and person, but he was not able to tell his date/year of birth, age, and full address correctly.

Serum uric acid level rose from 544 to 638 µmol/L. Blood cultures were negative.

Question 5: Which of the following is the most appropriate management of the agitation in Mr Z?

a. Application of restraints.
b. Dim ambient lighting and enforce low noise in the room.
c. Recurrent orientation by staff, bedside boards with dates/location.
d. Regular haloperidol (PO/IM/IV).
e. Rivastigmine patch.

Question 6: What is the next most appropriate course of action if both joint aspiration and MRI cannot be performed?

a. Continue colchicine and wait for improvement.
b. Continue colchicine and add prednisolone.
c. Continue antibiotics and refer to orthopaedic surgery for joint washout.
d. Continue antibiotics and colchicine and request for CT or alternative imaging.
e. Replace cefazolin with a broader-spectrum antibiotic like meropenem.

Patients with delirium can improve with environmental changes such as quiet surroundings, well-lit rooms, music therapy, and regular orientation by doctors, nurses, and allied health professionals. Unless absolutely necessary to prevent falls or dislodgement of therapeutic devices, the use of restraints should be avoided as it may exaggerate the delirium.

Should patients remain aggressive, agitated, and combative despite the use of non-pharmacological measures, certain medications may be used such as anti-psychotics (haloperidol, risperidone, quetiapine, olanzapine) and benzodiazepines (lorazepam). However, these medications should only be used on an ***as-needed*** basis at the lowest dose and for the shortest duration possible.

Haloperidol can be used via enteral or parenteral routes. Benzodiazepines should be avoided as studies have shown that these may precipitate or worsen delirium. These are only indicated if antipsychotics are contraindicated and patients are also at risk of other conditions such as alcohol withdrawal. Cholinesterase inhibitors have no role in the treatment or symptom management of delirium.

USG and MRI both have high sensitivity for diagnosis of effusion. USG can diagnose synovial oedema, effusion, and joint involvement. While inferior to MRI, it is cheaper and more easily available.

It is not advisable to wait and watch when septic arthritis is a suspicion as it can potentially damage the joint if suboptimally treated and can progress to the cortical and medullary bone resulting in osteomyelitis. It is also not advisable to add a systemic corticosteroid unless a clear diagnosis of crystal arthropathy or reactive arthritis is made as it may cause lymphopenia at the site of infection, thus exacerbating the infection.

Joint washout is an acceptable intervention if the infection is responding poorly to antibiotics and there is a high suspicion of atypical organisms as the pathogenic cause. It should, however, be attempted once the involvement of the joint has been confirmed by imaging.

****

USG of the left wrist was performed and showed diffuse skin and subcutaneous oedema in the forearm, dorsal wrist, and hand, in keeping with cellulitis. Diffuse synovial thickening with increased vascularity in the dorsal aspect of the radiocarpal, inter-carpal, and distal radioulnar joints was also noted in keeping with synovitis. There was no fluid collection or significant joint effusion.

Mr Z was continued on intravenous cefazolin and colchicine with trending of inflammatory markers and white counts as follows:

CRP (mg/L) 195 → 356 → 135 → 158 (day 7)
WBC {x10^9/L} 10.62 → 8.42 → 5.16 (day 7)

One week after admission, Mr Z's mentation improved considerably but he developed another spike of fever. He mentioned improvement in pain over his wrist and hand and had no other systemic complaint. On examination, the erythema was noted to extend from the left wrist/hand to the left forearm/elbow. There was significant synovitis over the left middle PIPJ and mild synovitis over the PIPJs of all other fingers on the left hand. There was no fluctuation over the wrist joint, with improved range of motion (45°). The elbow joint had full range of motion with no clinical effusion.

Repeat blood and urine cultures were negative. Antibiotics were escalated to intravenous crystalline penicillin and ceftazidime plus clindamycin.

Question 7: What is the most appropriate next course of action?

a. Refer to orthopaedic surgery for joint washout.
b. Refer to orthopaedic surgery for surgical exploration.
c. Refer to physiotherapy for gentle rehabilitation.
d. Suspend all antibiotics and observe the fever trend.
e. Work up reactive arthritis and evaluate for atypical microorganisms.

As Mr Z continued to be febrile despite antibiotic treatment, he should be investigated for atypical organisms, resistant organisms, or disseminated infection with high load of causative organisms. Rapidly progressing erythema and extensive soft tissue infection will require surgical exploration and debridement for source control, as well as to complement the medical antibiotic therapy. Joint washout should be performed if the patient has significant effusion to provide a culture for organism identification, source control, and adequate drainage.

****

Urethral swabs for chlamydia PCR and gonorrhea PCR were negative. Transthoracic echocardiography showed no vegetation, normal left ventricular ejection fraction 54%, mild diastolic dysfunction, no mitral valve stenosis or regurgitation, and mild aortic sclerosis. Mr Z declined MRI wrist under sedation. Orthopaedic consult observed a limited role of joint washout in the absence of significant joint effusion. Mr Z was continued on triple antibiotics for two weeks followed by single intravenous cefazolin for four weeks via central catheter. Inflammatory markers were trended as follows:

CRP (mg/L) 158 → 42.6 → 244.8 → 162 → 26.5 → 6.3 (day 21)
WBC {x10^9/L} 5.16 → 5.62 → 9.85 → 6.20 → 5.80 (day 21)

On discharge, the mini mental state examination score was 22/30.

Questions 8: What advice would you give to the patient and family upon discharge?

In our patient, the diagnosis of septic arthritis was made in retrospect. His symptoms improved with prolonged broad-spectrum antibiotic therapy for clinical septic arthritis in the absence of fluid aspirate and cultures and diagnostic imaging. The patient was reviewed outpatient for resolution of symptoms and functional assessment.

This case highlights the delirium caused by septic arthritis in the elderly. Septic arthritis should be treated aggressively with antibiotics (broad-spectrum followed by targeted therapy based on culture results), covering common organisms such as *Staphylococcus aureus*, group A *Streptococci*, and gram-negative bacilli; atypical organisms may need to be covered in patients with risk factors. Most cases of septic arthritis in the elderly have radiologic evidence of pre-existing joint disease in the affected joint, and the commonest joint involved is the knee. Although crystal arthropathies and septic arthritis may cause chronic pain, the commonest cause of any joint pain in the elderly, nevertheless, is still osteoarthritis.

Key messages

1. When evaluating an infectious cause for delirium in the elderly, take care to examine the joints carefully. The elderly with septic arthritis may not be febrile!
2. Septic arthritis is diagnosed with joint aspirate for analysis and culture. For smaller joints such as MCPJs and PIPJs that may not be aspirated, a diagnosis can be made on MRI or USG.
3. Consider atypical organisms, resistant organisms, or disseminated bacterial infection in cases of septic arthritis which apparently respond suboptimally to initial antibiotic therapy.

Answer key

1. Characterise the joint pain: first or multiple episodes, previous gouty attacks and joints involved, frequency of attacks per year, and medications;

   Characterise the fever: with chills, precedes or occurs after the joint swelling, any treatment other than paracetamol (e.g., antibiotics, colchicine);

   Determine his functional capacity (cognition): underlying cognitive decline, history of short-term memory loss, apraxia, aphasia, agnosia, executive dysfunction, previous episodes of delirium, episodes of wandering;

   Establish his social support (caregiver, environment): designated caregiver, home care availability or support services such as meals on wheels etc., home environment such as lift landing, attached toilets, sitting commodes, bathroom adjustment as per elderly care needs.
2. 12.
3. Bedside swallowing test (swallowing impairment may suggest new stroke, intracranial lesions, and risk for aspiration leading to pneumonia);

Post void residual urine by bladder scan or physical examination (suggests tendency for urinary retention and urinary tract infection);

Per rectal examination (look for impacted stools that may suggest constipation);

Sitting and standing postural BP change (suggests tendency for falls, imbalance, and impaired posture reflexes).

4. A.
5. C.
6. D.
7. E.
8. Mr Z should be reviewed in the outpatient clinic for functional limitation of the affected joints, as septic arthritis of the wrist can lead to long-term functional restrictions or osteomyelitis may develop subsequently. For Mr Z's cognitive decline, he should receive a geriatrician's assessment and be advised to avoid precipitating causes such as dehydration, infection, constipation, and anticholinergic medication. Furthermore, he should have a designated caregiver (or caregivers) to assist with medications, meals, and mobility to prevent falls. Future financial and healthcare planning should also be discussed.

References

Sendi P, Kaempfen A, Uckay I, Meier R (2020) Bone and joint infections of the hand. *Clin Microbiol Infect* **26**(7): 848–856.

Vincent GM, Amirault JD (1990) Septic arthritis in elderly. *Clin Orthop Relat Resp* **251**: 241–245.

Wei LA, Fearing MA, Sterberg EJ, Inouye SK (2008) The Confusion Assessment Method: A systematic review of current usage. *J Am Geriatr Soc* **56**(5): 823–830.

8 Delirium II (Medication)

Cheong Li Anne, Jessica Chen Weizhen

Mdm D is an 85-year-old lady who was brought in by her family members to the emergency department with change in behaviour over the past three days. The family reported her appearing anxious, removing her clothing, and passing urine in the corridor. She has a known history of hypertension, hyperlipidaemia, lumbar spondylosis, and osteoarthritis of the knee. Prior to this admission, she was independent with her activities of daily living and able to ambulate with a point stick in the community.

Further history from the family revealed that Mdm D had been experiencing knee pain for the past two weeks. She saw her family doctor, who prescribed tramadol 50 mg TDS and Anarex (paracetamol/orphenadrine) 2 tablets TDS. She has not opened her bowels in the past three days. Reduced urine output was also observed. There was no report of fever, cough, dysuria, or abdominal pain.

On examination, Mdm D was oriented to time, place, and person but was distractible and could not follow a proper conversation. Cardiorespiratory examination was unremarkable. Abdominal examination revealed a palpable bladder while digital rectal examination showed faecal impaction. The right knee was swollen and mildly tender, with crepitus elicited over passive range of motion. Neurological examination was unremarkable.

Question 1: Identify Mdm D's clinical syndrome and its aetiology.

Question 2: Outline an initial management plan.

Delirium is an acute, fluctuating syndrome of altered attention, awareness, and cognition precipitated by an underlying condition or event in vulnerable persons. It can be diagnosed using the Confusion Assessment Method criteria:

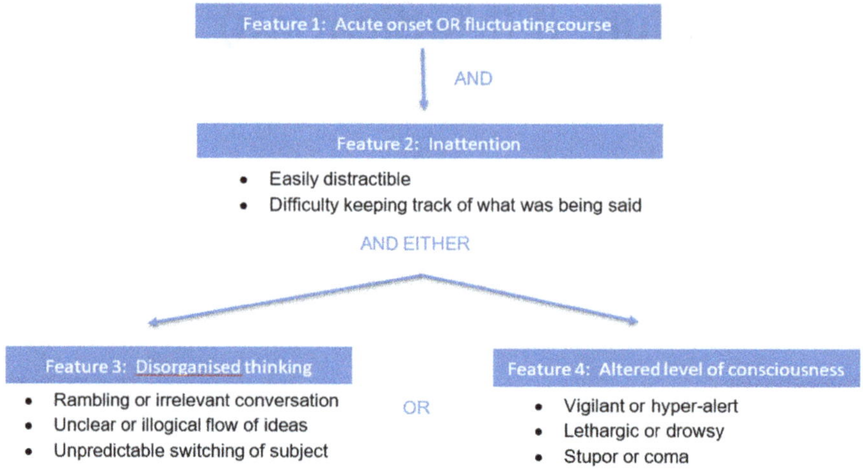

There are three subtypes of delirium:

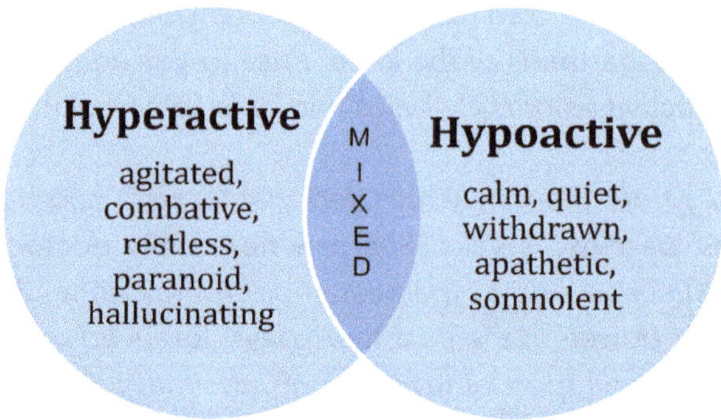

Though more common, the hypoactive form is harder to detect in older adults and is often under-recognised. Patients with delirium carry an overall high morbidity due to falls, pressure sores, malnutrition, and continence problems in addition to the underlying precipitant which is often a serious condition (coronary event, stroke, infection). Furthermore, delirium adds to caregiver stress, increases hospital length of stay, and increases the risk of further functional decline and need for long-term institutionalised care.

It is important to note that delirium should not be viewed as a standalone diagnosis but instead act as a cue to the clinician to search for possible underlying precipitating and predisposing causes. A thorough history and physical examination is key.

Causes of delirium are described in Table 8.1 — you can appreciate why the elderly are particularly vulnerable to developing delirium!

Table 8.1. Aetiologic considerations in Delirium.

Predisposing factors	**Precipitating factors**
Demographic characteristics – age >65 years – male sex Cognitive status – Previous history of delirium – Depression – Underlying dementia Visual and hearing impairment Malnutrition Drugs – Polypharmacy – Treatment with psychoactive drugs – Alcohol abuse Medical history – Multiple coexisting conditions – Chronic renal or hepatic disease – History of stroke or neurologic disease – Recent trauma or surgery Functional status – Dependence, immobility	Intercurrent illnesses – Infections, e.g., pneumonia, urinary tract infection (***also look for less common sources — skin esp. sacrum in bed-bound, joints***) – Hypoxia – Acute organ dysfunction, e.g., myocardial infarction, heart failure, acute renal failure, hepatic failure – Urinary retention – Faecal impaction Metabolic – Anaemia – Electrolyte derangements – Hypoglycemia – Hypothyroidism/hyperthyroidism – Vitamin deficiencies: thiamine, – Poor nutritional status Neurological conditions – Meningitis or encephalitis – Cerebrovascular accident – Intracranial bleed – Seizure/epilepsy Drugs – Sedatives, narcotics, anticholinergic drugs, anticonvulsants Environmental issues – Use of physical restraints – Bladder catheterisation – Multiple procedures – Prolonged sleep deprivation – New environment – Pain
Useful mnemonic for *common* causes of delirium: "**PINCH ME**" – Pain Infection Nutrition Constipation Hydration – Medication Environment	

Prescribing for the older adult can be challenging. With age, there are changes with drug distribution, metabolism, and excretion (Table 8.2).

Table 8.2. Pharmacokinetic considerations in drug prescribing in the older adult.

Absorption	– ↑ gastric pH and ↓ gastric emptying → changing net absorption – ↓ splanchnic blood flow → delaying peak effects – ↓ bowel motility → altering peak effects
Distribution	– ↑ adipose tissue → ↑ accumulation and duration of effect for lipophilic medications – ↓ total body water → lower required loading doses for hydrophilic medications
Metabolism	– ↓ phase one metabolism (modification reactions usually occurring within the liver) → ↑ of phase-1-dependent medications – ↓ hepatic blood flow → altered metabolism
Elimination	– ↓ glomerular filtration rate. ***Important to renal dose adjust drugs accordingly***.

The altered physiology of the elderly results in increased risk of drug side-effects. Table 8.3 discusses some common classes of drugs which predispose to delirium in the older adult.

Basic laboratory workup for older adults presenting with delirium would include full blood count, renal function and electrolytes, liver function test, and electrocardiogram. Further evaluation should be individualised according to the patient's presentation, medical history, and physical examination. While neuroimaging is not routinely required, it should be considered with patients with focal neurological deficits, a history of head trauma, systemic anticoagulation, or elevated risk of intracranial processes such as metastatic malignancy.

Management should be focused on identifying and treating precipitating factors of delirium. Supportive measures are also important in both the prevention and management of delirium. These include ensuring adequate nutrition and hydration, adequate analgesia, encouraging mobilisation, avoiding sleep disruption, and ensuring regular emptying of bladder and bowels. Physical restraints and bladder catheterisation should be avoided if possible. Patients with visual or hearing impairment will benefit from having their spectacles and hearing aids with them. The presence of a familiar caregiver at the bedside is also very useful in patients who are at risk or who are already delirious. In the inpatient setting, it is important to identify hospitalised patients who are at risk of delirium (see predisposing factors in the above table) and put in place measures to reduce that risk.

Occasionally agitation and behavioural issues may be dangerous or disruptive of essential medical care and chemical restraints may be required. Typical

Table 8.3. Common Drugs Predisposing to Delirium in the older adult.

Therapeutic class	Rationale	Remarks
Anticholinergic drugs		
First generation antihistamines, e.g., hydroxyzine (Atarax), chlorpheniramine (Piriton), diphenhydramine (Benadryl)	Highly anticholinergic: risk of confusion, dry mouth, constipation, and urinary retention.	Consider second-generation antihistamines, e.g., loratadine, cetirizine.
Antispasmodics, e.g., atropine, hyoscine butylbromide (Buscopan)	Highly anticholinergic.	
Anti-emetics, e.g., prochlorperazine (Stemetil), promethazine	Risk of anticholinergic side-effects.	Consider metoclopramide.
CNS		
Benzodiazepines, e.g., lorazepam (short-acting), diazepam (long-acting)	Increased sensitivity and decreased metabolism of long-acting agents. Increased risk of cognitive impairment, delirium, and falls.	
Non-benzodiazepine hypnotics, e.g., zaleplon, Zolpidem (Stilnox)	Increased risk of sedation and delirium.	
Tertiary tricyclic antidepressants, e.g., amitriptyline, imipramine	Highly anticholinergic.	Consider alternatives, e.g., for depression: SSRI or SNRI. For neuropathic pain: SNRI, gabapentin, pregabalin, Lidocaine patch.

(Continued)

Table 8.3. *(Continued)*

Therapeutic class	Rationale	Remarks
Analgesia		
Opioids, e.g., oxycodone, morphine, tramadol	Risk of sedation, urinary retention, constipation; Risk of serotonin syndrome when used with SSRI; Reduced seizure threshold.	Use only in moderate to severe pain; Start at lower dose; Avoid long duration or sustained release formulations.
Muscle relaxant orphenadrine (Anarex)	Highly anticholinergic.	Avoid use.
Others		
Corticosteroids	Psychiatric side-effects such as mania, depression, psychosis, and delirium are common.	When indicated, use lowest dose and shortest required duration. Dose in the morning.

Note: Adapted from the American Geriatrics Society Beer's Criteria List.

antipsychotics (e.g., low dose haloperidol 0.5 mg Q8h PRN) or atypical antipsychotics (e.g., olanzapine 2.5–5 mg ON, risperidone 0.5–2 mg ON) are most commonly used. Care should be taken to check for a ***prolonged QT interval*** which is a known side-effect. Benzodiazepines should be considered in patients with alcohol withdrawal or when Lewy body dementia is suspected.

It is important to note that the clinical course of delirium may be protracted in some patients, lasting from weeks to months. Post-discharge follow-up is important to track a patient's cognitive recovery after an acute precipitating event as these patients are at risk of cognitive decline.

****

Question 3: How should Mdm D's pain be assessed and managed?

Pain is a highly prevalent and often under-treated clinical problem in older adults. Poor pain control can contribute to poor nutrition, hydration, delirium, and functional decline. Identifying pain can be challenging due to physicians' and patients' misconception that pain is an expected part of ageing. Communications of symptoms may also be poor due to hearing, visual, or cognitive impairment. Physicians are justifiably concerned about the potential side-effects of analgesia.

Pain assessment can be done using unidimensional scores such as numeric rating scales or visual analogue scales. Multi-dimensional measures such as the Pain Assessment IN Advanced Dementia (PAINAD) score can also be used for cognitively impaired older adults. Anxiety and mood as well as their impact on function and sleep should be evaluated as part of a comprehensive geriatric pain assessment.

Non-pharmacological measures such as exercise interventions should form a core component of a patient's treatment plan. Primary components include training in balance, flexibility, endurance, and strengthening. Prescription of a brace and orthosis by a therapist can also be helpful.

In terms of pharmacological treatment, the WHO analgesia pain ladder Table 8.4 can be used as a guide. However, clinicians should bear in mind nuances in treatment.

Table 8.4. Prescribing considerations of analgesia in the older adult.

	WHO pain ladder	Considerations in older adults
Mild pain	Paracetamol	Risk of liver toxicity at higher doses. Risk of unintentional overdose.
	Non-steroidal anti-inflammatory drugs (NSAID)	More prone to gastrointestinal bleeding. Reduced GFR may also preclude use. Consider use of topical NSAIDs as an alternative. If systemic NSAIDs need to be used, use the lowest dose for the shortest duration possible.
Moderate pain	Weak opioids, e.g., codeine and tramadol	More sensitive to sedative effects with increased risk of delirium, constipation, and urinary retention. May be considered in patients who do not respond to first-line analgesia. Start low and go slow (e.g., tramadol 25 mg TDS/PRN).
Severe Pain	Strong opioids, e.g., morphine, oxy-codone, fentanyl	Used in severe pain or when functioning or quality of life is impaired. Side-effects (e.g., sedation) may limit use. Start at a lower dose (e.g., mist morphine 2.5 mg Q6-8H) and gradually titrate upwards.

For neuropathic pain, consider adjuvants such as anticonvulsants (e.g., gabapentin, pregabalin) and avoid tricyclic antidepressants (TCAs) in view of anticholinergic side-effects.

In appropriate patients with sub-optimally controlled pain, consultation with a pain specialist should be considered. Options of minimally invasive procedures may be considered in specific patient groups (e.g., intra-articular injections in rotator cuff injuries or osteoarthritis, lumbar epidural steroid injection in lumbar stenosis).

Key messages

1. Delirium is an acute, fluctuating syndrome of altered attention, awareness, and cognition precipitated by an underlying condition or event in vulnerable persons.
2. Common precipitating causes of delirium include:

   Pain **I**nfection **N**utrition **C**onstipation **H**ydration

   Medication **E**nvironment
3. Prescriptions in the elderly have to be taken with care in view of differences in drug absorption, distribution, metabolism, and elimination. This can make them more prone to drug side-effects.
4. Drugs such as first-generation antihistamines and tricyclic antidepressant hypnotics (benzodiazepines and non-benzodiazepines) should be avoided in the elderly in view of elevated risk of delirium.
5. Pain management in the elderly requires a holistic approach starting with a comprehensive geriatric pain assessment. Pharmacological measures follow the WHO pain ladder but with attention to higher risk of side-effects of certain drug classes. Consider minimally invasive procedures for pain management in appropriate patients.

Answer key

1. Hyperactive delirium likely due to recent intake of analgesic drugs (tramadol and orphenadrine) which led to constipation and acute urinary retention.
2. Basic investigations, e.g., full blood count, renal panel, liver panel, electrocardiogram;

   Suspend Anarex and tramadol;

   Intermittent catheterisation for urinary retention;

Clear bowels with oral laxatives;

Early mobilisation with physiotherapist;

Optimise environmental factors: keeping calm, quiet environment, minimised sleep disruption, ensuring adequate hydration and nutrition.

3. Comprehensive geriatric pain assessment: use pain score (e.g., visual analogue, numeric rating); assess mood, anxiety, and their impact on function and sleep;

   Non-pharmacological strategies: physiotherapy, knee guard;

   Pharmacological treatment: topical NSAIDs, regular paracetamol, can restart tramadol at lower dose of 25 mg TDS PRN or codeine 15 mg TDS PRN;

   Consider referral for intra-articular injections for pain relief;

   Consider outpatient referral to Orthopaedics for consideration of knee replacement.

References

American Geriatrics Society Beers Criteria® Update Expert Panel (2019) American Geriatrics Society 2019 updated AGS Beers Criteria® for Potentially Inappropriate Medication Use in Older Adults. *J Am Geriatr Soc* **67**(4): 674–694.

Hanlon JT, Semla TP, Schmader KE (2015) Alternative Medications for Medications in the Use of High-Risk Medications in the Elderly and Potentially Harmful Drug-Disease Interactions in the Elderly Quality Measures. *J Am Geriatr Soc* **63**(12): e8–e18.

Kalish VB, Gillham JE, Unwin BK (2014) Delirium in older persons: Evaluation and management. *Am Fam Physician* **90**(3): 150–158.

Oh ES, Fong TG, Hshieh TT, Inouye SK (2017) Delirium in Older Persons: Advances in Diagnosis and Treatment. *JAMA* **318**(12): 1161–1174.

Reid MC, Eccleston C, Pillemer K (2015) Management of chronic pain in older adults. *BMJ* **350**: h532.

9 Behaviour Disturbances (Dementia)

Deanna Lee Wai Ching, Anupama Roy Chowdhury

Mr A is a 90-year-old gentleman who used to work as a bus driver prior to his retirement. He is ambulant with the aid of a walking frame, but he requires assistance for his other activities of daily living. He was still largely continent at home and was able to go to the toilet supervised. His past medical history includes hyperlipidaemia, paroxysmal atrial fibrillation (CHA_2DS_2-VASc 2–3, ejection fraction 60% on echocardiogram in 2013), and bilateral cataracts (not operated on). Mr A is on regular follow-up with a geriatrician for the problems of Alzheimer's dementia with behavioural and psychological symptoms of dementia (BPSD) and frequent falls. One of his falls resulted in a small subdural haematoma in the frontal region.

His regular medications include aspirin 100 mg OM, diltiazem-SR 90 mg OM, famotidine 20 mg OM, fluvoxamine 25 mg OM, quetiapine 6.25 mg ON/PRN for agitation, and hypromellose 0.3% eye-drops.

Mr A currently presents to the emergency department with behavioural change of 3 days' duration, where he has been noted to be more aggressive than usual. He has been shouting at his family members, threatening to hurt them using knives, and even threatening to commit suicide. He has not been able to sleep, and his family members were not able to cope with his behaviour. Prior to admission, he was found on the floor of his home and was unable to get up due to bilateral lower limb weakness. There was no recent change in medications.

Question 1: What additional history would you like to ask?

Patients with cognitive impairment and dementia are vulnerable and have increased risk of delirium. The acute change in behaviour in Mr A is due to delirium.

As Fig. 9.1 illustrates, the more vulnerable an older person is, the smaller the insult required to precipitate a delirium. For example, in a patient with moderate to severe dementia, constipation or even just a change in their familiar environment or caregiver may precipitate delirium.

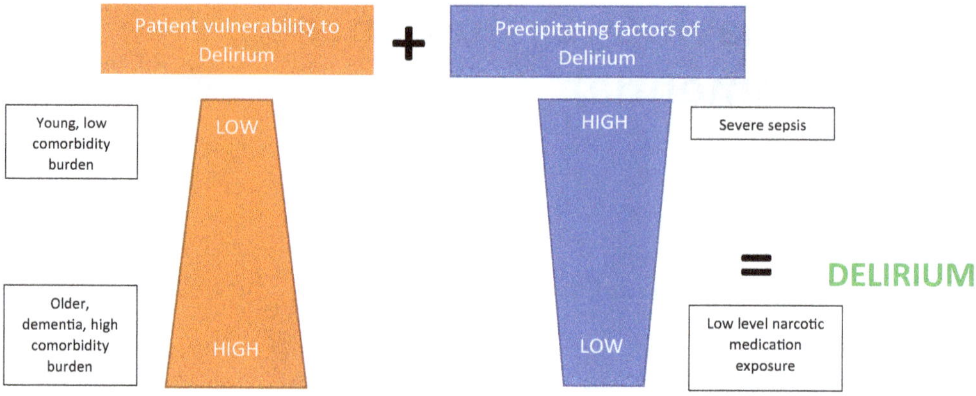

Fig. 9.1. Model adapted from Inouye, *et al.* (2014) Delirium in elderly people. *Lancet* **383**(9920): 911–922.

****

Mr A does not have any infective symptoms; his bowel and bladder habits were normal. He reports low mood but no hallucinations. At baseline, Mr A has short-term memory loss but is able to recognise family members and hold a simple coherent conversation. He has difficulty keeping track of days and dates but has no disorientation to time of day. His appetite has reduced in the past two days.

On physical examination, his vital signs were temperature 37.2°C, blood pressure 116/78 mmHg with no postural drop, heart rate 96/min, and respiratory rate 20/min with SpO_2 98% on room air. Mr A was disorientated to time, place, and person. He was inattentive during the consult. There was no conjunctival pallor, scleral icterus, cervical lymphadenopathy, or pedal oedema. Heart sounds were dual, lung fields were clear, and abdomen was soft and non-tender. Per rectal examination revealed an intact anal tone with unimpacted brown stool. Post-void residual urine (PVRU) was 230 mL. Neck was supple. Neurological examination showed facial symmetry, normal extraocular moments, slightly reduced power in all four limbs, normal tone and reflexes including Babinski's, and intact cerebellar function. Bilateral cataracts were noted and hearing was impaired. Mr A was unable to cooperate with the Abbreviated Mental Test.

Question 2: What are the most likely causes of the altered behaviour in this patient?

Delirium often occurs in cognitively compromised patients and hence it must be recognised in Mr A. He also has several other predisposing factors for delirium including advanced age, functional impairment, sensory impairment, and baseline use of psychoactive drugs. Other predisposing factors include severe underlying illness and malnutrition. ***Identification of delirium must be followed by a search for the aetiology*** so that it can be addressed. A meticulous physical examination will identify easily treatable causes such as faecal impaction and urinary retention. In cases where a fall is suspected, all the joints and bones — especially the hip joints — must be palpated and gently ranged to identify fractures.

Often even after a detailed history and physical examination, the cause of the delirium may be unclear and investigations would be needed to identify the cause. Blood, urine, electrocardiogram (ECG), and simple radiological investigations would be reasonable for a start. Neuroimaging is not required for all delirious patients but should be considered if there is a neurological deficit, suspected stroke or bleed, increased bleeding risk (antiplatelet or anticoagulant, low platelet count etc.), or unresolving delirium with no apparent cause.

****

Laboratory investigations showed:

WBC count	*9.83 x 10^9/L*	*(4–10)*
Haemoglobin	*11.9 g/dL*	*(12–16)*
Platelet count	*167 x 10^9/L*	*(140–440)*
Blood urea	*7.8 mmol/L*	*(2.7–6.9)*
Sodium	*123 mmol/L*	*(136–146)*
Potassium	*4.3 mmol/L*	*(3.5–5.1)*
Serum creatinine	*89 umol/L*	*(45–84)*
Calcium	*2.63 mmol/L*	*(2.09–2.46)*
Phosphate	*0.89 mmol/L*	*(0.94–1.5)*
Magnesium	*0.78 mmol/L*	*(0.75–1.07)*
Lactate	*0.9 mmol/L*	*(0.2–2.2)*
C-reactive protein	*81 mg/L*	*(0.2–9.1)*
Serum procalcitonin	*1.0 mcg/L*	*(<0.49)*
Total protein	*64 g/L*	*(68–85)*
Serum albumin	*36 g/L*	*(40–51)*
Total bilirubin	*8 μmol/L*	*(7-32)*
Serum ALT	*36 U/L*	*(6–66)*
Serum AST	*40 U/L*	*(12–42)*
Serum ALP	*90 U/L*	*(39–99)*
Gamma-GT	*84 U/L*	*(9–53)*
Serum TSH	*3.7 mIU/L*	*(0.45–4.5)*
Free T4	*10.8 pmol/L*	*(10–20)*
Trop I	*Normal*	
HbA1c	*6.9%*	

Urine dipstick: Leucocyte negative, nitrite positive, ketones negative, protein trace, glucose positive UFEME: WBC 700, RBC 80, epithelial cell 7.

Chest X-ray: No consolidation or pleural effusion and no air under diaphragm.

ECG: Atrial fibrillation with rate of 80/min and no acute ST changes. QTc within normal range.

CT brain: Stable resolving right anterior parafalcine subdural haematoma measuring up to 2–3 mm in thickness. Also chronic microvascular ischaemia and age-related involutional changes.

Question 3: What would be the working diagnoses for this patient?

Atypical presentations are a hallmark feature of illness presentations in the elderly. Age-associated changes in physiology coupled with the presence of multiple comorbidities and polypharmacy influence the presentations of disease in the older patient. Infections may not present with classical symptoms of fever or symptoms pointing toward a source. The older patient may present with a geriatric syndrome instead such as falls, altered mental state, or functional decline.

****

Mr A was started on antibiotics for his urinary tract infection. During the admission, he repeatedly called the nurses. During diaper change, he would hit, scratch, and pinch them. He was spitting out his food which further contributed to his poor oral intake. At night, he repeatedly tried to climb out of bed, leading to him being physically restrained for fall prevention.

Question 4: How would you manage this patient?

The underlying cause of the delirium, which is often a medical cause, must be addressed. In this situation, the urinary tract infection (UTI) must be treated, and imaging may be considered if there is recurrent UTI or if a structural abnormality is suspected. A digital rectal exam to assess prostate size, consistency, and tenderness is useful. Electrolytes need to be corrected as well.

Mr A is in an unfamiliar environment in the hospital. This in itself can worsen confusion and agitation in patients with significant cognitive compromise. Having a caregiver at the bedside at all times provides a familiar face to the person with dementia and can reduce agitation. Persons with dementia often eat better when a familiar person feeds them. His family can be encouraged to bring his favourite food and assist with feeding at meal times. As the older, confused patient often will not be able to voluntarily pour water into a cup and drink, the caregiver can assist with scheduled feeding of fluids in small amounts through the day to ensure adequate hydration.

As Mr A was not used to wearing diapers at home, this may cause discomfort in the hospital. He may not be able to pass urine and motion in the diaper, which is likely the reason for the repeated attempts to get out of bed at night. Some patients tend to tear off their diapers at night as well. Due to the underlying dementia, patients often cannot express their needs clearly, leading to a breakdown in communication, increased frustration, and agitation. It is important to find out the patient's usual habits at home as this would enable the healthcare team to deliver individualised, person-centred care. Providing a routine with scheduled voiding in the toilet or on a commode every few hours as well as taking him to the toilet at night may lead to improvement in the agitation.

Non-pharmacological measures are the first line of management for patients with behavioural disturbances. Behaviours such as agitation and aggression are often the result of unmet needs that the person with dementia has difficulty expressing. These needs may include hunger, thirst, feeling too warm or too cold, needing to go to the toilet, and fear with need for reassurance and comfort. For example, patients may not understand why they are being sponged or why their parameters are being taken. Explaining the activity in a calm and gentle tone before it is done may alleviate distress and reduce agitation. For stable patients, avoiding night disturbances (e.g., minimising the checking of parameters during sleeping hours, reducing noise and light) is helpful too. Many behaviours settle with non-pharmacological measures and do not require the addition of psychotropic agents.

However, in some patients, behavioural disturbances persist with risk of harm to themselves and others. In such cases, medications may be needed and a time-limited trial may be undertaken at the lowest effective dose with a view to discontinuation once the behaviours are manageable. Oral haloperidol 0.25–0.5 mg ON (available as a liquid in some formularies), quetiapine 6.25–12.5 mg ON, or olanzapine 2.5 mg ON may be used if deemed to be necessary. Liquid and orodispersible formulations may increase ease of administration. ***ECG should be done at baseline for the QTc as these drugs may prolong it.*** When used in an acutely delirious patient, these drugs must be reviewed prior to discharge and must be discontinued if not needed. If they are continued on discharge, early review should be scheduled.

In patients who need pharmacological agents but cannot be given antipsychotics due to contraindications, a low dose benzodiazepine (e.g., lorazepam

0.25–0.5 mg ON) may be used — again for the shortest duration required. Beware that benzodiazepines can cause dependence, falls, and depression.

****

Mr A's agitation settled with treatment of his UTI and institution of non-pharmacological measures. His helper was allowed to stay by his bedside to assist with reorientation, daytime activities, toileting and feeding. His restraints were removed. Prior to discharge, his caregiver was educated on good perineal hygiene, prevention of constipation, encouragement of adequate voiding of his bladder, and maintenance of adequate hydration.

Mr A was reviewed in the geriatric clinic three months post-discharge. His family and helper reported gradually increasing agitation at home with restlessness and pacing up and down. He was hitting out at the helper more and had on one occasion injured her. He was sleeping in the day and staying up at night. He was also disinhibited at times, making sexual remarks towards the helper.

After excluding the presence of a superimposed delirium, these behaviours may be attributed to BPSD. Once again, non-pharmacological measures are the mainstay of management. Persons living with dementia do well with routine where the events of the day are predictable. Engaging in meaningful activities targeted at the patient's abilities and interests during the day would prevent excessive daytime sleeping. Many undesirable behaviours stem from lack of engagement and boredom. Activity engagement can also be provided in dementia day care centres. Physical activity in the form of a walk or exercises and getting adequate sunlight will aid in promoting night sleep. Caffeinated drinks and limitation of fluids after the early evening also help reduce nocturia and sleep disturbance.

In patients who exhibit aggression with risk of harm to self or others, the environment needs to be modified to make it as safe as possible. Dangerous objects including knives and scissors need to be kept out of reach. Caregiver education is very important to enable and empower the caregiver to cope with the challenges of living with someone with dementia. Avoiding arguments, verbal de-escalation, and remaining calm often help to ease tense situations.

In selected cases, pharmacological agents may be required to aid in the management of BPSD. Drug classes used include antidepressants (e.g., selective serotonin reuptake inhibitors), antipsychotics, mood stabilisers (e.g., valproate), and benzodiazepines. Treatment is individualised considering the patient's behaviours, timing, distress to patient and caregiver, and side-effect profile. Side-effects of the aforementioned drug classes include but are not limited to cardiovascular risks, sedation, increased risk of falls, worsening of cognition, and functional decline. It involves a risk-benefit assessment and discussion with the family and caregiver.

Recognising that dementia is of increasing prevalence in an ageing population, there have been several services set up to support caregivers and persons living with dementia. Dementia Singapore (www.dementia.org.sg) is one such organisation that has a suite of services including caregiver support services (e.g., home support team, caregiver support groups and networks, Eldersit services that provide home-based engagement), dementia day care, arts and dementia programmes, and self-advocacy programmes (e.g., Voices for Hope). They also provide training programmes for professionals, family caregivers, and foreign domestic workers. Several other organisations provide similar services and more information may be obtained from the AIC website (www.aic.sg). Another website that provides useful tips and personal stories by and for caregivers of persons with dementia is www.forgetusnot.sg.

Mr A was enrolled into a dementia day care centre near his house. His fluvoxamine dose was increased to 50 mg ON as his hypersexuality was causing distress to the helper. On review in two months, his family reported that he enjoyed the activities in the day care centre and had also made new friends. They were happy that he was now sleeping better at night and there was a decrease in the hypersexuality and agitation.

Key messages

1. Behaviour change in geriatric patients is a common presentation and it is important to perform a holistic assessment to ascertain the diagnosis of the behaviour change, be it delirium, dementia, or depression. This assessment often includes a comprehensive geriatric assessment and the complications of behavioural change.
2. Behavioural change is often multifactorial. Its management requires a multi-pronged approach including treating the underlying cause, prevention of precipitation, non-pharmacological interventions, and pharmacological measures.
3. It is crucial to discriminate between the differential diagnoses of behavioural change: delirium, dementia, and depression. In first presentation, we would need to treat reversible causes.

Answer Key

1. As this is an acute change from baseline behaviour, it is necessary to approach this situation as how you would approach a delirious patient — whereby it is crucial to assess the situation holistically and in entirety. Additional history would need to include the duration of the behaviour change, progression, identifying

the cause as well as addressing the complications. The present situation should be compared with his previous baseline cognition and function. To assess all these, a comprehensive geriatric assessment would be ideal.

In terms of causes, the evaluation approach will start by eliminating the common causes which can be quickly brought to mind with one of two useful mnemonics, **VITAMIN C** or **DELIRIUM.**

V	**Vascular** = stroke/acute intracranial event	**D**	**Drugs**
I	**Infection/Inflammation** = focal (e.g., septic arthritis) or general (e.g., pyelonephritis with bacteraemia)	**E**	**Electrolytes** and physiologic abnormalities
T	**Trauma** = esp. intracranial (e.g., after a recent fall)	**L**	**Lack of drugs** (non-compliance)
A	**Autoimmune** = quite rare in elderly	**I**	**Infection**
M	**Metabolic** = electrolytes, endocrine-related (e.g., glucose, thyroid), organ related (e.g., liver, kidney)	**R**	**Reduced sensory input**
I	**Iatrogenicity, infarction** = polypharmacy, drug–drug interactions, myocardial infarction/pulmonary embolism/any embolic event	**I**	**Intracranial problems**
N	**Neoplastic** = malignancy of primary or metastatic cancers, paraneoplastic syndromes	**U**	**Urinary retention and faecal impaction**
C	**Constipation!**	**M**	**Myocardial problems** (e.g., myocardial infarction, heart failure, arrhythmias)

Complications evaluation is always required in the management of behavioural change. For example, complications of severe sepsis include haemodynamic dysfunction and incontinence which can lead to imbalance and instability and ultimately present as a fall in the elderly.

2. Based on the initial clinical assessment of Mr A, the following differential diagnoses should be entertained:

   ? Occult infection — very common in the elderly

   ? Metabolic cause, especially of electrolyte imbalances related to poor appetite

   ? Neurological cause — acute intracranial event (background of paroxysmal atrial fibrillation), non-convulsive seizure (cerebral insult in previous frontal subdural haematoma)

   ? Acute coronary event

3. Acute delirium on background of dementia with BPSD and previous subdural haemorrhage precipitated by
   - Occult infection likely urinary tract infection;
   - Hyponatraemia and hypercalcaemia from poor oral intake

4. Treat the cause of delirium, i.e., send urine for culture and begin empirical antibiotics, and encourage oral intake especially hydration which will improve delirium;

   Non-pharmacological measures, e.g., minimising night disturbances, having a caregiver at the bedside, avoiding restraints, engaging in daytime activities etc.;

   Pharmacological agents if patient causes significant distress to himself or carers.

Reference

Kratz T (2017) The diagnosis and treatment of behavioral disorders in dementia. *Dtsch Artebl Intl* **114**(26): 447–454.

10 Depressive Symptoms

Tan Boon Hian, Anupama Roy Chowdhury

Mdm A is an 83-year-old lady who was electively admitted for a hernia operation. The surgical team had made a medical referral for evaluation of amnesia.

According to the daughter and helper, Mdm A has been repetitive when asking questions and dwelling on the same topic in conversations. She had been calling people on the telephone repeatedly up to five times a day. She also seemed to lose track of the time of the day and kept asking her helper about it. She kept forgetting recent events like breakfast, but her long-term memory appeared to be intact. Her highest educational level was pre-university.

The daughter additionally shared concerns about her mood. Mdm A could be temperamental at times, worried over all kinds of small things, and was more apathetic at other times. When confronted, the patient denied that she had low mood, attributing her behaviour to her old age.

Functionally, she was independent in her basic activities of daily living. During the COVID pandemic, she hardly went out and hence stopped social interactions with people. She was still able to cook and make her own porridge should her helper become busy. She was able to communicate to her daughter her needs and wants. She could use the telephone and could manage a small budget of money. Her medications were supervised.

Her appetite was generally poor and for a long time she had difficulty sleeping at night and resorted to short naps when tired in the day. When unable to sleep, she would watch television. In fact, she spends most of the day watching television and occasionally washing vegetables in preparation for meals.

Mdm A stayed with her daughter and helper. She has been widowed with two daughters and three sons for many years.

Clinical examination showed no neurological abnormalities. Abbreviated mental test score was 10/10. The Chinese Mini Mental State Examination score was 25/28. There was no agnosia, aphasia, apraxia, or decline in attention or social cognition.

Question 1: There are few possibilities for this clinical presentation, but what is the differential diagnosis to rule out as soon as possible?

Question 2: After having ruled that out, what preliminary investigations would you order to aid with the diagnostic process?

Possible differential diagnoses to consider in this setting include delirium, mild cognitive impairment, dementia, and depression (pseudodementia).

Differential diagnoses	**Delirium**	**Mild cognitive impairment**	**Dementia**	**Depression**
Timeline	Acute	Chronic	Chronic	Subacute (>2 weeks) to chronic
Cognitive domains affected	Predominantly ***attention*** but may be global	Usually single domain, especially ***memory or executive***, but may also be multi-domain	Can be single but progresses to multi-domain with severity of disease	***Low mood*** predominates. Usually attention loss dominant and cognitive performance is both mood- and effort-dependent
Sensorium	Impaired; drowsy in hypoactive delirium	Normal	Normal in early stage; chronic loss in late stages	Normal
Function	Global acute decline	No functional decline	May be cognitive initially, but global chronic decline eventually	Global decline, affects social functioning as well
Cognitive test pattern	Global loss temporarily and gets better as medical illnesses improve	Mild objective deficits	Deficits in certain domains initially and eventually global; does not get better	Variable; random or no answers due to lack of effort

(*Continued*)

Differential diagnoses	**Delirium**	**Mild cognitive impairment**	**Dementia**	**Depression**
Clinical status	Unwell, usually with many or severe medical issues	Usually well	Usually well but geriatric syndromes develop as dementia progresses	Unwell only if suicidal, psychotic, or catatonic
Mood	Mostly normal	Mostly normal	Variable; can range from normal to anxious/depressed	Prominently low; ***vegetative symptoms*** (e.g., loss of appetite and weight, fatigue, low energy, insomnia) occur; may be agitated
Natural history	Fluctuating and will mostly resolve if underlying cause treated; may be superimposed on other three underlying differential diagnoses	May improve, stay the same, or deteriorate (depending on aetiology)	Defined by its progression and deterioration	Waxes and wanes; 70% of depressed elderly relapse
Curable?	Yes	Depends on underlying aetiology	No	Yes

The table highlights the importance of a good clinical history (including reviewing old notes), ascertaining the timeline, progression, and predominance of symptoms, and assessment of any confounding medical illnesses which suggest a component of delirium that may be treatable. The history should be taken from a reliable and consistent informant. A holistic assessment is made from the history with objective clinical assessments of both cognition and mood. As dementia is a progressive disease, longitudinal observation may be required to differentiate between the differential diagnoses.

Pitfalls of diagnosing depression in the elderly:

— *It is sometimes mistaken for dementia ("pseudodementia") because the cognitive impairment may occur in the absence of typical symptoms of depression, thus masquerading as dementia. Conversely, many patients in the early stages of dementia retain insight and become depressed. Clues that depression may be the cause of cognitive impairment include decline over weeks to months rather than years, apathy, significant life events or social stressors preceding the cognitive decline, and associated disturbances in appetite or sleep.*

— *Many elderly patients with depression exhibit atypical features and may occasionally manifest as a geriatric syndrome (see table below).*

— *Medical causes manifesting as depression include symptomatic anaemia, obstructive sleep apnoea, vitamin B12 deficiency, organ problems (cardiac disease, lung/liver/renal failure), endocrine problems (hypocortisolism, hypo/hyperthyroidism, hypo/hypercalcaemia), chronic infections, cancers, and neurodegenerative disease. Depression can manifest prior to and during these disease states.*

— *Drug effects that mimic depression include benzodiazepines and drugs for Parkinson disease (levodopa, dopamine agonists), antihypertensives (beta-blockers, methyldopa, hydralazine), corticosteroids, and hormones (oestrogens, progesterone, tamoxifen).*

****

Laboratory investigations were essentially normal. CT brain showed old infarcts in the thalami and caudate heads as well as mild diffuse volume loss with a frontal and temporal lobar predilection.

In a subsequent visit, Mdm A continued to maintain her previous function. Her family shared that she was becoming increasingly attention seeking — wanting to speak to family members all the time despite their various commitments. They also observed increasing irritability and agitation, with the emergence of various somatic complaints such as abdominal discomfort and generalised body aches culminating in the patient scolding her children for not taking her to see a doctor for all her complaints. Yet when Mdm A was brought to see the doctor, she would scold the daughter as well. Suicide was threatened during her bouts of anger. The patient expressed fears of abandonment. The patient would also alternate this with bouts of apathy during which she refused to be engaged in activities at home and had no motivation to do anything at all. She had lost interest in cooking and her sleep became increasingly difficult and disrupted with night-time awakenings. There were no complaints of panic, palpitation, nor tremors. When approached individually, the patient denied all of the abovementioned symptoms.

Question 3: Is Mdm A likely to have depression or not?

Table 10.1. Clinical Features of Depression.

Typical features (Need to be pervasive and happen nearly every day, all day)	Atypical features in the elderly (Best illustrated in the Cornell scale for depression in dementia)
1. Depressed mood 2. Marked diminished interest or pleasure 3. ***Significant weight loss or gain (>5%)*** 4. ***Insomnia or hypersomnia*** 5. ***Psychomotor agitation or retardation*** 6. ***Fatigue or loss of energy*** 7. Feelings of worthlessness or excessive guilt 8. Diminished ability to think or concentrate 9. Suicidal ideation	More functional impairment More ***vegetative symptoms (symptoms 3–6)*** Less likely to express sadness More likely to manifest as irritability More likely to have hypochondriasis Early morning awakenings Mood-congruent delusions of poverty, illness, or loss May manifest as a geriatric syndrome, e.g., recurrent falls, delirium, functional decline, malnutrition, elder abuse, frailty, incontinence

Question 4: Suggest a suitable pharmacologic treatment for Mdm A.

The DSM-5 diagnostic criteria for major depressive disorder (i.e., depression) are as follows:

(a) ≥5 symptoms (see typical features in table below) have been present during the same 2-week period and represent a change from previous functioning; at least one of the symptoms is either (1) depressed mood or (2) loss of interest or pleasure.

(b) Functional: the symptoms cause clinically significant distress or impairment in social, occupational, or other important areas of functioning.

(c) Absence of dementia, delirium, medication use, or other psychotic disorders (e.g., schizophrenia or mania).

The screening of depression is dependent on (a) the choice between self-rated or observer-rated scales, (b) the presence of cognitive impairment, (c) the amount of contact time with the patient, and (d) the personal preferences of the physician requesting the screening.

Common user-rated scales include:

- The geriatric depression scale (GDS) which comes in various question number formats but the most commonly used is the 15-question format. The GDS can be used in patients with or without cognitive impairment but the patient must reliably self-report. One can download a free app called "Geriatric Depression Test: Geriatric Self-harm Tracker" which, upon completing the questions, will automatically compute the GDS score and interpret the severity of depression.
- The PHQ9 which can be used in both elderly and non-elderly patients without dementia.
- The Cornell scale for depression in dementia (CSDD) which is an observer/caregiver-rated scale used to screen for patients with dementia who cannot self-report reliably.
- The Montgomery–Åsberg depression rating scale which is an alternative to the CSDD.

The above scales usually take 10–15 minutes to complete. It should be emphasised that screening scales are meant for screening and thus results need to take into account the patient and their symptoms. For example, Mdm A had a GDS of 4 but exhibited symptoms of depression, and she responded well to subsequent antidepressant treatment.

In the event of lack of time (e.g., busy clinic consult or large scale screening), one can consider just asking the Yale single question, "***Do you often feel sad or depressed?***" or the PHQ2 (which comprises of the first two questions of the PHQ9).

Prior to starting any treatment, ***suicide risk assessment*** is important as the safety of the patient should be prioritised and this affects the disposition of the patient and subsequent management. One should ask the patient if they have any suicidal thoughts or have made any plans to end their life, as well as their caregivers if the patient exhibited any evidence of self-harm, self-neglect, or harm towards others. Patients with multiple illnesses and those who are socially isolated would be at increased risk.

The management of depression, like any other geriatric syndrome, is divided into non-pharmacological and pharmacological management.

Non-pharmacological management, in essence, is to individualise multidisciplinary case management (psychological and social support) to fit the person and his/her interactions with family, as well as to optimise the environment. This is in line with the goals to avoid triggers and reinforce the activities and settings that improve mood. Psychological therapies are often employed as well — cognitive behavioural therapy is the intervention which has shown the most evidence of efficacy in the elderly. Exercise is an important intervention that is known to help with depression and other geriatric syndromes comorbid with or resultant from this condition. The senior activity centres as well as the day care centres are important community services (homage.sg/resources/) that create a warm and familiar environment for the elderly to socialise through various programmes and activities and seek social support. For home-bound seniors, CREST (Community Resource Engagement and Support Team) services (awwa.org.sg) and Befriender services (aic.sg/care-services/befriending-service) can be considered.

Pharmacological management in patients with depression is often used in tandem with non-pharmacological measures.

Antidepressants can be classified in Table 10.2. The ability to cause sedation can occur via multiple mechanisms, such as through serotoninergic receptor antagonism, melatonin receptor agonism, or anticholinergic effects.

Table10.2. Classification of Antidepressants.

Antidepressant class	Sedating	Non-sedating ("activating"; i.e., cause patient to improve attention or alertness but may have insomnia as a side-effect)	Important side-effects
(1) Selective serotonin reuptake inhibitor (SSRI)	Fluvoxamine, paroxetine	Fluoxetine, escitalopram ($1.73 per 5 mg), sertraline	Hyponatraemia (syndrome of inappropriate ADH secretion); increased risk of gastrointestinal bleeding (serotonergic mechanisms); QT prolongation
(2) Serotonin and norepinephrine reuptake inhibitor (SNRI)		Venlafaxine, duloxetine ($3.17 per 30 mg)	Can aggravate hypertension; increased risk of gastrointestinal bleeding (serotonergic mechanisms); liver derangement (dual-acting antidepressant)
(3) Monoamine oxidase inhibitor (MAOI)	Neutral effects on sedation		Hardly used due to potential for serotonergic syndrome (even with foods like cheese) and limited efficacy
(4) Noradrenergic and specific serotonergic antidepressant (NaSSA)	Mirtazapine at low doses (7.5 mg ON) is sedating, but higher doses (>15 mg ON) may be over-stimulating as norepinephrine effects overwhelm the sedating effects of serotonin		Liver derangement (dual-acting antidepressant); weight gain
(5) Norepinephrine-dopamine reuptake inhibitor (NDRI)		Bupropion	Seizures, hallucinations

(*Continued*)

Table10.2. *(Continued)*

Antidepressant class	Sedating	Non-sedating ("activating"; i.e., cause patient to improve attention or alertness but may have insomnia as a side-effect)	Important side-effects
(6) Melatonin receptor agonist	Agomelatine (not widely available)		
(7) Serotonin antagonist and reuptake inhibitor (SARI)	Trazodone		Seizures, priapism
(8) Tricycylic antidepressant (TCA)	Nortriptyline		Potent anticholinergic and arrhythmogenic properties
(9) Serotonin modulator and stimulator (SMS)		Vortioxetine ($1.71 per 5 mg)	

In terms of relative efficacy, most antidepressants have near-equal efficacy and therefore its use is often determined by its side-effect profile, which may limit its use in a patient or may be sometimes beneficial to the patient. For example, we often use fluvoxamine for its sedating effects and efficacy on obsessive–compulsive behaviours. In the elderly, we often use mirtazapine because it increases appetite and improves sleep. In patients with apathy, escitalopram or sertraline can be used. In palliative care, TCAs such as nortriptyline are used for its additional ability to treat neuropathic pain (at lower doses). Duloxetine, an SNRI, has been used for urinary incontinence and neuropathic pain. In general, the SSRIs are often used as first line in the older patient due to their favourable safety profile. Doses are started low with gradual escalation and close monitoring.

In cases whereby we are unable to distinguish between depression and dementia but the patient's symptoms are impairing function and causing distress, sometimes a trial of treatment with an antidepressant may be used to see if cognition improves before labelling a patient with dementia.

Apart from exploiting the likely side-effect profile, the other considerations for prescribing antidepressants in the elderly include symptoms which the patient presented with, their comorbid medical conditions, and potential for polypharmacy and drug–drug interactions. We also plan for ease of taper in the event of complications (hence, fluoxetine is not preferred for use due to difficulties in taper) as well as cost (latest costs are mentioned for the more expensive drugs in the table).

An antidepressant often takes four to eight weeks to take effect — this information should be factored into the counseling process with the patient and family. Doses are started low with regular review every few weeks for tolerance to the medication prior to increasing the dose.

When an antidepressant fails, one should (a) check compliance to non-pharmacological and pharmacological therapy, (b) exclude a delirious process which is a medical emergency, and (c) revisit the history to ascertain if there is truly a depressive disease or a differential condition such as psychosis or dementia. One should consider assessing the safety of the patient and consider admission if delirium is a possibility.

Once (a–c) have been ruled out, treatment-refractory depression may be managed with the following strategies:

- dose escalation
- switching antidepressants with consideration of cross taper
- augmentation by dual antidepressants or other medications such as antipsychotics (in agitated depression), methylphenidate, and lithium
- electroconvulsive therapy can be, and has been, employed in the elderly with refractory or complicated depression (e.g., concomitant catatonia), psychosis, treatment resistance, or refusal of oral intake

If in doubt, multidisciplinary management in conjunction with relevant subspecialities (e.g., psychiatry) would benefit the patient. Treatment-resistant cases as well as cases assessed to be suicidal or with high suicide risk must be referred to a psychiatrist for evaluation and management.

****

The Geriatric Depression Scale score was 4/15. Mdm A was started on mirtazapine at night and she was concurrently enrolled at a senior activity centre. Upon review in two months, her mood and social interactions have significantly improved.

Key messages

1. Depression and cognitive impairment are common comorbid diseases in the elderly.
2. Depression is a treatable condition, with non-pharmacological and pharmacological treatments; the choice of antidepressant is based on the comorbidities and side-effects of the antidepressant.
3. Diagnosis of depression involves thorough clinical history and physical assessment and may involve observation over a period of time and therapeutic trials.

Answer key

1. Delirium. It is a medical emergency and needs to be first assumed, ruled out, and addressed (see other chapters with discussions on delirium). Obtaining the time line of cognitive and behaviour change is important as a fairly acute presentation would suggest a delirium.
2. As cognition is the main presenting complaint in this patient, laboratory investigations in this patient should include thyroid function, vitamin B12 level, and folate and calcium levels. Neuroimaging in the form of either CT brain or MRI brain dementia protocol is also recommended. (If stroke is suspected in a patient, an MRI stroke protocol may be used instead.)
3. Mdm A fulfills the DSM-5 criteria for depression, exhibiting both typical and atypical features (refer to Table 10.1).
4. A suitable antidepressant to start for Mdm A is mirtazapine 7.5 mg ON. Review in four to eight weeks and titrate accordingly.

References

Allan CL, Ebmeier KP (2013) Review of treatment for late-life depression. *Adv Psychiatr Treat* **19**(4): 302–309.

Cipriani A, Furukawa TA, Salanti G, *et al.* (2018) Comparative efficacy and acceptability of 21 antidepressant drugs for the acute treatment of adults with major depressive disorder: a systematic review and network meta-analysis. *Lancet* **39**(10128): 1357–1366.

Kok RM, Reynolds CF 3rd. (2017) Management of Depression in Older Adults: A Review. *JAMA* **317**(20): 2114–2122.

McGovern AR, Kiosses DN, Raue PJ, Wilkins VM, Alexopoulos GS (2014) Psychotherapies for late-life depression. *Psychiatr Ann* **44**(3): 147–152.

11 Psychotic Symptoms

Anupama Roy Chowdhury

This chapter is a compilation of two clinical scenarios of psychotic symptoms in the elderly.

CASE 1

Mr K is a 77-year-old man who was transferred from the Institute of Mental Health (IMH) for pneumonia. He has no significant past medical history. He has been admitted to IMH for about a month. Prior to that, he has had multiple visits to the emergency department and admissions to several hospitals for multiple somatic symptoms that he blames his neighbour for. His neighbour is a 45-year-old lady who lives with her husband and two children. His relationship with the neighbour was good until two years ago when he started to believe that she was casting spells on him and spraying toxic gas into his house. He then attributed his shortness of breath, chest pains, and giddiness to the toxic chemicals. He had never seen her actually coming near his house or smelt anything unusual, but he firmly believed that she was responsible for him feeling unwell. This had resulted in him calling the police on several occasions, which eventually led to the IMH admission.

Question 1: How would you best describe what Mr K had been experiencing?

a. Cognitive decline
b. Delusions
c. Depression
d. Hallucinations
e. Somatisation

Question 2: What relevant further history would you like to elicit given this man's age?

Hallucinations are described as an experience involving the apparent perception of something that is not present. It may manifest as a sound, sight, smell, touch, or taste that the affected person perceives but does not actually exist. Delusions on the other hand are described as firm unshakeable beliefs that the person believes to be real despite being contradicted by reality or rational argument. These are different psychotic symptoms with multiple causes in the older patient including an underlying neurological disorder, substance abuse, and delirium. Psychosis may also manifest as disorganised speech and behaviour. Psychotic symptoms are not uncommon in the older patient, so having knowledge of their causes and a basic approach would be beneficial for any medical professional involved in the care of the older patient.

History is crucial in aiding diagnosis of the underlying aetiology. Establishing the timeline of the psychotic symptoms — onset and duration — would help ascertain whether it is of acute onset or part of a more chronic disorder such as late-onset schizophrenia or dementia.

A psychosis of acute onset must be treated as delirium. Other features of delirium include a fluctuating course, inattention, disorganised thought, and altered level of consciousness. However, the key feature is its acute onset. Once delirium is identified, the underlying cause must be looked for (e.g., infection, stroke, adverse effects of drugs especially those with anticholinergic effects, substance abuse, urinary retention) and treated as it may be potentially life-threatening. Neurological conditions such as encephalitis and temporal lobe epilepsy may also manifest as psychotic disturbances.

Causes of chronic persistent psychotic symptoms would include neurodegenerative disorders (e.g., Alzhemier's dementia, vascular dementia, Lewy body dementia, Parkinson disease) and primary psychotic disorders (delusional disorders, late-onset schizophrenia, or affective disorders).

After obtaining a history of the duration of the psychotic symptoms in the older patient, a good cognitive history must be obtained. This helps to ascertain whether the psychotic symptoms are part of a neurocognitive disorder. A history suggestive of cognitive decline over time with significant interference in their daily life would suggest a major neurocognitive disorder or dementia. Persons with Alzheimer's disease may have paranoid delusions that people within the household are stealing their things. Due to poor memory, they misplace their belongings and then start believing that others have taken them. Even when they find the missing item, they may believe that someone hid it. They often also have delusions of infidelity where a female patient may believe her spouse is having an affair with the neighbour or helper. Persons with Lewy body dementia may have visual hallucinations where they see animals or people. Asking about the mood of the patient over time is also important to identify an underlying mood disorder with secondary psychotic features.

A physical examination including a neurological exam is essential to identify Parkinsonism and deficits from a previous stroke. Patients with Parkinson disease often have psychotic symptoms due to the dopaminergic effects of drugs used to treat the underlying condition. A recent increase in dosing of their dopaminergic agents may precipitate a psychotic episode.

Investigations should be tailored to the suspicion of the underlying aetiology based on history and physical examination. Full blood count, renal panel, liver panel, thyroid panel, and calcium and vitamin B12 levels are reasonable initial blood investigations as they may identify medical conditions amenable to treatment. If infection is suspected, C-reactive protein and procalcitonin level may be added as well as other investigations to identify the source. A baseline 12-lead ***electrocardiogram (ECG)*** must be obtained as drugs used in the treatment of psychosis may have effects on cardiac conduction.

Neuroimaging is useful to identify stroke disease, tumours, and brain atrophy. Persons with Alzheimer's disease may have hippocampal and medial temporal lobe atrophy. In patients with suspicion of epilepsy, an electroencephalogram should be obtained. A lumbar puncture is useful in the diagnosis of intracranial infections and autoimmune or paraneoplastic encephalitis. It is often performed when initial investigations are unyielding. The acutely psychotic patient may not be able to cooperate with a lumbar puncture and may need to be sedated. Additionally, the presence of lumbar spondylosis and osteophytes in the elderly can make the procedure challenging.

****

Further history was obtained from Mr K's brother, his next-of-kin. Mr K had lost his wife to cancer ten years ago and had been living alone since. His brother visited him fortnightly and spent the day with him. They seldom spoke over the phone due to Mr K's hearing impairment (and his refusal to use his hearing aid). Mr K was still able to manage his daily affairs including buying his own food, withdrawing money from the automated teller machine, keeping his house clean, and shopping for his daily needs. He was able to take public transport to nearby malls and return home safely. His brother had not noted any decline in his memory, language, or planning abilities. He also seemed to be in good spirits except when he spoke about his neighbour. His brother was unable to understand why Mr K had developed this paranoia towards his neighbour. On examination, he had no evidence of Parkinsonism or other abnormal neurology.

Question 3: What is the most likely diagnosis?

a. **Alzheimer's dementia**
b. **Autoimmune encephalitis**
c. **Delusional disorder**
d. **Dementia with Lewy bodies**
e. **Psychotic depression**

Question 4: Which of the following drug classes is the most appropriate first-line treatment for Mr K?

a. **Acetylcholinesterase inhibitors**
b. **Antidepressants**
c. **Antipsychotics**
d. **Benzodiazepines**
e. **N-methyl-D-aspartate receptor antagonist**

Mr K was diagnosed by his psychiatrist as having a delusional disorder. A possible differential to consider is a very late-onset schizophrenia. There was no history of cognitive decline or mood disturbance to suggest an underlying dementia or depression. The duration of his symptoms was also prolonged for consideration of autoimmune encephalitis, which usually has a subacute onset of a few weeks to months with accompanying working memory deficits, facial dyskinaesias, altered mental status, and seizures.

Late-onset schizophrenia is defined as onset after 40 years of age and very late-onset schizophrenia is defined as onset after 60 years of age. This term has been used to describe a schizophrenia-like illness that occurs in the later years of life in the absence of an amnestic syndrome or any organic brain disease. When compared with early- or late-onset schizophrenia, very late-onset schizophrenia (onset >60 years of age) is more prevalent in females, with affected patients often having sensory impairment and being socially isolated. They have a greater likelihood of visual hallucinations and a greater risk of tardive dyskinaesia, but a lesser likelihood of family history of schizophrenia, formal thought disorder, and affective blunting.

Psychotic disorders can be very distressing to both the patient and caregiver. If left uncontrolled, they can lead to neglect and abuse of the older person, as well as institutionalisation.

Antipsychotic medications have been shown to improve acute symptoms and reduce relapse in chronic psychotic disorders. However, the older patient is more vulnerable to adverse effects of these medications due to age-related effects of pharmacokinetics and pharmacodynamics. One of the principles in prescribing for the older patient is to "start low, go slow" with regular monitoring for adverse effects. Depot antipsychotic medications are useful in older patients who may have difficulty with medication compliance.

Potential side-effects include extrapyramidal side-effects (Parkinsonism, akathisia, tardive dyskinaesia), anticholinergic effects (blurred vision, constipation, dry mouth), postural hypotension and sedation (increased risk of falls), as well as abnormalities of liver function tests and QTc prolongation on the ECG.

The newer atypical antipsychotic medications (Table 11.1) have a better side-effect profile when compared to conventional antipsychotics. Clozapine use is limited by the need to monitor white cell counts due to the risk of agranulocytosis which may occur more frequently in the older patient. In contrast to other antipsychotics that prolong QTc, aripiprazole is the least likely to do so. It is also less likely to cause extrapyramidal side-effects, weight gain, and sedation.

Table 11.1. Recommended Doses for the Most Frequently Prescribed Antipsychotics.

Atypical antipsychotics	Starting dose (mg/day)	Maximum dose (mg/day)
Quetiapine	6.25–12.5	100–200
Olanzapine	2.5	10–15
Risperidone	0.25–0.5	2–3
Aripiprazole	5 ($5.66 per 10 mg tablet)	30

The choice and dose of antipsychotic will depend on the underlying aetiology of the psychosis and patient profile. As in all other areas of medicine, a holistic and individualised approach is required. In selected patients, cognitive behavioural techniques, social skills training, and occupational therapy may be of benefit alongside pharmacological treatment.

****

Mr K was started on intramuscular zuclopenthixol 200 mg every 28 days as he started becoming paranoid towards healthcare staff, believing they were poisoning him. He gradually improved with less hostility towards healthcare staff and less resistance to eating his meals and medications.

<u>CASE 2</u>

Mr T is an 80-year-old man who presented with a one-year history of increasing agitation associated with visual hallucinations. He lives with his son and grandson, who are finding it increasingly difficult to manage him at home. He often sees people whom he believes are his enemies and waves knives around trying to fight them. He gets upset when he is interrupted and then threatens to hurt his family or himself. These episodes were noted to be more prominent towards the late afternoon to early evening with him subsequently bearing no recollection of the episodes.

On taking a detailed cognitive history, his family reports that he has gotten lost in his neighbourhood on a few occasions and recently has had trouble finding the bathroom within the house. He stands on the side of the wash basin to brush his teeth instead of the front. He has been repetitive but otherwise he does not forget major events. He has trouble recognising relatives who do not frequently visit. He has had a long-standing history of acting out his dreams in his sleep, hence his bed is padded against the wall and installed with rails to prevent injuries.

Mr T is independent in his basic activities of daily living but has been requiring assistance in his instrumental activities of daily living for the last two to three years due to his deteriorating memory, sense of direction, and ability to plan.

Question 5: What is the most likely diagnosis?

a. Alzheimer's dementia (AD)

b. Autoimmune encephalitis

c. Dementia with Lewy Bodies (DLB)

d. Major depressive disorder (MDD)

e. Very late-onset schizophrenia

Question 6: Which of the following drugs is the most appropriate first-line treatment for Mr T?

a. Donepezil

b. Fluvoxamine

c. Haloperidol

d. Lorazepam

e. Risperidone

Mr T presents with psychotic symptoms (visual hallucinations) on a background of cognitive decline. Cognitive history reveals global cognitive decline with prominent visuospatial dysfunction as evidenced by him getting lost in his neighbourhood and now having difficulty finding his way around the house. The sleep disturbances described are suggestive of a rapid eye movement (REM) sleep disorder. Core clinical features of DLB include fluctuations in cognition, attention and arousal, visual hallucinations, REM sleep behavior disorder, and Parkinsonism. Not all features are present at diagnosis in all individuals. A diagnosis of DLB must be considered in Mr T given his presentation.

Other supportive features for DLB include sensitivity to neuroleptics, postural instability, falls, syncope, autonomic dysfunction (constipation, postural hypotension), hypersomnia, hyposmia, apathy, anxiety, depression, and hallucinations in other modalities.

Cholinesterase inhibitors including donepezil and rivastigmine (Table 11.2) may improve visual hallucinations and agitation in DLB. Donepezil is available in oral formulation (once-daily dosing) and rivastigmine is available in oral (twice-daily dosing) and transdermal patch formulations. Side-effects of cholinesterase inhibitors include slowing of heart rate, nausea, vomiting, and diarrhea. A baseline ECG is useful in identifying underlying heart blocks and bradycardia prior to initiation of treatment.

Patients on rate control agents (e.g., beta blockers, digoxin) should have their heart rate monitored at visits and counselled with regards to symptoms of bradycardia and when to seek medical attention. Gastrointestinal side-effects are often mild and transient. In order to maximise tolerance, these drugs are started at low doses and gradually up-titrated every few weeks.

Table 11.2. Recommended Doses for the Most Frequently Prescribed Cholinesterase Inhibitors.

	Starting dose	Maximum dose
Rivastigmine patch	4.6 mg/24 hr ($4.84 each)	13.3 mg/24 hr
Rivastigmine oral	1.5 mg BD	6 mg BD
Donepezil	2.5 mg once/day	10 mg once/day [doses beyond 10 mg are seldom tolerable by the elderly patient]

As patients with DLB are very sensitive to antipsychotics which can trigger a worsening of their condition, these must be avoided if possible. However, in cases with severe and disturbing psychotic symptoms, quetiapine may be trialed starting at 6.25 mg/day and gradually titrated upwards with close monitoring of the patient. Hallucinations that are not disturbing to the individual or others do not require treatment with medication.

****

On taking a more detailed social and lifestyle risk history, Mr T's son informs the medical team that he has been drinking alcohol since the age of 40 when he stopped his regular job, and this has gotten worse over the last few years. He drinks an average of three bottles of beer in the evenings. Though they try to control his alcohol intake, they suspect he sneaks out in the daytime to the coffee shop on certain days to drink as the neighbours have reported seeing him downstairs with few bottles of beer on the table. They also observed that his hallucinations and agitation appear to settle for a while after he drinks a bottle of beer.

With this new piece of information about the alcohol, it is plausible that Mr T's agitation and hallucinations are related to his alcohol use. He may also have a concomitant dementia, but alcohol withdrawal must be considered given his history of significant alcohol intake and the improvement in agitation and hallucinations with ingestion of alcohol.

It cannot be assumed that the older person does not drink alcohol or use controlled drugs. The older person may also be struggling with addiction problems to alcohol, benzodiazepines, opioids etc. Patients and families may not volunteer this information and hence it must be asked in a polite and sensitive manner.

Patients suspected of having alcohol withdrawal, such as Mr T, can be started on thiamine and a regimen involving benzodiazepines that are gradually tailed down to aid with the withdrawal. Withdrawal symptoms can be monitored using the revised Clinical Institute Withdrawal Assessment of Alcohol Scale (CIWA-Ar) chart. This scoring tool is also available on a free mobile app called "CIWA Score". Patients can be referred to a formal de-addiction programme subsequently.

****

Mr T was started on a tailing dose of lorazepam with improvement in his agitation and hallucinations. On review two months later in the clinic, his family reported some persistence in his hallucinations with continued cognitive decline. He was subsequently started on a trial of rivastigmine.

Key messages

1. Psychosis in the elderly is not uncommon.
2. A detailed and comprehensive history of the nature and duration of the psychosis, cognition, and other associated symptoms is valuable in differentiating the different causes of psychosis in the elderly.
3. In patients with visual hallucinations, a diagnosis of DLB must be considered and other supporting features must be looked for as these patients are very sensitive to neuroleptics.
4. History of alcohol and substance use must be routinely asked for even in the older patient.

Answer key

1. B. If Mr K had reported being able to smell the toxic gas, it may point to olfactory hallucinations. However, despite not seeing his neighbour coming near or smelling anything suspicious of toxic gas, he still believes she is poisoning him — hence he is having delusions.
2. Cognitive and functional history.
3. C.
4. C.
5. C.
6. A.

References

Karim S, Byrne EJ (2005) Treatment of psychosis in elderly people. *Adv Psychiatr Treat* **11**: 286–296.

McKeith IG, Boeve BF, Dickson DW, *et al.* (2017) Diagnosis and management of dementia with Lewy bodies: Fourth consensus report of the DLB Consortium. *Neurology* **89**: 88–100.

12 Giddiness I (Anaemia)

Denise Tan Yan, Alvin Tan Wee Beng

Mr T is a 75-year-old retired shopkeeper with a significant past medical history of hypertension, hyperlipidemia, diabetes mellitus, and ischaemic heart disease for which he is on lifelong aspirin 100 mg OM. He also has an active smoking history of 30 pack-years. He drinks alcohol on social occasions, and does not binge drink.

Over the past few weeks, Mr T has been experiencing episodes of non-vertiginous giddiness which mostly coincide with changes in posture, especially when he gets up suddenly. He has had a couple of episodes of near falls as a result of the giddiness. Prior to this, he was ambulating independently in the community without aids and had no significant history of falls. However, he noted occasional and very short-lived episodes of giddiness that were similar to this presentation for the past few years, although he had brushed it off as transient moments of imbalance.

On examination, Mr T was alert and fully oriented but had significant pallor. His vitals were heart rate 90/min regular, blood pressure 115/81 mmHg lying down and 86/69 mmHg after standing up for three minutes, and SpO_2 98% on room air. Small ecchymoses were present over his arms. There was no peripheral lymph adenopathy. Heart and lungs sounds were normal. Abdominal examination was unremarkable; in particular, there was no hepatosplenomegaly and no ballotable kidney. Per rectal examination revealed black tarry stools. His gait was normal, but it was noted that he was initially unsteady upon being asked to stand up from a sitting position and had verbalised non-vertiginous giddiness that went away after a short while. Limb power was full.

Question 1: What are some initial investigations to order for work up of the giddiness?

The clinical presentation suggests that the patient is anaemic and is experiencing symptomatic postural hypotension. There is a clinically significant postural drop (20 mmHg drop in systolic blood pressure and/or 10 mmHg drop in diastolic blood pressure, associated with non-vertiginous giddiness that is worse on upright posture and better on recumbency.

In considering the causes of postural hypotension, one important question to ask is whether there is an appropriate tachycardia in response to the decrease in blood pressure.

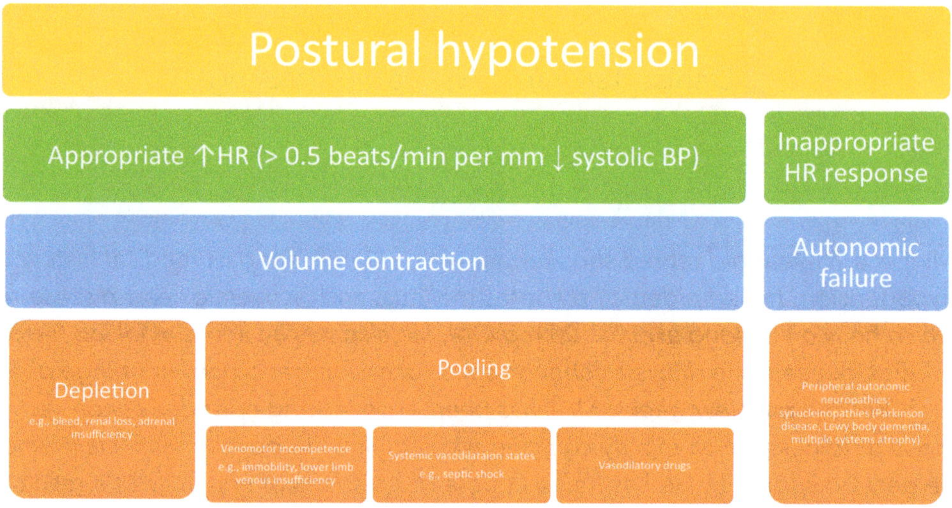

****

The results of his full blood count (FBC) are:

Haemoglobin (Hb)	*5.2 g/d*	*(12–16)*
White blood cell	*4.77 x 10^9/L*	*(4–10)*
Platelet	*700 x 10^9/L*	*(140–440)*
Red blood cell	*3.8 x 10^{12}/L*	*(4.2–5.4)*
Haematocrit	*34.7%*	*(36–46)*
MCV	*74.3 fL*	*(78–98)*
MCH	*20.6 PG*	*(27–32)*
MCHC	*27.7 g/dL*	*(32–36)*
Red cell distribution width	*23.4%*	*(10.9–15.7)*
Reticulocyte count	*1.48%*	*(0.2–2.0)*

White cell differential counts normal

Question 2: There are a few differential diagnoses for Mr T's anaemia based on this full blood count. Postulate the most likely one and explain your answer.

Mr T has a microcytic and hypochromic (MCHC) anaemia. The differential diagnoses for MCHC anaemia are iron deficiency, thalassemia, anaemia of inflammation, and sideroblastic anaemia. If we have the benefit of a previous normal FBC, then we will know that this is likely acquired (i.e., iron deficiency or anaemia of inflammation, not congenital such as thalassemia).

How to interpret the iron panel:

- Serum iron: has considerable variation within a day — when used alone, has little clinical value.
- Transferrin: iron is bound to transferrin in the plasma. Transferrin levels are reduced in inflammation.
- Total iron binding capacity (TIBC): a direct measure of the level of transferrin available to bind to iron.
- Transferrin saturation (TF sat): a measure of the amount of iron bound to transferrin.
- Ferritin: reflects body iron stores — the most sensitive indicator of iron deficiency in an otherwise well patient. It is also an acute phase reactant and can be raised in liver disease, inflammation (e.g., infection), and malignancy. ***Levels <15 μg/L usually indicate iron deficiency, whereas levels >100 μg/L usually exclude iron deficiency.***

A guide to the interpretation of the iron panel, with the more useful tests in bold, is shown in this table:

	Iron deficiency	**Anaemia of inflammation**	**Iron deficiency AND inflammation**	**Iron overload**
Iron	↓	↓	↓	↑
TIBC	↑	↓	↔ or ↓	↔ or ↓
TF sat	↓	↓	↔ or ↓	↑
Ferritin	↓↓	↔ or ↑	↔	↑

In a patient with chronic iron deficiency, where there is a lack of iron for adequate erythropoiesis, the reticulocyte count will be low or normal. Conversely, in acute blood loss or haemolysis, we can expect a marked increase in red cell production by a healthy bone marrow, reflected in a marked increase in the reticulocyte count.

Screening for thalassemia is done using Hb electrophoresis to identify the relative proportions of HbA, HbA2, and HbF. It can also identify the presence of any additional abnormal haemoglobins such as HbH. In some centres, the Hb electrophoresis test is conducted together with a special stain (brilliant cresyl blue or methylene blue stain) to identify HbH inclusion bodies in the red cells that are present in varying proportions in patients with α-thalassemia.

Generally speaking, we will make sure a patient is iron replete before sending them for Hb electrophoresis. This is because iron deficiency and α-thalassemia will show the same findings on Hb electrophoresis (i.e., all types of haemoglobin are decreased in equal proportion).

Anaemia of inflammation can result from a variety of diseases that are associated with acute or chronic immune activation. Previously, it was thought to be associated mainly with malignancies, chronic infections, and inflammatory diseases. However, we now know that it can occur with other common chronic conditions like obesity, diabetes, and heart failure. The anaemia is a result of increased hepcidin, an important regulator of iron synthesis, causing decreased iron absorption from the gastrointestinal tract and reduced iron release from the macrophages of the reticuloendothelial system.

Sideroblastic anaemia is the least common of the four causes of MCHC anaemia. It results from a defect of erythropoiesis and can be acquired (e.g., drug-induced or due to copper deficiency) or inherited and is usually regarded as a differential for unexplained anaemia after more common causes such as iron deficiency and thalassemia have been ruled out. Diagnosis is made by identifying ringed sideroblasts in a bone marrow aspirate.

****

Further laboratory investigations revealed the following:

Iron panel		
Transferrin saturation	*3.5%*	*(12–15)*
Iron	*3 μmol/L*	*(7.7–32)*
Transferrin	*3.40 g/L*	*(2.00–3.31)*
Ferritin	*1.6 μg/L*	
Total iron binding capacity	*85 μmol/L*	*(39–60)*
Hb electrophoresis		
HbA	*97%*	*(97–99)*
HbA2	*2.7%*	*(1–3)*
HbF	*0.3%*	*(0.1–1.4)*

Peripheral blood film: microcytic hypochromic red blood cells with few target cells.

Question 3: What are some possible explanations of Mr T's anaemia?

One should consider these three aetiologic categories of iron deficiency anaemia in adults:

(1) Decreased dietary intake

Note that while decreased dietary intake does contribute to iron deficiency, it is ***often not*** the main cause especially if the anaemia is severe and a patient's diet is not completely void of iron. We still have to investigate for other more sinister causes of iron deficiency! While meat contains haem iron, non-haem iron can be found in green leafy vegetables (e.g., spinach, kale) and supplemented grains. However, absorption of haem iron is more efficient (15–35% of intake versus 10–20%).

(2) Impaired absorption

Non-haem Fe^{3+} iron is solubilised from food within the acidic gastric environment. It is then converted to Fe^{2+} and absorbed in the duodenum and upper jejuneum as non-haem Fe^{2+} or as haem. Atrophic gastritis and chronic *Helicobacter pylori* infection can cause hypochlorhydria which in turns affects iron absorption due to decreased stomach acidity. Other gastrointestinal conditions affecting the stomach, duodenum, and jejuneum such as inflammatory bowel disease, celiac disease, or gastric bypass surgery can also affect iron absorption.

(3) Blood loss

This is the most common cause of iron deficiency in adults and can be overt or occult. Sources of overt bleeding are usually evident from history taking, while occult bleeding usually occurs from the gastrointestinal tract. Common causes include upper or lower gastrointestinal malignancies, peptic ulcer disease, oesophageal varices, and diverticular disease. Sometimes, the source is not identified on both upper and lower gastrointestinal endoscopies. This may be the case in small bowel lesions such as arteriovenous malformations or smaller lesions that may be missed especially if there is poor bowel preparation.

****

On further history, Mr T shared that he has had difficulty with his bowel movements. He sometimes has loose stools and at other times has had to strain at his stools. His stools are sometimes mixed with a small amount of blood which he had attributed to his haemorrhoids. He also has upper abdominal pain associated with taking food, as well as nausea but no vomiting. This has contributed to a recent loss of appetite along with some loss of weight which he was unable to quantify. He denies any difficulty swallowing solids or liquids and there is no abdominal pain.

Mr T was transfused with two units of packed red blood cells, each unit over 2–3 hours. Four hours after the transfusion was complete, he developed breathlessness with desaturation.

His vital signs were temperature 37.5°C, heart rate 100/min, blood pressure 180/100 mmHg, respiratory rate 24/min, and SpO_2 90% on room air (increased to 95% on 2 L of O_2). Mr T was able to speak in short sentences. Bibasal crepitations were heard over the posterior chest.

Question 4: What are your differential diagnoses? Prioritise them.

Question 5: Outline your immediate management based on the most likely diagnosis.

Patient blood management guidelines generally recommend a restrictive haemoglobin transfusion threshold of 7–8 g/dL for asymptomatic adults, as outcomes are similar and patients are less exposed to risks of transfusion.

However, there is no established specific guideline on haemoglobin targets in elderly patients who not only have age-related physiological changes in their cardiovascular and pulmonary systems but who often have comorbidities such as cardiovascular disease. Hence, the decision to transfuse should be contextualised to the individual patient, such as deciding whether to use a higher transfusion threshold of 8 g/dL.

Transfusion-associated circulatory overload (TACO) is an under-recognised complication of transfusion. It occurs when the volume of transfused blood products is more than what the patient's circulatory system can tolerate, resulting in congestive cardiac failure. Risk factors for this include extremes of age, patients with diminished cardiac reserves and chronic kidney disease, or patients who already have a positive fluid balance before the transfusion.

It usually occurs within hours of transfusion (usually within six hours) and is associated with hypertension, tachycardia, and desaturation, together with signs of congestive cardiac failure — raised jugular venous pressure, pulmonary crepitations, and possibly an S3 gallop rhythm.

Transfusion-related acute lung injury (TRALI) is the main differential for TACO. It is an immune-mediated acute transfusion reaction due to donor antibodies against the patient's leukocyte antigens, resulting in non-cardiogenic pulmonary oedema. It can be distinguished from TACO by the absence of physical signs of congestive cardiac failure, as well as hypotension rather than hypertension. A transient mild fever may also be present. Unlike TACO, the pulmonary oedema in TRALI will not respond to diuretic therapy (the hypotension commonly seen in TRALI also precludes the use of it).

Transfusion-related anaphylaxis would more likely result in hypotension rather than hypertension, and rhonchi (from bronchoconstriction) rather than bilateral crepitations.

The correction of iron deficiency usually takes the form of oral iron in divided doses (e.g., Iron polymaltose 100 mg BD) or intravenous iron (e.g. IV Ferric carboxymaltose 500 mg) if a person is intolerant to oral iron, has gastrointestinal malabsorption, or a short timeline before surgery.

****

Mr T subsequently underwent endoscopic evaluation and was found to have peptic ulcer disease with a 2 cm Forrest 2c ulcer in the antrum. Gastric mucosal biopsy showed the presence of H. pylori infection. He was prescribed a course of H. pylori eradication therapy as well as oral haematinics, and aspirin was suspended.

On a subsequent review, Mr T's haemoglobin level remained stable and aspirin was restarted without complications. However, he continued to be aware of occasional episodes of postural giddiness. Further history at this point showed that he had been on amlodipine 5 mg OM, enalapril 5 mg BD, and atenolol 50 mg OM for hypertension. Atenolol was discontinued without significant worsening of hypertension control and he reported a resolution of his postural giddiness thereafter.

Question 6: In situations like Mr T's, where the cause of postural hypotension is poorly reversible and the patient continues to have symptoms, what are some management options?

This would be a good time to refresh your memory by referring to the discussion on management of orthostatic hypotension in Chapter 1 on Falls I (Blood Pressure Changes).

Key messages

1. Orthostatic hypotension can result in quality of life impairment as well as significant morbidity and mortality in the event of injurious falls. Thus, it should be evaluated carefully, even in a patient with a clearly acute cause, as there may be underlying chronic issues that predispose to its development.
2. Iron deficiency in an elderly patient is most commonly due to occult or overt blood loss. Hence, we must investigate for an underlying malignancy, usually from the gastrointestinal tract.

3. Elderly patients, with reduced cardiovascular reserves or chronic renal impairment, are at higher risk of transfusion-associated circulatory overload. Hence, transfusions should be given judiciously and, where appropriate, can be given at a slower rate or together with diuretics.

Answer key

1. Full blood count (do note that pseudo-normal MCV can occur in iron-deficient patients who have concomitant causes for macrocytosis; e.g., concomitant folate and vitamin B12 deficiency, liver and thyroid dysfunction, chronic alcohol use);

   Coagulation profile (given history of black tarry stools, aspirin intake, and postural hypotension);

   Renal panel (a disproportionately raised urea will support bleeding from the upper gastrointestinal tract; chronic kidney disease with decreased erythropoietin production can also cause anaemia and should also be considered where appropriate);

   Group and cross match (essential in preparation for potential blood transfusion);

   Cardiac enzymes and electrocardiogram (look for any myocardial ischaemia).
2. The constellation of MCHC anaemia, raised RDW, and mild thrombocytosis is classical for iron deficiency anaemia (with reactive thrombocytosis).
3. Decreased iron intake (e.g., vegan);

   Impaired iron absorption from the gastrointestinal tract (e.g., inflammatory bowel disease, atrophic gastritis);

   Occult blood loss especially gastrointestinal.
4. Most likely diagnosis: transfusion-associated circulatory overload (TACO).

   Main differential diagnoses: transfusion-related acute lung injury (TRALI), desaturation unrelated to the transfusion (e.g., hospital-acquired pneumonia);

   Least likely: transfusion-related anaphylaxis with bronchoconstriction.
5. Stop the transfusion or slow the rate.

   Supportive management viz. supplementary oxygen, close monitoring of intake and urine output;

   Intravenous diuretics (e.g., furosemide);

   Notify the hospital's blood bank about the transfusion reaction.
6. Non-pharmacological management may be classified as follows:

Non-pharmacological strategy	What to advise	What to avoid
Lifestyle modifications	Regular exercises — can be done in seated or recumbent positions if standing is poorly tolerated.	Hot showers and saunas (can cause peripheral vasodilation); Long or frequent short periods of bed rest (can cause cardiovascular deconditioning); Eating large meals or meals with high glycaemic index and/or carbohydrate load (increased splanchnic diversion of blood flow).
Volume expansion	Aim for daily fluid intake of 2 to 2.5 L (challenging in patients with medically indicated fluid restriction; e.g., congestive cardiac failure, chronic kidney disease); Increase salt intake (also challenging in some patients).	Caffeinated beverages and alcohol (have diuretic effects).
Physical counter-manoeuvres	Some manoeuvres can be done during daily activities which can help maintain blood pressure when standing: leg crossing, standing on tiptoe, stooping, squatting, and buttock clenching; Change positions (e.g., seated to standing) in a gradual manner.	Straining and other Valsalva-like manoeuvres.

(Continued)

(*Continued*)

Non-pharmacological strategy	**What to advise**	**What to avoid**
Compression garments	Elastic compression stockings and abdominal binders [main issue is that of compliance due to difficulty with putting them on and the discomfort of wearing them due to the tightness of application].	
Sleeping with head of bed raised	Elevate head up 30° to 45° when lying in bed (helps mediate supine hypertension as well as reduces nocturnal polyuria from supine hypertension — nocturnal polyuria increases risk of falls at night due to frequency and also contributes to postural hypotension in the day due to volume depletion).	

Pharmacological management can be considered for recalcitrant postural hypotension that does not respond to non-pharmacological strategies viz. midodrine, fludrocortisone.

References

Cascio MJ, DeLoughery TG (2017) Anemia: Evaluation and Diagnostic Tests. *Med Clin North Am* **101**(2): 263–284.

Goodnough LT, Schrier SL (2014) Evaluation and management of anemia in the elderly. *Am J Hematol* **89**(1): 88–96.

Peixoto AJ (2022) Evaluation and management of orthostatic hypotension: Limited data, limitless opportunity. *Cleve Clin J Med* **89**(1): 36–45.

Semple JW, Rebetz J, Kapur R (2019) Transfusion-associated circulatory overload and transfusion-related acute lung injury. *Blood.* **133**(17): 1840–1853.

13 Giddiness II (Pancytopenia)

Richard Yiu Cheung, Alvin Tan Wee Beng

Mr Y is a 72-year-old retired engineer with a background history of chronic hepatitis B infection, diabetes mellitus, and hypertension. He complained of intermittent giddiness of one month's duration. His giddiness was non-vertiginous and sometimes related to posture, lasting only a few seconds each episode. His giddiness occurred more frequently in the recent one week which prompted him to see his general practitioner.

He also experienced shortness of breath on exertion. He used to be able to ride a bicycle for two hours continuously. However, during the past two weeks, he would get tired after fifteen minutes of cycling. He would also suffer from shortness of breath and chest tightness after climbing two flights of stairs. He was still able to manage his usual housework. He did not have any numbness or weakness.

Mr Y does not smoke or drink alcohol. Apart from his medications for diabetes mellitus and hypertension, he did not take any other medication or traditional herbal medicine. He was not a vegetarian. He denied any gastric or bleeding symptoms. There was no family history of cancer or blood disorder.

On physical examination, he looked pale but was fully alert and oriented. Blood pressure was 145/75 mmHg with no significant postural drop. Pulse rate was regular at 85 beats per minute. Small ecchymoses were present over his arms. There was no peripheral lymphadenopathy. Heart and lungs sounds were normal. Abdominal examination was unremarkable; in particular, there was no hepatosplenomegaly and no ballotable kidney. Per rectal examination revealed brownish stool. His gait was normal and limb power was full.

Laboratory results from the general practitioner showed:

WBC count	*3.90 x 10^9/L*	*(4–10)*
Absolute neutrophil	*2.10 x 10^9/L*	*(2.00–7.50)*
Haemoglobin	*6.2 g/dL*	*(12–16)*
MCV	*112 fL*	*(78–98)*
Platelet count	*63 x 10^9/L*	*(140–440)*

Question 1: What are the next most appropriate laboratory investigations?

The full blood count showed macrocytic anaemia and thrombocytopenia. Although the total white blood cell (WBC) count was marginally low, there was no neutropenia at this point. A number of differential diagnoses need to be entertained at this stage, specifically vitamin B12 deficiency, Evans syndrome, bone marrow failure syndrome (e.g., aplastic anaemia, myelodysplastic syndrome, myelofibrosis), and thrombotic thrombocytopenic purpura (TTP).

Relevant initial investigations would be required to look for haemolysis and vitamin B12 deficiency.

Haematological and biochemical markers for haemolysis include reticulocytosis, hyperbilirubinaemia (unconjugated), elevated lactate dehydrogenase (LDH), and decreased haptoglobin level. If there is evidence of haemolysis, a direct Coombs test would be necessary to determine if the haemolysis is immune or non-immune in nature. Blood film is useful to look for any polychromasia, spherocytosis, and red blood cell (RBC) fragments. When there is evidence of haemolysis together with a significant amount of RBC fragments present on blood film suggestive of microangiopathic haemolysis, the possibility of TTP should immediately be considered because TTP is a fatal disease if left untreated. Other features of TTP include fever, renal failure, and neurological involvement such as confusion, numbness, weakness, and seizure — all of which were absent in Mr Y.

****

Further investigations revealed:

Reticulocyte	*3%*	*(0.5–2.0)*
Haptoglobin	*0.8 g/L*	*(0.3–2.0)*
Blood urea	*5 mmol/L*	*(2.7–6.9)*
Serum creatinine	*63 µmol/L*	*(62–106)*
Serum calcium	*2.22 mmol/L*	*(2.09–2.46)*
Total protein	*60 g/L*	*(68–85)*
Serum albumin	*35 g/L*	*(40–51)*
Total bilirubin	*15 µmol/L*	*(7–32)*

Serum ALT	*45 U/L*	*(6–66)*
Serum AST	*32 U/L*	*(12–42)*
Serum ALP	*50 U/L*	*(39–99)*
Serum LDH	*203 U/L*	*(135–350)*
Ferritin	*385 μg/L*	*(30–400)*
Folate	*10.5 nmol/L*	*(10.4–78.9)*
Vitamin B12	*95 pmol/L*	*(145–569)*

Peripheral blood film: macrocytic red blood cells, no nucleated RBC, and no RBC fragment; no early white blood and no platelet clump seen

ECG: normal sinus rhythm

CXR: normal cardiac size, no pulmonary congestion or mass

Question 2: Based on the findings so far, what other investigation(s) would you order?

Vitamin B12 deficiency commonly causes macrocytic anaemia. Other haematological manifestations include neutropenia, thrombocytopenia, pancytopenia, and intramedullary hemolysis due to ineffective erythropoiesis.

Detection of vitamin B12 deficiency prompts the question of the cause of its deficiency (nutritional deficiency versus pernicious anaemia). In pernicious anaemia which is an autoimmune condition with atrophic gastritis, there is vitamin B12 malabsorption.

Auto-antibody to intrinsic factor is highly specific to pernicious anaemia and, if present, is considered confirmatory for diagnosis of pernicious anaemia; however, the sensitivity of anti-intrinsic factor antibody is relatively low. Antiparietal cell antibody is present in the majority of patients with pernicious anaemia, but it is less specific and can be seen in simple atrophic gastritis and in autoimmune thyroid disease.

****

Mr Y's blood results are as follows:
Antiparietal cell antibody positive
Anti-intrinsic factor antibody negative

Question 3: Which of the following is/are appropriate management for Mr Y?

i. Packed cell transfusion	**Appropriate/not appropriate**
ii. Oral vitamin B12 replacement	**Appropriate/not appropriate**
iii. Intramuscular vitamin B12	**Appropriate/not appropriate**
iv. Gastroscopy	**Appropriate/not appropriate**

When faced with any patient with symptomatic anaemia, the first question to ask is whether any immediate treatment with blood transfusion is required. The answer depends on a discussion on the pros and cons of blood transfusion. While many local hospital guidelines allow blood transfusion for patients with Hb less than 7 g/dL, the important factors for consideration of immediate blood transfusion are:

- the severity of the patient's symptoms
- the patient's concurrent medical conditions
- the underlying aetiology of the anaemia
- the chronicity of the anaemia
- the availability of alternative effective treatment

Mr Y's vitamin B12 deficiency can be addressed with the options of oral versus parenteral replacement. Given the degree of his symptomatic anaemia, we would suggest considering parenteral administration upfront with intramuscular (or subcutaneous) vitamin B12 injection 1 mg daily for 3 to 5 days, followed by once-weekly administration for the next three weeks. Subsequent frequency of vitamin B12 administration will depend on the response to treatment.

After adequate parenteral replacement of vitamin B12, blood tests including full blood count and serum vitamin B12 level should be repeated to monitor for response.

****

As Mr Y was symptomatic with exertional breathlessness and chest pain, a decision was made to transfuse him with two units of red blood cell transfusion. His haemoglobin level increased to 8.5 g/dL post-transfusion. Intramuscular vitamin B12 was concomitantly commenced. He was discharged from hospital and continued to receive parenteral vitamin B12 replacement at his general practitioner clinic.

After four weeks, Mr Y's repeat blood tests are as follows:

WBC count	*2.90 x 10^9/L*	*(4–10)*
Absolute neutrophil	*1.32 x 10^9/L*	*(2.00–7.50)*
Haemoglobin	*7.3 g/dL*	*(12–16)*
MCV	*110 fL*	*(78–98)*
Platelet count	*42 x 109/L*	*(140–440)*
Reticulocyte	*3.9%*	*(0.5–2.0)*
Vitamin B12	*420 pmol/L*	*(145–569)*

Question 4: What is the most likely consideration at this point?

a. **Aplastic anaemia**
b. **Chronic lymphocytic leukaemia**
c. **Myelodysplastic syndrome**
d. **Myelofibrosis**

Although the vitamin B12 had been fully repleted after a month of replacement, the full blood count continued to show pancytopenia. This warrants a formal haematology referral.

Bone marrow aspirate and biopsy should be considered to diagnose a bone marrow failure syndrome. Several differential diagnoses that should be considered include aplastic anaemia, myelodysplastic syndrome, and myelofibrosis.

We commonly see reticulocytopenia in aplastic anaemia, though reticulocyte count may be normal in non-severe aplastic anaemia. Bone marrow biopsy will show hypocellular marrow without any abnormal infiltration or marrow fibrosis.

Myelofibrosis can lead to pancytopenia and often manifests with a leucoerythroblastic picture (with immature RBC and WBC — sometimes myeloblasts may be seen in the peripheral blood, usually less than 5% of the total WBC count). Although marked splenomegaly is a hallmark of primary myelofibrosis, it can be absent in a minority of cases. In this case, Mr Y did not have any splenomegaly and thus myelofibrosis was a less likely diagnosis.

The median age of onset of myelodysplastic syndrome (MDS) is between 65 and 70 years. The persistent pancytopenia with macrocytosis despite repletion of vitamin B12 makes this diagnosis more likely for Mr Y. The bone marrow of a MDS patient is usually hypercellular or normocellular and shows dysplasia in any of the three cell lineages (at least 10% of dysplasia in one cell lineage as part of the minimal diagnostic criteria).

The prognostic scoring system for MDS has evolved over time and the one most commonly used today is the Revised International Prognostic Scoring System (IPSS-R) which comprises of five prognostic variables: cytogenetics (bone marrow karyotype), bone marrow blast percentage, haemoglobin level, platelet count, and absolute neutrophil count. It allows patients to be stratified into five prognostic risk categories: very low, low, intermediate, high, and very high.

The treatment of MDS can range from aggressive therapy such as allogeneic stem cell transplant to best supportive care with blood transfusion support only. Clinical assessment of the patient's eligibility for intensive therapy would be needed. Sometimes, it can be quite obvious that in some patients with multiple comorbidities and/or organ failures, disease-modifying intensive therapies such as stem cell transplant and intensive chemotherapy may not be suitable. However, the decision is not easy to make. With the introduction of allogeneic stem cell transplantation with reduced intensity conditioning (RIC) regimen, elderly patients who were traditionally excluded from conventional myeloablative allogeneic stem cell transplantation may now be offered this potentially curative treatment option.

Several patient factors including the performance status and comorbidities of the patient also need to be assessed. Commonly used tools to assess performance status include the Eastern Cooperative Oncology Group and Karnofsky performance scores. Should time and resources permit, tools to identify frailty including performing a comprehensive geriatric assessment may help to risk-stratify and tailor suitable therapies for older patients. In addition, certain interventions targeted at identified deficits can be put in place to improve the patient's condition and reduce the risk of toxicities and other adverse outcomes. This often involves referrals to various members of a multidisciplinary team which is integral to the holistic care of a geriatric patient (e.g., physiotherapist for physical function, dietician for nutrition, medical social worker for social and psychological support).

Major comorbidities such as stroke, heart disease, and renal failure are negative predictive factors for the success of intensive therapy. While RIC allogeneic stem cell transplant presents a possible curative option for elderly patients with MDS, the paucity of suitable stem cell donors could be a realistic limiting factor as their siblings are often elderly themselves and may no longer be suitable to donate stem cells.

****

Mr Y was referred to the haematology clinic. Bone marrow studies showed hypercellular marrow with erythroid and megakaryocytic dysplasia (>10% dysplasia) and 4% myeloblasts — the bone marrow morphology was diagnostic of MDS. The cytogenetic studies reported the presence of monosomy 7 which was an adverse karyotypic abnormality in MDS. The IPSS-R category was very high risk, which conferred a median survival of 0.8 years if the MDS disease was left untreated.

Mr Y's medical conditions were stable and his major organ functions were normal. He was therefore referred to a tertiary hospital for chemotherapy and assessment for allogeneic stem cell transplant.

Key messages

1. Look for vitamin B12 deficiency and haemolysis in patients with macrocytic anaemia with or without other cytopenia.
2. Parenteral vitamin B12 replacement is the preferred treatment in pernicious anaemia.

3. After excluding the common peripheral causes of pancytopenia in an elderly patient, one should consider the possibility of bone marrow failure syndrome such as MDS, aplastic anaemia, and myelofibrosis.

Answer key

1. Serum vitamin B12 level and haemolytic screen.
2. Diagnostic tests for pernicious anaemia:

	Sensitivity	**Specificity**
Anti-intrinsic factor antibody	Low	High (confirmatory)
Antiparietal cell antibody	High	Low (also present in simple atrophic gastritis, autoimmune thyroid disease)

3. i. Appropriate.
   ii. Not appropriate.
   iii. Appropriate.
   iv. Not appropriate. *Although pernicious anaemia is associated with increased risk of gastric malignancy, the diagnosis of pernicious anaemia was not confirmed at that point in time. As Mr Y did not have any gastric symptoms and he had normal iron store, gastroscopy was not indicated.*
4. C.

References

Andres E, *et al.* (2012) Optimal management of pernicious anemia. *J Blood Med* **3**: 97–103.
Platzbecker U (2019) Treatment of MDS. *Blood* **133**: 1096–1107.

14 Giddiness III (Vestibular Disorder)

Tay Sok Boon, Cedric Koh Chien Hsiang,
Anupama Roy Chowdhury

Mr L is a 75-year-old Chinese gentleman with a history of diabetes mellitus, hypertension, benign prostate hypertrophy, and atrial fibrillation. He presented to the Emergency Department with intermittent vertiginous giddiness that worsens on head movement for the last 24 hours. These episodes were accompanied by vomiting. He has been compliant with his medications, which include rivaroxaban, amlodipine, losartan, tamsulosin, metformin, and glipizide.

Question 1: What is your diagnostic thought process as you take a more comprehensive history with respect to Mr L's giddiness?

Question 2: What aspects of physical examination are important?

HISTORY

The sole presence of giddiness (synonymous with "dizziness") in the elderly is a powerful predictor of falls, and falls are the leading cause of accidental death in the elderly. Hence, giddiness must never be taken lightly. Unlike younger patients, history is often difficult to ascertain as patients frequently have difficulty describing the sensation of giddiness. Determining if it is vertiginous or non-vertiginous is often an important first step and while it is often difficult in the elderly, every attempt must be made to try to elicit this in the history. Many older patients also use the word "giddy" when they feel unwell, so it is necessary to clarify what exactly one means by this — is it true dizziness or something else such as headache, light-headedness, stress etc.? Timing and triggers are very helpful.

Intermittent episodes of vertigo that last for few seconds to a few minutes triggered by head movement are often all one needs to make a diagnosis of **benign paroxysmal positional vertigo** (BPPV). The duration of the average episode of BPPV is less than a minute, though it often recurs. However, be aware that most patients with vertigo will give a history of worsening with head movement; the critical distinction to be made is whether the head movement ***triggers*** the vertigo (i.e., with complete resolution of vertigo between episodes) or whether the head movement ***exacerbates*** the vertigo that is ongoing. The former would be suggestive of BPPV while the latter would certainly warrant greater clinical concern.

Alternatively, if the patient presents with acute onset of vertigo lasting more than 24 hours, the diagnosis of **acute vestibular syndrome** needs to be considered. Common associated symptoms include nausea, vomiting, and gait instability. These symptoms, again, will often worsen with head movement but are typically continuously present at baseline. In this situation, the diagnosis of peripheral vestibulopathy with either vestibular neuronitis or labyrinthitis (if there is hearing loss, tinnitus, or fullness in the ear) are the usual causes. Recurrent and progressive episodes that last from 20 minutes to 24 hours are suggestive of Meniere disease.

However, a proportion of these patients have underlying dangerous posterior circulation strokes that can mimic the diagnosis of a vestibulopathy. For instance, an anterior inferior cerebellar artery stroke may present with unilateral ipsilateral deafness and vertigo from labyrinthine artery ischaemia. Hence, a high index of suspicion is required in the older patient, especially one with vascular risk factors and those on antiplatelets or anticoagulants (increased risk of bleed). Symptoms such as diplopia, dysarthria, dysphagia, limb ataxia, and limb weakness would raise concern for a posterior circulation stroke. The history must be meticulous and thorough as it may be challenging to elicit signs of a posterior circulation stroke in an older patient.

A history of migraine with associated symptoms (throbbing unilateral headache, photophobia, phonophobia, or aura) during episodes of vertigo may lead one to consider the diagnosis of vestibular migraine.

With polypharmacy becoming more prevalent in the elderly, it would be paramount to look through Mr L's medication list. Was the antihypertensive up-dosed recently? When was the α-blocker for his benign prostate hypertrophy started? Or perhaps did he skip his breakfast due to a busy morning but yet had already taken his glipizide? Is a diary of blood pressure and capillary blood glucose available for review?

Finally, don't forget that giddiness can also be the presenting complaint of non-neurological diseases. Symptomatic anaemia may present with giddiness without the classical symptoms of chest pain or breathlessness on exertion. Arrhythmias may also induce symptoms of giddiness and syncope — in Mr L, differentials of slow atrial fibrillation, sick sinus syndrome, and long pauses may need to be considered.

PHYSICAL EXAMINATION

Start with assessment of the vital signs. Bradycardia might be suggestive of underlying arrhythmia while tachycardia might suggest atrial fibrillation with rapid ventricular response. Postural blood pressure at 1 and 3 minutes should be taken.

A full neurological examination, particularly paying attention to the cranial nerves and cerebellum, would be needed. Examination of the cerebellar system should start with examination for nystagmus. Look first for spontaneous nystagmus on central gaze and subsequently test for nystagmus in all directions. The direction of nystagmus is named based on the direction of the fast phase. A peripheral cause of nystagmus should beat in the same direction regardless of the direction of eye movement (unidirectional nystagmus), and it is more pronounced when the patient looks in the direction of the fast phase. It commonly manifests as horizontal nystagmus.

Meanwhile, torsional or vertical nystagmus is more consistent with a central cause. Multidirectional nystagmus which changes on direction of eccentric gaze is concerning for a central cause.

This should be followed by examination of eye movements with both saccades and pursuit. Hypermetric or hypometric saccades and the loss of smooth pursuit may point towards a cerebellar lesion as well.

For more evidence of cerebellar disease, examination of the peripheries should focus on the presence of intentional tremor, past pointing, and dysdiadochokinesia. Axial instability of the trunk may be present. Pendular knee reflexes (>4 swings)

Tips and precautions for performing the Dix–Hallpike manoeuvre in the elderly person:

- *Many elderly patients have cervical spine problems (e.g., spinal stenosis, cervical radioculopathy) or vascular problems (e.g., vertebrobasilar insufficiency, orthopnoea) which limits the use of this manoeuvre.*
- *As the procedure can be intimidating and traumatic, always explain what you are about to do and stress the importance of keeping the eyes opened (or else you can't see the nystagmus!) during the manoeuvre.*
- *You may find it helpful to get the patient to fold his/her arms before you perform the manoeuvre.*
- *Consider performing on the asymptomatic side first.*
- *The "loaded" Dix–Hallpike test is a modification to increase the sensitivity of the test. With the head turned to the side that you are testing, flex the head (or lean the body forward) by 30° for about 30 seconds before performing the manoeuvre.*
- *If the head of the bed is against a wall so there is no space to dangle the head, you can modify the procedure by placing a pillow or rolled blanket under the thoracic spine.*

are a rare finding. Lastly, if the patient can stand, a gait examination may reveal a broad-based gait with unsteadiness.

For patients with intermittent episodes of vertigo, the Dix–Hallpike manoeuvre is the test of choice and is particularly helpful for diagnosis of posterior BPPV. Observable nystagmus after a brief delay and lasting **up to one minute** would constitute a positive result. The Dix–Hallpike test may not be positive if the lateral canal is involved.

In patients whom you suspect as having acute vestibular syndrome, a 3-step bedside oculomotor examination (HINTS: Head Impulse, Nystagmus, Test of Skew) has good sensitivity for ruling out a stroke. This is meant to be performed in currently symptomatic patients who have continuous symptoms as opposed to the Dix–Hallpike test for patients with acute and intermittent symptoms.

	Signs	
Steps of HINTS examination	**Peripheral lesion**	**Central lesion**
Head impulse: Ask the patient to fixate his/her gaze on your nose. Gently move the patient's head left and right to relax the neck muscles. Many older patients may have cervical spondylosis affecting their neck movements due to stiffness and pain. Once the patient is relaxed, rapidly move the patient's head back to the central position.	Abnormal with a corrective saccade	Normal with no corrective saccade (because the vestibular-ocular reflex is preserved)
Nystagmus: (discussed above)	Horizontal, unidirectional	Vertical or torsional, multidirectional
Test of Skew: Ask the patient to fixate his/her gaze on your nose and shine a light source. Looking at the reflection of the light source can help one appreciate if there is ***vertical*** misalignment. This should be followed by alternatively covering each of the patient's eyes.	No skew deviation	Positive for skew deviation: deviation of the eye while it is covered with its corrective movement during uncovering

This link brings you to an excellent instructional Youtube video on the HINTS examination by Medmastery with real-life illustrations.

Lastly, examination may reveal a non-neurological cause or contributing factor for giddiness. Conjunctival pallor and/or pallor in the palmar creases may suggest anaemia as a cause. Digital rectal examination may be needed to ensure that the patient is not actively bleeding. Auscultation of the carotids may reveal bruits that suggest carotid stenosis. Examination of the ear and otoscopy may also reveal evidence of otitis media contributing to peripheral vestibulopathy. The presence of vesicles in the external auditory canal may suggest Ramsay–Hunt syndrome which can present with vertigo, hearing impairment, and otalgia. Examination of the heart may reveal an aortic stenosis murmur. A general comprehensive exam may also reveal an acute medical illness (e.g., infection, heart failure) which may manifest as giddiness — such atypical presentations are not uncommon in the elderly!

****

There were no focal motor or sensory deficits noted on physical examination. Mr L's initial blood tests and an electrocardiogram (ECG) were normal. CT brain was unremarkable apart from mild cerebral atrophy. A review of his drug chart did not reveal any culprit medications. The first HINTS test done by the on-call doctor was negative for a central lesion. Mr L was thought to have benign paroxysmal positional vertigo and was prescribed betahistine. However, he did not experience any relief in symptoms after 48 hours. You repeated the HINTS test and noticed the absence of corrective saccade.

Question 3: What is the next most important investigation?

a. Electroencephalogram

b. Lumbar puncture

c. MRI brain

d. Telemetry monitoring

e. Tilt table test

When investigating an elderly person with giddiness, full blood count is helpful to assess for anaemia. Hyponatraemia is a common cause of giddiness in the elderly and is easily picked up with a renal panel. Extended electrolyte panel looking at calcium, magnesium, and phosphate need not routinely be ordered as these are usually not associated with giddiness unless there is an underlying arrhythmia.

ECG may reveal evidence of an underlying arrhythmia or a myocardial infarction causing giddiness. β-blockers are common medications used in older patients and can cause bradycardia. Heart blocks can occur *de novo* in the elderly or following inferior myocardial infarcts. The elderly patient may also be on multiple drugs that prolong QTc and cause an arrhythmia.

CT brain is insufficient to fully exclude posterior circulation stroke as early lesions or small lesions may be missed. In fact, a negative HINTS exam done by an ***experienced*** operator rules out stroke better than a negative MRI with diffusion-weighted imaging in the first 24 to 48 hours of symptom onset. However, if the index of suspicion is high for a cerebrovascular event due to persistence of symptoms, unsteady gait, or presence of risk factors, then further neuroimaging with an MRI should be undertaken.

A screen for infection with a chest X-ray and urinalysis may be needed in cases where the cause of giddiness is unclear after the above investigations.

****

The ward doctors ordered an MRI brain which showed a small acute cerebellar infarct. Mr L was started on an antiplatelet agent and he made excellent neurological recovery.

Key messages

1. Giddiness has a wide range of differential diagnoses, and the clinical presentation may be atypical in the elderly.
2. Reconsider your diagnosis if your patient does not demonstrate improvement to your initial treatment. The HINTS test, like all other tests, can give a false-negative result.
3. Have a high index of suspicion for central causes in patients with persistent symptoms and gait instability, as well as in those with cardiovascular risk factors.
4. Thorough history taking, good physical examination techniques, and an open mind are key to caring for the giddy elderly so as to not miss potentially life-threatening and treatable aetiologies. Giddiness left unaddressed is a common cause of falls and can cause a downward spiral of functional decline with subsequent low mood and loss of confidence due to the persistent symptoms.

Answer key

1. There is no model answer for such a question as different physicians will have their own clinical approaches. Your preferred approach should be sensible and immediately practical, but the most important thing is that it always works for you. Our thought process for giddiness in the elderly is usually but not always in the following sequential order:
   a. Is it true giddiness (vertigo = illusion of motion) or something else such as unsteadiness (balance issue), light-headedness (presyncopal issue), or non-specific (a state of unwellness)?
   b. If vertiginous, can it be stroke (risk factors, brainstem symptoms, and/or limb weakness)?
   c. If not stroke, is it peripheral syndrome (nausea/vomiting)?
   d. If peripheral, which syndrome [BPPV: position triggered, vestibular neuronitis: viral infection, labyrinthitis (with auditory symptoms): bacterial infection]?
   e. Contribution from medical comorbidity (e.g., hypertension/postural hypotension, hypoglycaemia, anaemia).
2. The following aspects of physical examination of a giddy elderly should be undertaken:
   a. Vital signs esp. temperature, blood pressure, and postural evaluation.
   b. Eyes esp. anaemia, HINTS.
   c. Cardiovascular system esp. heart rate and rhythm, auscultation of carotid and aortic areas.
   d. Neurological examination esp. cranial nerves, cerebellar, gait.
   e. Otoscopy.
3. C.

References

Bhattacharyya N, Baugh RF, Orvidas L, *et al.* (2008) Clinical practice guideline: Benign paroxysmal positional vertigo. *Otolaryngol Head Neck Surg* **139**(5 Suppl 4): S47–S81.

Kattah JC, Talkad AV, Wang DZ, Hsieh YH, Newman-Toker DE (2009) HINTS to diagnose stroke in the acute vestibular syndrome: three-step bedside oculomotor examination more sensitive than early MRI diffusion-weighted imaging. *Stroke* **40**: 3504–3510.

Ohle R, Montpellier RA, Marchadier V, Wharton A, McIsaac S, Anderson M, Savage D (2020) Can Emergency Physicians Accurately Rule Out a Central Cause of Vertigo Using the HINTS Examination? A systematic review and meta-analysis. *Acad Emerg Med* **27**(9): 887–896.

15 Stroke (Atrial Fibrillation)

Kaavya Narasimhalu, Melvin Chua Peng Wei

Mrs X is a 76-year-old Chinese female who needs minimal assistance in basic activities of daily living (ADLs) and ambulates with a quad stick. She has a past medical history of diabetes mellitus, hyperlipidaemia, hypertension, Parkinson disease, and ischaemic heart disease. Her medications include aspirin 100 mg OM, bisoprolol 2.5 mg OM, atorvastatin 40 mg ON, losartan 75 mg OM, metformin 500 mg TDS, glipizide 2.5 mg BD, empagliflozin 10 mg OM, levodopa 62.5 mg TDS, lactulose 10 mL TDS, Senna 2 tabs ON, and omeprazole 20 mg OM. She has no drug allergy. She is admitted to the ward with a transient episode of right-sided weakness associated with difficulty speaking which lasted for one to two hours. The electrocardiogram done in the emergency department showed atrial fibrillation.

Question 1: What important aspects of history would you like to ask for concerning her premorbid state?

Mrs X does have mild cognitive difficulties, but can manage most of her basic ADLs independently. According to her family and caregiver, she occasionally forgets what she has eaten for breakfast and lunch, but she is able to recognise family members, count money, call her children, and hold a meaningful conversation. She still goes to the market with her dedicated caregiver so as to keep herself active.

Her last fall was approximately three months ago and happened when she was exiting her bathroom after showering. She had slipped and fallen forwards, landing on her hands. She did not suffer major injuries from the fall. The family has thereafter ensured that there are anti-slip mats in place in the bathroom. Her Parkinson disease is mild and well controlled with her medications. She takes her medications at least 30 minutes before meals. She does not have freezing episodes or postural giddiness.

On examination, Mrs X is alert and not in visible distress. Her vital signs are temperature 37.2°C, blood pressure 116/78 mmHg with no postural drop, heart rate 96/min and irregularly irregular, and respiratory rate 20/min with SpO_2 98% on room air. She is oriented to time, place, and person. There is no conjunctival pallor, scleral icterus, cataracts, cervical lymphadenopathy, or pedal oedema. Cardiopulmonary and abdominal examinations were normal. Neurological examination revealed mild bradykinesia and cog-wheel rigidity over the wrists which was more prominent on the right. There was no pill-rolling tremor or mask-like facies. She had full power in all four limbs and preserved reflexes. Her gait was characterised by small shuffling steps, turning in numbers, and poor arm swing. There were no clinical signs to suggest vestibular dysfunction. Her score on the abbreviated mental test was 9/10. Both knees had crepitus on passive movements. No spinal tenderness was elicited.

Laboratory investigations showed:

WBC count	*9.83 x 10^9/L*	*(4–10)*
Haemoglobin	*10.9 g/dL*	*(12–16)*
Platelet count	*167 x 10^9/L*	*(140–440)*
Blood urea	*7.8 mmol/L*	*(2.7–6.9)*
Sodium	*134 mmol/L*	*(136–146)*
Potassium	*4.3 mmol/L*	*(3.5–5.1)*
Serum creatinine	*89 μmol/L*	*(45–84)*
Calcium	*2.14 mmol/L*	*(2.09–2.46)*
Phosphate	*0.89 mmol/L*	*(0.94–1.5)*
Magnesium	*0.78 mmol/L*	*(0.75–1.07)*
Lactate	*2.4 mmol/L*	*(0.2–2.2)*
Total protein	*64 g/L*	*(68–85)*
Serum albumin	*36 g/L*	*(40–51)*
Total bilirubin	*8 μmol/L*	*(7–32)*
Serum ALT	*36 U/L*	*(6–66)*
Serum AST	*40 U/L*	*(12–42)*
Serum ALP	*161 U/L*	*(39–99)*
Gamma-GT	*84 U/L*	*(9–53)*
Serum TSH	*3.7 mIU/L*	*(0.45–4.5)*
Free T4	*10.8 pmol/L*	*(10–20)*
HbA1c		*6.9%*

Chest X-ray: no consolidation or cardiomegaly
ECG: atrial fibrillation, rate 62/minute

Question 2: Based on the information thus far, what factors would you consider before discussing anticoagulation with her?

Any patient with complaints suggestive of a transient ischaemic attack (TIA) should be assessed for possible aetiology of the TIA. Here, there is a suggestion of a *cortical* TIA given that she had expressive dysphasia during the event.

A new diagnosis of atrial fibrillation in an elderly patient often causes considerable concern as the risk of recurrent stroke needs to be weighed against the risk of bleeding complications. Treatment decisions are often tailored to the individual, so the risks and benefits must be individualised. Other comorbidities need to be considered to determine the fall risk before deciding on whether to anticoagulate the patient.

Even if the eventual decision is for anticoagulation, the choice of anticoagulation should also be individualised. Polypharmacy is common in older patients as many of them have multiple medical conditions. It is therefore important to review the medication list to optimise the management of medical conditions and minimise the risk of drug–drug interactions. Additionally, the delivery routes of the various options must also be considered as not all anticoagulation options can be crushed for delivery via nasogastric tubes.

Given that she has atrial fibrillation (AF), her risk of recurrent strokes is high. The following tools are extremely useful at this stage and the interpretation of the results should be explained to the patient.

		CHA_2DS_2-VASc score	**HAS-BLED score**
Purpose		Calculates stroke risk for patients with AF	Estimates risk of major bleeding for patients with AF on anticoagulation
How to perform the assessment (links lead to MD+Calc)			
Illustration (Mrs X)	Calculation	2 (age) + 1 (gender) + 1 (hypertension) + 2 (TIA) + 1 (diabetes) = 7	1 (age) + 1 (hypertension) + 1 (medication predisposing to bleeding) = 3
	Interpretation	11.2% annual risk of stroke	3.7–5.8% annual risk of bleed

Part of the assessment particularly in the elderly would entail her fall risk status. At present, Mrs X is ambulant, and while she does have mild cognitive deficits, she is fairly independent in her basic ADLs (showering, dressing, toileting, feeding). Her Parkinson disease is well controlled as well. As such, the benefits of anticoagulation appear to outweigh the risks.

The main unaddressed issue in this elderly patient, however, is an unexplained anaemia. An attempt should be made to ascertain the cause of the anaemia prior to starting anticoagulation therapy.

Colonoscopy and upper gastrointestinal (GI) endoscopy can allow visualisation of mucosal lesions like ulcers, polyps, inflammation, or malignancy, and biopsies should be taken for histological examination. Alarm features that warrant endoscopic investigation are rectal bleeding (haematochezia), heme-positive stool, iron deficiency anaemia, significant weight loss, obstructive symptoms, recent onset of constipation without an obvious explanation, and family history of colorectal cancer or inflammatory bowel disease. These need to be evaluated in Mrs X.

In patients with unexplained iron-deficiency anaemia, it would be prudent to undertake endoscopic evaluation before starting anticoagulation. Most procedures under sedation are low-to-moderate risk after a stroke or TIA in the absence of large vessel occlusions or intracardiac thrombus. As such, one should consider inpatient colonic and upper GI endoscopic evaluation prior to commencing anticoagulation for Mrs X if she is agreeable. Optimal timing of the procedure can be discussed with a neurologist should there be any concerns.

****

Question 3: How would you specifically discuss anticoagulation with Mrs X and her family?

Key points to discuss in this case would be:

A. Risk of recurrent stroke without anticoagulation

Based on Mrs X's CHA_2DS_2-VASc Score, her risk of having a stroke each year is about 11.2%.

B. Risk of bleeding if treated with anticoagulation

Based on Mrs X's HASBLED score, her risk of having a major bleeding event is 3.7–5.8% per year.

C. Risk of falls, and how to mitigate these

Mrs X is at risk of falls both from frailty and from her Parkinson disease. Advice should be given to look for symptoms suggestive of postural giddiness which is commonly associated with Parkinson disease and its treatment, as well as to mitigate it. Antihypertensive agents and autonomic dysfunction from long-standing diabetes may further potentiate postural hypotension. Advise her that she should not rush when moving from a seated or lying position to a standing position, and that she should let half to one minute pass to ensure her blood pressure equilibrates before ambulating.

Patients with Parkinson disease are advised to go for walks on a daily basis as deconditioning happens quickly in those who are immobile. For preventive measures, her footwear should be evaluated for a tight fit (less likely to trip) and her home environment reviewed for hazards. For example, anti-slip mats should be put in place in areas that are commonly wet.

D. Evaluation of GI system prior to commencing anticoagulation

Patient and family should be informed that most major bleeding episodes tend to involve the GI system. Given that the anticoagulants can cause internal bleeding, it would be advisable to examine the stomach and colon prior to starting powerful blood thinners, especially in cases of unexplained anaemia or where there is clinical suspicion of potential pathology. Mrs X should be counselled about the risks of perforation (1/1,000 for colonscopy and 1/2,500 for upper GI endoscopy) and major adverse cardiovascular events due to intravenous sedation (you may access this link for calculating the revised cardiac risk index for pre-operative risk of cardiac complications after non-cardiac surgery) before deciding on whether to proceed.

E. Choice of anticoagulation if she were to start

Mrs X can be offered either warfarin or a novel anticoagulant like rivaroxaban or apixaban for anticoagulation. Arrange for the pharmacist to discuss interactions with diet and other medications. She should be reminded also to ensure compliance, and that while anticoagulation is one part of secondary prevention, good blood pressure control (systolic BP <140 mmHg, diastolic BP <80 mmHg) and good lipid control (LDL <2.5 mmol/L) would also be needed to help prevent further cardiovascular events.

Key messages

1. AF is a common condition in elderly patients.
2. Treatment of AF needs to be individualised, based on the risk/benefit ratio in each individual patient.

3. Consider whether the patient requires endoscopic evaluation prior to commencement of anticoagulation.
4. Consider the feasibility of different anticoagulants.

Answer key

1. Determine her physical, mental, and functional baseline status;

   Evaluate her fall risk (particularly in relation to her Parkinson disease and its control).
2. Evaluate the risk versus benefits of anticoagulation with prognostication tools and fall risk assessment;

   Workup (and management) of anaemia.
3. Explain to Mrs X and her family that she has a 1 in 10 chance of having a stroke every year;

   Explain to Mrs X and her family that a "blood thinner" is used to prevent a second stroke *and* inform them that she has a 1 in 20 chance of having a major bleeding episode while on it;

   Discuss with her the choice of anticoagulants (as her renal function is adequate, rivaroxaban is a good choice — 15 mg BD is appropriate as this patient is above 75 years old and her HASBLED score is 3);

   Refer her for upper and lower GI endoscopy, explaining the rationale for it and the attendant risks;

   Reinforce compliance to medication.

Reference

Sharrief A, Grotta JC (2019) Stroke in the elderly. *Handb Clin Neurol* **167**: 393–418.

16 Vomiting (Multifactorial)

Clarence Kwan Kah Wai, Anupama Roy Chowdhury

Mrs X is a 76-year-old Chinese female who is community ambulant. She has a past medical history of diabetes mellitus, dyslipidaemia, hypertension, and osteoporosis. Her medications include atorvastatin 40 mg ON, hydrochlorothiazide 25 mg OM, metformin 250 mg BD, glipizide 2.5 mg BD, risedronate 35 mg once a week, and cholecalciferol 1,000 units OM. She has no drug allergy. She does not smoke or drink.

She is admitted to the ward with a complaint of nausea and vomiting for the past few days. She highlights that her appetite has reduced for several months and this was associated with some weight loss which she estimates to be about 5 kg. She also finds that it is harder to move her stools, and following a bout of colicky abdominal pain a few days ago, she took painkiller medications which was left over from a previous prescription.

Question 1: In the process of discovering the cause of her problems, what aspects of a directed history would you further obtain?

Mrs X has been taking the same medications for her chronic medical conditions, but recently her metformin dose was increased from 250 mg to 500 mg BD. One week ago, she saw her general practitioner for abdominal bloating and poor appetite, and was started on esomeprazole 20 mg BD. In addition, she was given a course of Augmentin (amoxicillin-clavulanate) because she also reported mild dysuria and tactile fever.

Since the general practitioner visit, her appetite worsened to the point of her being able to take only a few spoonfuls of rice at each meal. The vomiting started after breakfast on the day she presented to the Emergency Department. The vomitus was non-bloody and composed of partially digested food. Mrs X felt much better after vomiting, but was brought to the hospital by concerned family members after another bout of vomiting at dinner.

Mrs X did not experience any headache, visual disturbance, or other neurologic symptoms. She noted that her urine had been fairly concentrated and she occasionally had a warm sensation when she passed urine. The rest of systemic review yielded negative answers.

****

On examination, Mrs X was alert and not in visible distress. Her weight was 40 kg. Vital signs were temperature 37.2°C, blood pressure 156/78 mmHg with no postural drop, heart rate 96/min, and respiratory rate 20/min with SpO_2 98% on room air. She was oriented to time, place, and person. There was no conjunctival pallor, scleral icterus, cervical lymphadenopathy, or pedal oedema. Her mucous membranes were dry. Dentition was poor with several loose teeth noted. Abdominal examination revealed an appendicectomy scar over the right iliac fossa. There was voluntary guarding and diffuse abdominal discomfort on deep palpation but no rebound tenderness. Bowel sounds were present but sluggish; no succussion splash was elicited. Per rectal examination revealed an empty rectum and intact anal tone. Neurological examination was unremarkable. Fundoscopy did not reveal papilloedema. No cataracts were seen and there were no clinical signs to suggest vestibular dysfunction or cranial nerve palsy. There was no evidence of peripheral neuropathy. Cardiopulmonary examination was normal.

Question 2: What are the key differential diagnoses that you would want to rule out at this stage?

Mrs X has a history of abdominal surgery and now presents with abdominal pain, vomiting, and sluggish bowel movements. This could potentially represent acute intestinal obstruction secondary to underlying adhesions. Examination of the abdomen in elderly patients can be challenging especially in this case because clinical signs can be masked or exaggerated by medications. Atypical presentations are more common in the older patient and they contribute to the lack of classical symptoms and signs. The older person with cognitive impairment also may not be able to express pain. Grimacing, facial expressions, groaning as well as the older person pushing the examining hand away may point to tenderness on palpation. An abdominal X-ray demonstrating dilated bowel loops and multiple air-fluid levels (erect posture) is a simple and rapid initial investigation to confirm the diagnosis. However, if there are clinical features of acute abdomen such as focal tenderness or peritonism, cross-sectional imaging would be the investigation of choice and may also allow identification of the transition point and underlying aetiology.

When managing elderly patients, it is good practice to review the chronic medication list physically rather than relying solely on clinical records. It is often helpful to seek corroboration with family members on the temporal sequence of medication use and symptom development, especially in the case of an elderly patient with cognitive or memory impairment. In Mrs X's case, a physical medicine reconciliation revealed that Mrs X had misunderstood her doctor's instructions and was taking *both* 250 mg and 500 mg of metformin BD. Additionally, the painkiller medications turned out to be Panadeine (paracetamol + codeine) which was previously prescribed for knee pain. Metformin, Augmentin, and codeine are associated with gastrointestinal (GI) side-effects such as nausea and vomiting.

Finally, elderly patients may not manifest the typical symptoms of infection such as fever. Additionally, ongoing infections may exacerbate the age-related physiologic decline of GI functions leading to GI symptoms which may confound the clinical picture. While the clinician has to be watchful for occult infections, the threshold for initiating antibiotic treatment should be a calibrated one with due consideration of the side-effects and potential harm of medications as mentioned above.

****

Laboratory investigations showed:

WBC count	*9.83 x 10^9/L*	*(4–10)*
Haemoglobin	*11.9 g/dL*	*(12–16)*
Platelet count	*167 x 10^9/L*	*(140–440)*
Blood urea	*7.8 mmol/L*	*(2.7–6.9)*
Sodium	*132 mmol/L*	*(136–146)*
Potassium	*4.3 mmol/L*	*(3.5–5.1)*
Serum creatinine	*89 μmol/L*	*(45–84)*
Calcium	*2.14 mmol/L*	*(2.09–2.46)*
Phosphate	*0.80 mmol/l*	*(0.94–1.5)*
Magnesium	*0.70 mmol/L*	*(0.75–1.07)*
C-reactive protein	*8.0 mg/L*	*(0.2–9.1)*
Serum procalcitonin	*<0.1 mcg/L*	*(<0.49)*
Total protein	*64 g/L*	*(68–85)*
Serum albumin	*36 g/L*	*(40–51)*
Total bilirubin	*8 μmol/L*	*(7–32)*
Serum ALT	*36 U/L*	*(6–66)*
Serum AST	*40 U/L*	*(12–42)*
Serum ALP	*80 U/L*	*(39–99)*
Gamma-GT	*84 U/L*	*(9–53)*
Serum TSH	*3.7 mIU/L*	*(0.45–4.5)*
Free T4	*10.8 pmol/L*	*(10–20)*
HbA1c	*6.6%*	

Urine dipstick: Leucocyte negative, nitrite positive, ketones negative, protein trace, glucose positive UFEME: WBC 20, RBC 10, epithelial cell 45

Chest X-ray: No consolidation or pleural effusion and no air under diaphragm

Abdominal X-ray (AXR): No dilated bowel loops, no faecal loading, and no air-fluid levels. (Note: even if the AXR shows significant faecal shadows, it is important to do a holistic assessment taking into account the entire clinical picture so as to not miss a more dangerous pathology such as an underlying tumour, diverticulitis, or ureteric stone that may co-exist with constipation)

Question 3: Outline an appropriate management plan for Mrs X in the acute setting.

In the acute setting, Mrs X should be given anti-emetics, preferably via the intravenous route if she is unable to even retain fluids. Common agents include:

- Metoclopramide which blocks the D2 receptors in the central chemoreceptor trigger zone. It also induces gastric emptying through its action on 5-HT4 receptors to stimulate cholinergic neural pathways in the stomach. (Note: use with caution in patients with Parkinsonism/Parkinson disease as the dopamine-antagonistic effect may worsen symptoms of Parkinsonism.)
- Ondansetron which blocks the 5-HT3 receptors in the central chemoreceptor trigger zone. It has a more potent anti-emetic effect but does not affect gastric emptying.

Intravenous hydration should be commenced until there is adequate resolution of nausea and vomiting. Elderly patients on intravenous hydration should be reviewed regularly for features of fluid overload, particularly if there is a history of ischaemic heart disease, renal failure, or cardiac insufficiency.

Don't forget to address precipitating factors too. Offending medications should be discontinued if they are not clinically indicated have been or substituted with a suitable replacement. Urine should be sent for cultures and empirical antibiotic treatment initiated for lower urinary tract infection.

****

After two days, Mrs X's appetite improved with supportive management, though she still experienced occasional vomiting. Repeat blood investigations showed:

Blood urea	*5.5 mmol/L*	*(2.7–6.9)*
Sodium	*136 mmol/L*	*(136–146)*
Potassium	*3.2 mmol/L*	*(3.5–5.1)*
Chloride	*101 mmol/L*	*(98–107)*
Bicarbonate	*22 mmol/L*	*(19–29)*
Serum creatinine	*48 µmol/L*	*(45–84)*
Calcium	*2.10 mmol/L*	*(2.09–2.46)*
Phosphate	*0.40 mmol/L*	*(0.94–1.5)*
Magnesium	*0.58 mmol/L*	*(0.75–1.07)*

Question 4: What is the most likely cause of the electrolyte abnormalities?

a. Continued upper GI electrolyte loss
b. Occult lower GI electrolyte loss
c. Hydrochlorothiazide use
d. Refeeding syndrome
e. Suboptimal oral intake

Question 5: What is the next investigation of choice for Mrs X?

a. Barium meal
b. CT abdomen
c. CT brain
d. Gastroscopy
e. 24-hour pH monitoring

The risk factors in Mrs X for refeeding syndrome are a ***protracted duration of poor intake*** (minimal oral intake for approximately a week prior to admission) as well as ***significant weight loss***. In such patients, it would be prudent to check and aggressively replace serum electrolytes as her oral intake improves. The electrolyte deficiencies — especially severe ***hypophosphataemia*** — can cause life-threatening arrhythmias, rhabdomyolysis, paresis, confusion, and respiratory insufficiency. Many of these symptoms are relatively non-specific and can go unrecognised especially in the frail elderly.

If Mrs X recovers completely after cessation of the offending medications and adequately addressing the other contributing factors for her GI symptoms, it is also reasonable to adopt a watchful monitoring strategy.

Persistent or recurrent vomiting is considered an alarm feature that warrants further investigation. Gastroscopy under sedation is a simple procedure and generally well tolerated by most patients. This can allow visualisation of mucosal lesions (e.g., polyps, inflammation, malignancy) which may occlude or narrow the GI lumen. Abnormal areas may be biopsied for histological examination. A barium meal is non-invasive and can allow for detection of mass lesions and/or luminal irregularities. It is reasonable if the clinical index of suspicion is low and the patient strongly prefers a non-invasive modality for investigation before consideration of gastroscopy should there be abnormal or equivocal findings.

In the appropriate clinical context, non-GI causes to be considered may include:

- **Central causes**. The vomiting centre and chemoreceptor trigger zone are located in the medulla oblongata, thus brainstem space-occupying lesions may cause persistent nausea and vomiting. Typically, the symptoms are worst in the morning and may respond better to anti-emetics rather than prokinetic agents. MRI of the brain is the investigation of choice if a central cause is suspected.
- **Diabetic gastroparesis**. Amongst comorbidities frequently encountered among older people, diabetes appears to have the greatest impact on gastric emptying. This differential should be considered particularly in patients with suboptimal glycaemic control and with evidence of end-organ damage such as peripheral neuropathy.
- **Poor dentition**. Patients with loose teeth may swallow larger pieces of food without chewing. The lack of proper mastication affects digestion and may lead to post-prandial bloating. Patients may report intermittent (often self-induced) vomiting to relieve such bloating. However, the occurrence of acute vomiting in this context should also prompt consideration of bezoar formation and super-imposed intestinal obstruction.
- **Cardiac causes**. A myocardial infarction or acute coronary syndrome may present atypically as just vomiting in the older individual without classical chest pain.

****

Mrs X underwent gastroscopy which was unremarkable except for a small hiatal hernia and mild oesophagitis. Random gastric biopsies showed minimal chronic inflammatory infiltrates without evidence of H pylori, intestinal metaplasia, or dysplasia. Her metformin was reduced to 250 mg BD and glipizide increased to 5 mg OM with reasonable glycaemic control. She was also fitted with dentures and normal diet was resumed shortly after discharge.

During clinic review three months later, she reported persistent post-prandial abdominal bloating. She also described occasional vomiting of small amounts of food especially after belching. She has tried to reduce her meal portions and she avoids lying down soon after her meals as she has found that this partially helps her symptoms. However, she is still significantly distressed by the post-prandial discomfort.

Question 6: What is the most appropriate management of Mrs X's persistent symptoms?

a. **Diet and lifestyle modification**
b. **Initiate ondansetron for functional nausea and vomiting disorder**
c. **Referral to surgical colleague for hiatal hernia repair**
d. **Trial of a few weeks of regular omeprazole for gastroestrophageal reflux with metoclopramide PRN**
e. **Trial of high-dose prednisolone for eosinophilic gastritis/enteritis**

It is important to distinguish between vomiting and regurgitation. Vomiting is described as a forceful and involuntary expulsion of gastric contents. Regurgitation is typically effortless and a non-forceful movement of gastric contents to the hypopharynx, during which patients may voluntarily expel the gastric contents.

Gastroesophageal reflux disease (GERD) is not only more common in the elderly, but its presentation is also often atypical. Regurgitation is a common symptom associated with GERD in the elderly (unlike the typical heartburn in younger patients) and is probably what Mrs X was describing as vomiting. Other atypical symptoms include dyspepsia, anorexia, dysphagia/odynophagia, belching, weight loss, and respiratory symptoms (chronic cough, hoarse voice).

A functional disorder would be exceedingly unlikely for first presentation in an elderly. Eosinophilic gastroenteritis is a rare condition which has been excluded from the gastric biopsies.

GERD can be treated with a combination of medical treatment options as follows:

A. Exercise and lifestyle modification.

- o Physical effects
  - General activity can improve gut motility
- o Gravitational effects
  - Keeping an upright posture after meals
  - Elevating the head of the bed (e.g., with pillows or a thick blanket)
- o Physiological effects
  - Diaphragmatic breathing exercises can help strengthen the lower oesophageal sphincter

- Losing weight in an obese patient can reduce abdominal pressure (which if increased tends to relax the lower oesophageal sphincter); however, exercise prescriptions in an older individual will need to take into account other comorbidities such as cardiac issues and osteoarthritis
- Avoidance of tight clothing
- Smoking cessation (smoking exacerbates GERD by directly provoking acid reflux and possibly by reducing lower oesophageal sphincter pressure)

B. Dietary modification.

- o Quality of food
  - Avoidance of foods with high fat content as this slows down gastric emptying
  - Avoidance of fizzy drinks as they induce bloating and belching
  - Avoidance of foods that precipitate reflux (e.g., citrus food, onions, garlic)
- o Quantity of food
  - Smaller meals are recommended
- o Timing selection
  - More frequent meals of smaller portions for caloric intake throughout the day
  - Avoidance of late evening meals

C. Pharmacologic management.

- o Avoidance of medications (where possible) that reduce lower oesophageal sphincter pressure/tone (e.g., anticholinergics, calcium channel blockers).
- o Proton pump inhibitors are an effective treatment for GERD by reducing the acidity of refluxate; however, many patients take it after symptom onset

Pitfalls of omeprazole use especially in the elderly:

— *Omeprazole may, by reducing the clearance, potentiate the effects of many common drugs like* ***warfarin****, nifedipine, carbamazepine, diazepam, methotrexate, and* ***phenytoin****.*

— *Omeprazole may, by enhancing absorption, potentiate the effects of digoxin.*

— *Continuous profound gastric acid suppression, especially in the elderly at risk of pernicious anaemia, may lead to vitamin B12 deficiency through the inability to release intrinsic factor.*

— *Hypomagnaesemia has been recognised as a side-effect of proton-pump inhibitors.*

— *Risks that need to be further verified through prospective studies: increased risk of osteoporotic fractures in postmenopausal women, cognitive impairment and dementia.*

— *Use esomeprazole in tube feeding as unlike omeprazole, it can be dispersed in water.*

expecting quick relief and it is important to highlight that they should be taken approximately 30 minutes before meals for maximal efficacy.

- o Be careful of antacid use in the elderly as it can interfere with the absorption of other essential medications, have undesirable effects on bowel habits (e.g., aluminium- and calcium-containing agents may worsen constipation), and increase overall salt intake (certain preparations contain sodium bicarbonate).
- o If persistent regurgitation is an issue, patients may benefit from baclofen which reduces the frequency of lower oesophageal relaxation and hence the episodes of reflux. This should be started at a low dose (5 mg TDS) with very gradual increments as it causes significant drowsiness especially amongst the elderly.

Key messages

1. Acute nausea and vomiting in the elderly is commonly due to medications or infections. However, surgical entities such as acute intestinal obstruction and life-threatening conditions such as acute coronary syndrome must be considered in the appropriate clinical context. Management is directed at the underlying aetiology and is largely supportive.
2. Where symptoms persist or recur episodically, further evaluation for an underlying aetiology is required. The choice of investigations is guided by the clinical context and index of suspicion.
3. Patients often confuse regurgitation with vomiting. When taking history from patients, it is good practice to get them to describe their symptoms in greater detail so as to make this distinction.

Answer key

1. Details on recent abdominal colic (including detailed constipation history);

   Infective symptoms;

   CNS symptoms suggestive of increased intracranial pressure or vestibular dysfunction;

   Medication changes/additions — a detailed drug history is crucial as this often reveals the cause of the underlying symptom.
2. Acute intestinal obstruction possibly due to adhesions, bezoar (improperly chewed food due to poor dentition), severe constipation and/or medications;

   Infection (e.g., urosepsis).

3. IV metoclopramide 10 mg TDS or IV ondansetron 8 mg TDS;
   IV dextrose saline drip and feeds as tolerated;
   Stop Augmentin and Panadeine (instruct not to consume on her own);
   Suspend metformin and monitor sugars;
   Single dose of oral fosfomycin 3 g dissolved in a savoury juice drink.
4. D.
5. D.
6. D.

References

Otaki F, Iyer PG (2021) Gastroesophageal reflux disease and Barrett esophagus in the Elderly. *Clin Geriatr Med* **37**(1): 17–29.

Ramirez FC (2000) Diagnosis and treatment of gastroesophageal reflux disease in the elderly. *Cleveland Clin J Med* **67**(10): 755–765.

17 Diarrhoea (Antibiotic Use)

Tey Tze Tong, Anupama Roy Chowdhury

This chapter is a compilation of two clinical scenarios of an acute diarrhoeal illness in the elderly, both of which are related to recent antibiotic use.

CASE 1

Mr T is an 85-year-old man who was admitted from a nursing home, of which he has been a resident for the past few years. He has a past medical history of hypertension, hyperlipidaemia, ischaemic heart disease, and osteoarthritis of the knees.

He presented to the Emergency Department with dysuria, fever, and right loin pain. His renal punch was positive on the right side. Urine microscopy showed 500 red blood cells, 800 leucocytes, and 3 epithelial cells. He was admitted to the ward for further management. Urine cultures grew Escherichia coli. The working diagnosis was pyelonephritis, and he was treated with intravenous tazobactam and piperacillin. Gradual improvement was observed and the fever subsided after five days of treatment.

On the seventh day of admission, Mr T developed five episodes of loose stool. He had no abdominal pain or vomiting. He was able to take full shares of his meals. Vital signs were temperature 36.8°C, blood pressure 103/69 mmHg, and heart rate 70/minute. Skin turgor was normal and mucous membranes were hydrated. The abdomen was soft and not guarded with normal bowel sounds. His stool was noted to be brownish and watery.

Question 1: What other essential physical examination should be performed?

Patients with severe constipation can develop stool that is too large to be expelled through the anus. The resultant rectal distension triggers a relaxation of the internal anal sphincter and the obstruction induces secretion proximal to the obstructing stool. Liquid stool leaks out as it seeps around the impaction. Unfortunately, patients with overflow diarrhoea are often inappropriately treated with anti-diarrhoeal agents which worsen the problem! Rectal examination or plain abdominal X-ray will show significant stool burden. Treatment is often a combination of manual evacuation of the impacted faeces, enemas, suppositories, and other laxatives.

****

Renal panel was organised and the patient was put on a stool chart to monitor stool consistency and blood. Hydration was optimised. Further investigations showed:

Stool for glutamate dehydrogenase (GDH): negative
Stool for Clostridioides difficile toxin: negative

Question 2: Which of the following is the most likely cause of his diarrhoea?

a. Antibiotic-associated diarrhea
b. *Clostridioides difficile* infection
c. *Escherichia coli* gastroenteritis
d. Ischaemic colitis
e. Norovirus gastroenteritis

This scenario is a common case of antibiotic-associated diarrhoea (AAD). Clinicians who are not aware of this condition will worry that there is unexplained diarrhoea in their patient and may be unable to offer a confident management plan. The clinical picture shows a patient who, apart from the presence of watery stools, was non-toxic and relatively well. Once *Clostridioides difficile* has been excluded based on stool studies, the diagnosis of AAD can be made. The mainstay of management is supportive, with the prompt cessation of antibiotics if it is clinically safe to do so. Hydration status should be ensured with oral or intravenous fluids and electrolyte abnormalities checked for and corrected.

In situations where patients are distressed by copious output, anti-diarrhoeal drugs such as loperamide 2–4 mg QDS may be prescribed for symptomatic relief, though these are to be used in a time-limited fashion with regular review so as to avoid constipation and ileus. Lomotil (diphenoxylate 2.5 mg/atropine 25 μg) is seldom used in elderly patients as it is frequently associated with acute cognitive changes and may also cause ileus.

Infectious causes of gastroenteritis are usually caught in the community. Given that this patient was admitted to hospital for pyelonephritis and the diarrhoea occurred during the hospital stay, it is unlikely that he caught a new pathogen, making *E coli* and Norovirus unlikely. Patients who have *Clostridioides difficile* infection are more unwell and may experience abdominal discomfort and reduced appetite. Stool colour may be slightly greenish to brown.

The underlying pathophysiology of AAD is thought to be related to disturbances in the gut microbiota caused by antibiotics. The chief differential of AAD is *Clostridioides difficile* colitis, which in fact is much less common. Data shows that only 10–25% of all antibiotic-associated diarrhoea is caused by *Clostridioides difficile*, whereas 70–90% are due to changes in the gut microbiota. AAD can last from days to weeks before normal stool consistency returns.

For elderly patients in the community presenting with acute diarrhoea, the following framework is useful. One can think about the causes of acute (<4 weeks' duration) diarrhoea in the elderly as the 4 "I"s: Infection, Iatrogenic, Ischaemic, and Impaction/Incontinence.

Infection: The elderly are particularly prone to infectious diarrhoea for various reasons: immunosenescence (reduction in secretory immunoglobulin A in the gut mucosa), changes in gut microbiota (less bifidobacteria and more bacteroides), and age-related reduction in gastric acid production. Elderly patients cohorted in hospitals and nursing homes encounter a higher risk of acquisition of enteric pathogens through faecal-oral exposure. Norovirus, in particular, is highly infectious and is associated with watery diarrhoeal outbreaks in nursing homes and communal residences. The vast majority of Norovirus-associated deaths occur in elderly patients!

Common medications associated with diarrhoea in the elderly:

— *drugs used to treat constipation viz. osmotic laxatives (lactulose, polyethylene glycol), stimulatory laxatives (bisacodyl, sennosides)*
— *anti-inflammatory drugs (NSAIDs)*
— *most antibiotics*
— *cardiac drugs (β-adrenergic receptor blockers, digoxin, quinidine, procainamide)*
— *gastric drugs (H2-receptor antagonists, proton pump inhibitors, magnesium-containing antacids)*
— *others (e.g., herbal products, vitamin and mineral supplements)*

Iatrogenic: Nearly half of the drugs listed in the pharmacopoeia cite diarrhoea as a common side-effect, and its incidence is even higher in the elderly due to polypharmacy for multiple medical problems.

It is important to recognise that tube feeding also commonly causes diarrhoea, most probably due to calorie-dense formulas infused directly into the small bowel, thus representing a form of dumping syndrome. This problem may be averted by slowing the rate of feeding, increasing fibre in the formula, and giving an anti-diarrhoeal drug such as loperamide.

Ischaemic colitis: Most often presenting in the elderly population, this is typically a dramatic but frequently self-limited presentation of acute severe abdominal pain (often left lower quadrant) and bloody stool on the background of a precipitating factor such as hypotension, vasculitis, thrombosis, or cancer. A few patients continue to develop peritonitis or gangrenous ischaemic colitis which requires segmental resection of the necrotic areas — this would be associated with a high risk of morbidity and mortality in the elderly.

Impaction/Incontinence: This has been addressed above.

****

CASE 2

Mdm L is a 72-year-old woman with a past medical history of Parkinson disease who was admitted for cough, shortness of breath, and fever for two days. Chest radiograph showed right lower zone opacification with a small pleural effusion. She required 2 L/min of oxygen via nasal prongs to maintain an SpO_2 of 95%. Intravenous ceftriaxone was started for treatment of community-acquired pneumonia. Blood cultures were negative after 48 hours and her intravenous antibiotic was changed to oral amoxicillin/clavulanate on the third day of admission. Due to prolonged bed rest, she experienced functional decline and she was transferred on the fifth day to a community hospital for physical rehabilitation.

In the first week of her stay in the community hospital, Mdm L complained of six episodes of loose watery stool. She had mild central abdominal pain but no vomiting. She was taking half shares of her meals. Vital signs were temperature 37.5°C, blood pressure 98/60 mmHg, and heart rate 90/min. Physical examination revealed a lethargic woman with a dry tongue. Her abdomen was soft and not guarded with hyperactive bowel sounds. Her stool was noted to be watery and greenish.

Total white cell count was 16 x 10^9/L (4–10). Renal panel was normal. Further investigations showed:

Stool for glutamate dehydrogenase (GDH): positive
Stool for Clostridioides difficile toxin: positive for toxin A and B

Question 3: What is your interpretation of the test results?

Question 4: What is the most appropriate treatment?

A. Intravenous metronidazole

B. Intravenous vancomycin

C. Oral probiotics

D. Oral rehydration solution

E. Oral vancomycin

GDH is a metabolite that is present in both toxigenic and non-toxigenic strains of *Clostridioides difficile*. As such, the test has high sensitivity but low specificity. This test is usually combined with Toxin A & B enzyme immunoassay (Toxin EIA), which has low sensitivity but moderate specificity. The nucleic acid amplification test (NAAT or PCR) has high sensitivity (as it detects genes not toxins) but low-to-moderate specificity. It is available as part of the stool gastrointestinal PCR test, or if the standard C Diff toxin/GDH test is equivocal, the lab will run PCR as a tie breaker.

This patient presents with *Clostridioides difficile* Infection (CDI) which was caused by her antibiotic treatment for pneumonia. The risk factors for infection include advanced age, duration of hospitalisation, and exposure to antibiotics. All antibiotics have the potential to cause CDI, but the ones with highest risk are the 3rd/4th generation cephalosporins, fluoroquinolones, carbapenems, and clindamycin. CDI can occur both during antibiotic treatment and up to 3 months after the end of the antibiotic course.

The CDI should be graded and managed accordingly:

Severity rating of CDI	WBC >15 × 10^9/L and/or serum creatinine >132 μmol/L	Hypotension/ shock, ileus, or megacolon	Recommended first-line treatment
Non-severe	0	0	• Oral metronidazole 500 mg TDS x 10d • Oral vancomycin 125 mg QDS x 10d
Severe	✓	0	• Oral vancomycin 125 mg QDS x 10d • Oral fidaxomycin 200 mg BD x 10d (presently not available in Singapore)
Fulminant	0	✓	• Oral vancomycin 500 mg 6H • Intravenous metronidazole 500 mg 8H • Consider adding rectal vancomycin if significant ileus is present

The patient should be transferred to an isolated room with a dedicated toilet to prevent transmission to other patients. Gloves and gowns must be worn by healthcare staff, and local hospital infection control protocols adhered to. ***Hand-washing with soap and water*** is essential to prevent spread as alcohol-based hand rubs are ineffective against Clostridioides spores. The duration of amoxicillin/clavulanate should be kept as short as possible as the ultimate goal of treatment is to discontinue it and allow the normal bowel microflora to restore itself.

Older individuals are not only more likely to contract CDI, but they are also more likely to contract relapsing and fulminant disease that can be fatal. Their mortality rate more than doubles in those above 80 years of age compared to those aged 61 to 70. This may be due to a combination of immunosenescence, medical comorbidities, and increased exposure to drugs that may predispose to infection (e.g., proton pump inhibitors) or drugs that predispose to more toxic strains of *C difficile* (e.g., fluoroquinolones). As such, prevention of CDI is key. This can be achieved through judicious use of antibiotics with adherence to local guidelines, stewardship programmes, and various institutional efforts to minimise horizontal transmission.

Key messages

1. Antibiotic-associated diarrhoea (AAD) is caused by disruption of the gut microbiota by antibiotics.
2. Clostridium difficile infection (CDI) should be excluded by stool testing before the diagnosis of AAD is made.
3. AAD may last from days to weeks but is ultimately self-limiting.
4. CDI may range from mild to fulminant in severity. Recommended therapy is guided by its severity.
5. CDI patients must be isolated and local infection control protocols adhered to.

Answer key

1. Digital recital examination to rule out constipation (as spurious diarrhoea is a very common cause of diarrhoea in the older patient!).
2. A.
3. Diarrhoea due to *C difficile* infection.
4. E (as patient has severe *C difficile* infection).

References

Kelly CR, Fischer M, Allegretti JR, LaPlante K, Stewart DB, Limketkai BN, Stollman NH (2021) ACG Clinical Guidelines: prevention, diagnosis, and treatment of *Clostridioides difficile* Infections. *Am J Gastroenterol* **116**(6): 1124–1147.

McDonald LC, Gerding DN, Johnson S, *et al.* (2018) Clinical practice guidelines for *Clostridioides difficile* infection in adults and children: 2017 update by the Infectious Diseases Society of America (IDSA) and Society for Healthcare Epidemiology of America (SHEA). *Clin Infect Dis* **66**(7): e1–e48.

Polage CR, Solnick JV, Cohen SH (2012) Nosocomial diarrhea: evaluation and treatment of causes other than *Clostridioides difficile*. *Clin Infect Dis* **55**(7): 982–989.

Pérez-Cobas AE, Gosalbes MJ, Friedrichs A, *et al.* (2013) Gut microbiota disturbance during antibiotic therapy: a multi-omic approach. *Gut* **62**(11): 1591–1601.

18 Abdominal Pain (Constipation)

Poojha Sachdeva, Melvin Chua Peng Wei

Mrs X is a 76-year-old Chinese female who needs minimal assistance in basic activities of daily living and ambulates with a quad stick. She has a past medical history of diabetes mellitus, hyperlipidaemia, hypertension, Parkinson disease, and ischaemic heart disease. Her medications include aspirin 100 mg OM, bisoprolol 2.5 mg OM, atorvastatin 40 mg ON, losartan 75 mg OM, metformin 500 mg TDS, glipizide 2.5 mg BD, empagliflozin 10 mg OM, levodopa 125 mg QDS, lactulose 10 mL TDS, Senna 2 tabs ON, and omeprazole 20 mg OM. She has no drug allergy. She was admitted to the ward with a complaint of abdominal pain over the left lumbar region for the past three days. The pain is constant, dull, and aching. It does not radiate, has no precipitating factors, and is relieved by passing motion. She had an episode of non-bilious vomiting on the morning of admission. There is no history of fever, chest pain, shortness of breath, cough, or rhinorrhoea. However, she noted a recent increase in urinary frequency for which she has started wearing diapers. Her stools have also been hard, for which she adds bisacodyl suppository PRN. Mrs X normally goes for daily walks two times a day and has a helper as a dedicated caregiver.

Question 1: What additional history would you like to ask?

Mrs X does not smoke and drink. She had been compliant to her medication but she ran out of it for three days. She has been well except for occasional rigidity at the end of the day. Three weeks ago, she suffered back pain after slipping in the toilet for which her general practitioner prescribed a fixed dose combination of paracetamol and codeine for a week. She also consumed traditional Chinese medicine for the back pain. Since the fall, she has stopped going for her daily walks.

According to her family and caregiver, she occasionally forgets what she has eaten for breakfast and lunch, but she is able to recognise family members, count money, call her children, and hold a conversation. She last opened her bowels two days ago; the stool was hard with some streaks of blood. She still passes flatus. Her appetite has reduced in the past two days. She had no dysuria or gross haematuria.

On examination, Mrs X is alert and not in visible distress. Her vital signs are temperature 37.2°C, blood pressure 116/78 mmHg with no postural drop, heart rate 96/min, and respiratory rate 20/min with SpO_2 98% on room air. She is oriented to time, place, and person. There is no conjunctival pallor, scleral icterus, cervical lymphadenopathy, or pedal oedema. Abdominal examination revealed tenderness on deep palpation over the right lumbar region, but renal punch was negative and there was no organomegaly, abdominal rigidity, or rebound tenderness. Per rectal examination revealed unimpacted brown stool, internal haemorrhoids at a 4 o'clock position, and intact anal tone. On neurological examination, she had mild bradykinesia and cog-wheel rigidity over the wrists which was more prominent on the right. There was no pill-rolling tremor or mask-like facies. She had full power in all four limbs and preserved reflexes. Her gait was characterised by small shuffling steps, turning in numbers, and poor arm swing. Her score on the abbreviated mental test was 9/10. Both knees had crepitus on passive movements. No spinal tenderness was elicited. No cataracts were noted and there were no clinical signs to suggest vestibular dysfunction. Her cardiopulmonary examination was normal.

Question 2: List the medical issues to be addressed.

Any patient with complaints of abdominal pain with tenderness should be worked up for acute surgical abdomen. It is particularly important to keep this in mind during medical or non-surgical rotations. Examination of the abdomen in the older person can be challenging due to inadequate history, paucity of signs, atypical presentations of disease, inability to cooperate, or underlying cognitive impairment.

Any fall in the older person requires full neurological, cardiovascular, and locomotor examination to diagnose causative and precipitating causes and to look for complications of the fall. It is imperative to work up for underlying osteoporosis in postmenopausal females and elderly males to prevent fractures.

Polypharmacy is common in older patients as many of them have multiple medical conditions. It is therefore important to review the medication list to optimise the management of medical conditions and to withdraw unnecessary medications so as to reduce pill burden and minimise the risk of drug–drug interactions.

****

Laboratory investigations showed:

WBC count	*9.83 x 10^9/L*	*(4–10)*
Haemoglobin	*11.9 g/dL*	*(12–16)*
Platelet count	*167 x 10^9/L*	*(140–440)*

Blood urea	*7.8 mmol/L*	*(2.7–6.9)*
Sodium	*134 mmol/L*	*(136–146)*
Potassium	*4.3 mmol/L*	*(3.5–5.1)*
Serum creatinine	*89 µmol/L*	*(45–84)*
Calcium	*2.14 mmol/L*	*(2.09–2.46)*
Phosphate	*0.89 mmol/L*	*(0.94–1.5)*
Magnesium	*0.78 mmol/L*	*(0.75–1.07)*
Lactate	*2.4 mmol/L*	*(0.2–2.2)*
C-reactive protein	*81 mg/L*	*(0.2–9.1)*
Serum procalcitonin	*1.0 mcg/L*	*(<0.49)*
Total protein	*64 g/L*	*(68–85)*
Serum albumin	*36 g/L*	*(40–51)*
Total bilirubin	*8 µmol/L*	*(7–32)*
Serum ALT	*36 U/L*	*(6–66)*
Serum AST	*40 U/L*	*(12–42)*
Serum ALP	*161 U/L*	*(39–99)*
Gamma-GT	*84 U/L*	*(9–53)*
Serum TSH	*3.7 mIU/L*	*(0.45–4.5)*
Free T4	*10.8 pmol/L*	*(10–20)*
HbA1c	*6.9%*	

Urine dipstick: Leucocyte negative, nitrite positive, ketones negative, protein trace, glucose positive UFEME: WBC 700, RBC 80, epithelial cell 7

Chest X-ray: No consolidation or pleural effusion and no air under the diaphragm.

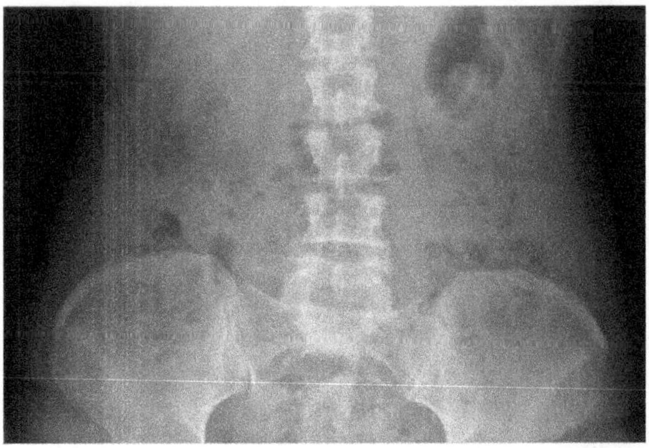

Fig. 18.1. Abdominal X-ray of Mrs X.

Question 3: Make three pertinent observations from the abdominal X-ray.

The laboratory works are to check for anaemia (can be associated with colon cancer presenting as constipation), diabetes (autonomic neuropathy leading to constipation), electrolyte abnormalities (hypercalcemia), and hypothyroidism (TSH) which may present as constipation. *Clostridium difficile* infection should be tested for patients who have a history of recent significant antibiotic use as they can present with toxic megacolon and ileus causing constipation.

Abdominal X-ray is performed at initial presentation to rule out intestinal obstruction. It is quick, non-invasive, and carries less radiation risk as compared to a CT scan.

Question 4: Would you consider colonoscopy and/or functional studies for Mrs X?

Colonoscopy can allow for visualisation of mucosal lesions like solitary rectal ulcer, polyps, inflammation, or malignancy, and biopsies should be taken for histological examination. It may be offered to all patients above 50 years of age who have not had colon cancer screening, as well as to those of younger age if there is a family history of colorectal cancer. Alarming features that warrant endoscopic investigation are rectal bleeding (haematochezia), heme-positive stool, iron deficiency anaemia, significant weight loss, obstructive symptoms, recent onset of constipation without any obvious explanation, and family history of colorectal cancer or inflammatory bowel disease. Endoscopy should also be done prior to surgical management for constipation.

Colonic transit studies are used in patients whose major complaint is infrequent defaecation and who are resistant to laxative treatment. Colonic transit time is defined as the time it takes for stool (faeces) to pass through the colon. It can be done using various methods such as scintigraphy, wireless motility capsules, or radiopaque markers.

An anorectal manometer can be used to diagnose dyssynergic defaecation, rectal sensory problems, and the assessment of response to biofeedback therapy. It studies the relaxation of the external and internal anal sphincter in response to increased rectal pressure. Colonic manometers help to identify sensory dysfunction and a neuropathic or myopathic colon.

Defaecography is a test for functional and anatomical abnormalities in the anorectal region — this investigation should be done in conjunction with manometric tests and not in isolation.

Question 5: What would you consider to be the MOST likely causes/risk factors of constipation in Mrs X? Select three options.

a. **Diabetes mellitus**
b. **Fluid restriction**
c. **Hypothyroidism**
d. **Limited mobility**
e. **Medications**
f. **Parkinson disease**

Mrs X is known to have Parkinson disease which itself is a risk factor for reduced gut motility. Two weeks prior to admission, she had a fall which reduced her mobility. The opiate analgesic (codeine) prescribed for her back pain can also reduce gut motility.

Mrs X did have reduced appetite for two days prior to admission which may have aggravated the constipation. However, the onset of abdominal pain preceded the reduced oral intake. The borderline low free T4 is unlikely to contribute to constipation. Diabetes mellitus can cause autonomic neuropathy which may affect gut contractions leading to constipation. However, her diabetic control is reasonably satisfactory (HbA1c 6.9%) with no signs of diabetic nephropathy (or retinopathy) to suggest the development of small vessel disease.

The final diagnosis for Mrs X was constipation (colic) secondary to codeine intake, reduced mobility, and Parkinson disease. It was complicated by a urinary tract infection (UTI).

Females are more prone to UTIs as compared to males due to anatomical differences in the urinary tract. In postmenopausal women, atrophic vaginitis may cause lower urinary tract symptoms similar to that of a UTI. In any older female with UTI, it is prudent to exclude underlying urinary retention which predisposes to development of a UTI. Causes of urinary retention include anticholinergic medications (antihistamines can have an anticholinergic effect!), neurogenic bladder (e.g., diabetic neuropathy), constipation, and poor mobility. This can be easily identified at the bedside by either physical examination (palpable bladder) or using a bladder scan (Figure 18.2) which will pick up a high post-void residual urine (PVRU). Finally, note that the intake of sodium glucose co-transporter-2 (SGLT2) inhibitors probably further increased the risk of UTI in Mrs X.

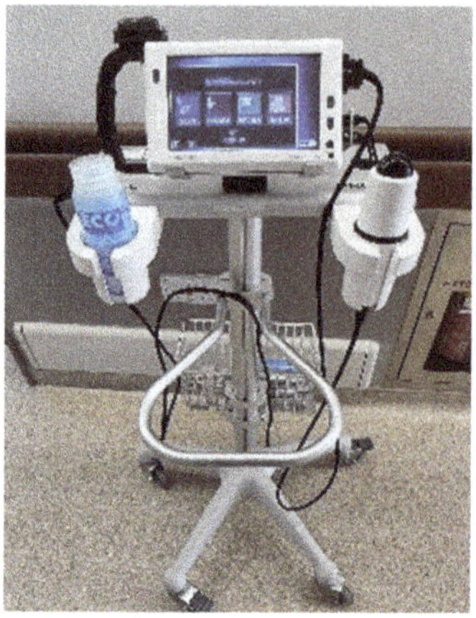

Figure 18.2. Bladder scan. The bedside ultrasound has replaced the conventional method of in-and-out catheterisation to assess residual urine in the bladder. It is easy and painless to use, providing accurate and reliable measurement of urine volume despite being operator-dependent. PVRU between 50 to 100 mL is considered normal (adequate bladder emptying) in the elderly.

Question 6: How would you address the problem of constipation in Mrs X?

Key management principles of constipation in the elderly are:

A. ***Lifestyle modifications.*** General activity can improve gut motility. Diaphragmatic breathing and posture can ease defaecation too. Patients should be advised to sit up, lean forward, and raise their feet 8 to 12 inches above the ground to improve defaecation dynamics.

B. ***Dietary modifications.*** Increased fibre intake of 20 to 25 g/day adds bulk to stool, leading to colonic distention and stool propulsion. Its effect may take weeks to manifest. Note that dietary fibre should be slowly increased over several weeks and must be accompanied by adequate fluid intake to decrease the risks of adverse effects such as bloating, gas, and paradoxical constipation!

C. ***Medication adjustment.*** Medications that reduce gut motility such as opioids and anticholinergics should only be prescribed for specific indications and individualised to the patient's needs. They must be reviewed regularly and stopped when not required.

D. ***Laxatives.*** Bulk (e.g., ispaghula husk), osmotic (e.g., lactulose, polyethylene glycol), and stimulatory (e.g., bisacodyl, sennosides) laxatives help to reduce constipation. Especially in the elderly, a stimulant laxative should be prescribed alongside opioids. Bulk-forming laxatives are generally less suitable for the older patient because of an associated need to increase fluid intake. For initial and short-term use, lubricant laxatives (e.g., liquid paraffin oral emulsion) can be helpful. Chronic use of bisacodyl or overuse may result in diarrhoea, causing water and electrolyte depletion, steatorrhea, and protein-losing enteropathy.

E. ***Novel pharmacologic agents.*** Selective 5-HT_4 receptor agonists (e.g., prucalopride 1–2 mg/day, $2.34 per 1 mg) have shown efficacy in reducing constipation in patients above 65 years of age. There is also evolving evidence of the role of dopamine 2 receptor antagonists (e.g., domperidone, $0.12 per 10 mg) in modulating gut motility. A trial of colonic secretagogues (e.g., lubiprostone which activates chloride channel protein 2 to promote water secretion into the intestinal lumen) may be considered for severe constipation that is refractory to all other treatment; however, the patient should be informed about the side-effect of nausea.

F. ***Biofeedback therapy.*** This is a painless method of retraining the pelvic floor and abdominal wall muscles to facilitate evacuation. It is particularly helpful for patients with pelvic floor dysfunction and rectal hyposensitivity.

G. ***Physical evacuation measures.*** Faecal impaction, if present, can be treated with mineral oil or warm water enemas. Manual evacuation may help too.

****

In addition to lactulose and senna, Mrs X was treated with per rectal bisacodyl suppository for bowel clearance. Domperidone 10 mg TDS was also added to help improve gut motility. She passed a large amount of brown stool on the second and third days of admission, but her right abdominal discomfort persisted. Blood cultures grew Escherichia coli, and abdominal ultrasound showed right perinephric fat stranding with no evidence of collection. She was treated with ten days of amoxicillin-clavulanate with gradual clinical improvement and reduction of inflammatory markers. She also underwent inpatient rehabilitation for her balance and muscle strengthening to prevent further falls. Upon discharge, she was referred for outpatient screening colonoscopy.

Key messages

1. Constipation is a common cause of abdominal pain in the elderly and can lead to many medical complications such as delirium, stool impaction, stercoral colitis, anorectal injuries, and UTIs.
2. Constipation is often multifactorial and its management requires a multi-pronged approach including lifestyle changes and pharmacological interventions.
3. Colonoscopy should be offered to suitable elderly patients with a favourable risk- benefit profile presenting with constipation with other red flag symptoms and signs.

Answer Key

1. a. Alcohol and smoking history [chronic pancreatitis, ischaemic bowel disease?]; history of atrial fibrillation
   b. Compliance to medications and drug history [diabetic ketoacidosis, over-the-counter medication and TCM?];
   c. Control and progression of Parkinson disease [postural hypotension, falls, cognition, gastrointestinal complaints?];
   d. Last bowel motion, passage of gas, loss of appetite, and urinary complaints such as dysuria, haematuria [constipation, bowel obstruction, systemic infection etc.]
2. a. Abdominal pain and tenderness to exclude acute abdomen;
   b. Elderly fall with OA knees, Parkinsonian gait;
   c. Possible osteoporosis and fragility fracture;
   d. Optimisation of chronic medical issues.
3. Faecal loading;
   Absence of dilated bowel loops;
   Absence of air-fluid levels.
4. Yes, colonoscopy should be offered to Mrs X as she has never had endoscopy before.
5. D, E, F.
6. First-line treatment: ensure adequate hydration and mobility; dietary modifications if possible with more fruits/vegetables; augment the laxatives (e.g., add another stimulant); try a different osmotic laxative, such as increasing lactulose dose or switching lactulose to Macrogol (polyethylene glycol);
   Second-line treatment: add a pharmacologic agent (e.g., prucalopride).

References

Emmanuel A, Mattace-Raso F, Neri MC, *et al.* (2017) Constipation in older people: A consensus statement. *Int J Clin Pract* **71**(1).

Kang SJ, Cho YS, Lee TH, *et al.* (2021) Medical management of constipation in elderly patients: systemic review. *J Neurogastroenterol Motil* **27**(4): 495–512.

19 Fever (Urinary Tract Infection)

Pushpalatha Bangalore Lingegowda, Zheng Shuwei,
Jade Soh Xiao Jue, Anupama Roy Chowdhury

Mr C is a 75-year-old Chinese man who has a known history of hypertension, paroxysmal atrial fibrillation, recurrent strokes with scar epilepsy, benign prostatic hypertrophy, and vascular dementia. Three years ago, he was placed on a long-term in-dwelling urinary catheter after hospitalisation for acute right middle cerebral arterial stroke complicated by acute retention of urine secondary to immobility and extended-spectrum beta-lactamases-producing Escherichia coli urinary tract infection. Functionally, he has been bed-bound and minimally communicative since. He has been taken care of by a domestic helper for the past three years and the helper was replaced two weeks ago. He has not required any hospitalisation for the past three years and has only been seeing a regular general practitioner every six months for follow-up of his chronic medical conditions. His medications are amlodipine 2.5 mg OM, terazosin 1 mg ON, and sodium valproate EC 200 mg TDS.

Mr C was brought to the emergency department for fever and poor oral intake over the past three days.

On clinical examination, Mr C was drowsy but opened eyes to call. He appeared clinically dehydrated. His vital signs were temperature 38.2°C, pulse rate 110/min, respiratory rate 17/min, blood pressure 133/89 mmHg, and oxygen saturation 97% on room air. Neck was supple. Heart sounds were dual without murmurs and there were no pulmonary crepitations. Abdominal examination revealed suprapubic tenderness on deep palpation without guarding. Bilateral limb contractures were present.

Question 1: What are your differential diagnoses?

Question 2: Outline your initial management plan.

This elderly patient presents with fever, poor oral intake, and lower abdominal tenderness. Clinical diagnosis is often made more challenging in patients who are unable to provide a direct history of presenting complaints. An acute febrile illness in older adults is most commonly infective in aetiology. While benign viral infections commonly affect the young, elderly patients often present with serious bacterial infections. The chest, genitourinary tract, and skin are common sources. The older vulnerable patients, especially those with cognitive impairment, often present with a change in mental status or delirium.

Because of limited available history, a thorough physical examination for potential sites of infection is necessary. If the initial history and examination does not reveal an obvious source, a less common source must be actively looked for. Palpation of the joints to exclude septic arthritis and inspection of pressure points including the sacrum in a poorly mobile patient are essential to avoid missing infected pressure sores. Ear infections can also be picked up by otoscopy. Examination for a stiff neck for meningitis may be confounded by pre-existing spinal pathology, and in cases where no other cause is found for an altered mental state, a lumbar puncture may be required to exclude intracranial infection.

While the presence of an in-dwelling catheter (IDC) in association with suprapubic tenderness raises the index of suspicion for catheter-associated urinary tract infection (CAUTI), careful consideration needs to be made for the presence of acute abdomen. Examination of the abdomen can be notoriously difficult in the older patient. Grimacing, facial expressions suggestive of pain, and pushing the examining hand away raise suspicion of significant pain in the abdomen. CAUTI should only be diagnosed in a catheterised patient with symptoms and signs suggestive of a urinary tract infection (UTI) or as a diagnosis of exclusion in a patient with otherwise unexplained systemic signs of infection.

The workup for CAUTI should include two sets of blood cultures. A pre-existing IDC will be colonised by bacteria, hence collecting urine cultures from the existing IDC will ***not*** reflect the true pathogens causing UTI. In a patient whom you suspect to have CAUTI, the IDC should ideally be changed before collecting urine for microscopy and cultures.

For all CAUTI, we should empirically cover for *Pseudomonas aeruginosa*. Intravenous cefepime would be an appropriate antibiotic to commence while awaiting culture result. However, patients with renal impairment must be monitored for onset of delirium and other neurological manifestations with the drug.

****

Laboratory investigations showed the following:

Haemoglobin	*12.1 g/dL*	*(14.0–18.0)*
WBC	*12.86 x10⁹/L*	*(4.00–10.00)*
Platelet count	*286 x10⁹/L*	*(140–400)*
Urea	*11.9 mmol/L*	*(2.7–6.9)*
Sodium	*144 mmol/L*	*(136–146)*
Potassium	*4.8 mmol/L*	*(3.5–5.1)*
Bicarbonate	*20.8 mmol/L*	*(19.0–29.0)*
Creatinine	*84 µmo/L*	*(59–104)*
C-Reactive Protein	*67.1 mg/L*	*(≤4.9 mg/L)*
Albumin	*30 g/L*	*(40–51)*
Bilirubin total	*23 µmol/L*	*(7–32)*
Alkaline phosphatase	*86 U/L*	*(39–99)*
Alanine transaminase	*9 U/L*	*(6–66)*
Aspartate transaminase	*9 U/L*	*(12–42)*
Troponin T	*19 ng/L*	*(≤ 29)*

Urine dipstick: Nitrite positive, leukocytes 3+, blood 2+, protein 1+

Electrocardiogram: Normal sinus rhythm

Chest radiograph: No consolidation

He was started on intravenous meropenem by the on-call team based on urine culture results from three years ago.

By the next morning, Mr C was less drowsy and able to open his eyes spontaneously. He was hemodynamically stable with resolution of tachycardia. He remained febrile with a temperature of 38°C. He was reviewed by the primary team consultant, who switched his antibiotics to intravenous cefepime.

48 hours into his admission, Mr C has remained clinically well. He remains febrile over the course of the past 24 hours with a maximum temperature of 38.6°C. Repeat full blood count showed resolution of leukocytosis. The blood culture susceptibility results returned as follows:

ORGANISM: Klebsiella pneumoniae

Ampicillin	*R*
Amoxicillin/Clavulanate	*S*
Piperacillin /Tazobactam	*S*

Cefazolin	*S*
Ceftriaxone	*S*
Cefepime	*S*
Aztreonam	*S*
Gentamicin	*S*
Ciprofloxacin	*R*
Meropenem	*S*
Ertapenem	*S*

Urine cultures grew the same bacteria with similar susceptibility patterns.

Question 3: What is your plan of action in the light of these findings?

This patient has not had significant healthcare contact for the past three years, so his risk of multi-drug resistant microorganisms is low. As he is also hemodynamically stable, the prior culture results from three years ago may not be clinically relevant in the initial management of this patient.

When commencing patients on new medications, it is important to check for any drug–drug interactions, especially for elderly patients who may be on multiple chronic medications. Specific to Mr C, one should note that concomitant carbapenem usage may decrease the serum concentration of sodium valproate, thus concurrent usage is not recommended. If concurrent carbapenem use is necessary, additional anti-seizure medication may be needed.

Mr C has *Klebsiella pneumoniae* bacteraemia secondary to bilateral pyelonephritis. Prolonged fever is sometimes observed in patients with pyelonephritis and in patients who are clinically improving. With positive culture and susceptibility to guide the team, antibiotic regimens can be simplified to ***narrower spectrum options***. In this case it would have been cefazolin, a first-generation cephalosporin. Subsequent oral antibiotic options would also be a first-generation cephalosporin like cephalexin rather than broader spectrum ones like amoxicillin-clavulanic acid. Intravenous to oral antibiotic switch can be attempted once the patient is haemodynamically stable and clinically improved.

Abdominal imaging would be useful in this poorly communicative patient with bacteraemia to exclude complicated urinary tract infections such as renal abscesses and to exclude perforated viscus. In a local study, 3.8% of patients with *K. pneumoniae* bacteraemia had endophthalmitis, with generally poor visual prognosis. In patients who are otherwise not able to provide reliable ocular symptoms, it may be prudent to seek an ophthalmologic evaluation.

****

In the light of bacteraemia and suspected urinary source of septicemia, Mr C underwent a computed tomography scan of the abdomen and pelvis to evaluate for presence of a complicated UTI. It revealed hypoenhancement of both kidneys and bilateral perinephric fat stranding suggestive of bilateral pyelonephritis. He continued to improve clinically following antibiotic de-escalation.

This patient has blood culture positivity and upper urinary tract involvement, suggesting the presence of a complicated UTI. Treatment is generally recommended for 10 to 14 days in such instances.

Mr C was discharged well after a week of hospitalisation. Three days later, he was seen again in the emergency department following accidental dislodgement of the IDC during transfer. A new urinary catheter was inserted and gross haematuria was noted. He was clinically well, afebrile, haemodynamically stable, and at baseline mentation. Clinical examination was otherwise unremarkable. Urine dipstick showed nitrite positive, leukocytes 3+, and blood 3+.

The general practitioner reviewed the urine culture result two days later:

ORGANISM: Escherichia coli
Viable count = 100,000 cfu/mL

Ampicillin	*R*
Amoxicillin/Clavulanate	*R*
Piperacillin/Tazobactam	*R*
Cefazolin	*R*
Ceftriaxone	*R*
Cefepime	*S*
Aztreonam	*R*
Gentamicin	*S*
Ciprofloxacin	*R*
Meropenem	*S*
Ertapenem	*S*

Question 4: What is the next most appropriate management?

a. Administer intramuscular gentamicin in the clinic and review again in two days.

b. Ask the patient's family to bring him back to the emergency department for admission for intravenous antibiotic as there is no oral antibiotic option.

c. Ask the patient's family to bring him back to the emergency department to change the IDC.

d. **Ignore the results since the patient is well, asymptomatic, and without clinical signs suggestive of CAUTI.**
e. **Refer to urologist for cystoscopy.**

General measures to decrease risk of CAUTI include the following:

- insertion of urinary catheters only for appropriate indications
- early removal of IDCs
- consideration of alternatives to in-dwelling catheterisation (e.g., intermittent catheterisation, use of condom catheters)
- aseptic techniques for catheter care, i.e., sterile insertion, maintenance of a closed drainage system, maintenance of gravity drainage

Specific to this patient who has a recent change in caregiver, assessment of his/her competency in sterile catheter care is important to address.

In a patient with a long-term IDC, pyuria and/or bacteriuria is almost always uniformly present, so the presence of either is unreliable in diagnosing CAUTI. Defining significant bacteriuria is also difficult since some level of bacterial colonisation is universal in urine from catheterised patients.

Asymptomatic bacteriuria refers to bacteriuria without signs or symptoms referable to the urinary tract. Asymptomatic bacteriuria or fungiuria rarely results in adverse outcomes such as pyelonephritis, renal abscess, or bacteremia and generally do ***not*** require treatment. Unfortunately, much of hospital antimicrobial misuse stems from such instances and every clinician has a role in recognising the distinction between symptomatic UTI versus asymptomatic bacteriuria.

This patient presented with accidental dislodgement of urinary catheter where gross haematuria from traumatic catheter removal is not unexpected and there is no clinical indication to screen this patient for bacteriuria. Based on the 2019 Infectious Disease Society of America clinical practice guideline for the management of asymptomatic bacteriuria, screening for or treating asymptomatic bacteriuria in patients with long-term IDCs is not recommended.

Key messages

1. Serious bacterial infections are common causes of elderly patients presenting with acute delirium.
2. CAUTI is diagnosed in the context of presence of signs or symptoms suggestive of a UTI or as a diagnosis of exclusion in patients who have unexplained signs of systemic infection.

3. Asymptomatic pyuria with or without bacteriuria may not be clinically significant and a careful clinical assessment for the presence of infection needs to be performed, rather than antimicrobial treatment of bacteriuria.

Answer key

1. CAUTI; need to rule out ascending infection resulting in pyelonephritis and bacteraemia. Other differential diagnoses include acute abdomen, meningo-encephalitis, and stroke.
2. Change urinary catheter, collect urine specimen for microscopy and culture; blood cultures x2 sets; empirical IV cefepime.
3. Switch the antibiotic to cefazolin as it has the narrowest spectrum amongst the usable antibiotics from the culture results. CT abdomen/pelvis in context of Klebsiella bacteraemia is often indicated to look for the presence of visceral organ abscesses. An ophthalmologic evaluation should be considered in patients with signs or symptoms of concern for endophthalmitis or in patients who are unable to provide a reliable history.
4. D.

References

Behr MA, Drummond R, Libman MD, Delaney JS, Dylewski JS (1996) Fever duration in hospitalized acute pyelonephritis patients. *Am J Med* **101**(3): 277–280.

Chenoweth CE, Gould CV, Saint S (2014) Diagnosis, management, and prevention of catheter associated urinary tract infections. Infect *Dis Clin N Am* **28**(1): 105–119.

Jang YR, Eom JS, Chung W, Cho YK (2019) Prolonged fever is not a reason to change antibiotics among patients with uncomplicated community-acquired acute pyelonephritis. *Medicine* **98**(43): e17720.

Nicolle LE, Gupta K, Bradley SF, *et al.* (2019) Infectious Disease Society of America clinical practice guideline for management of asymptomatic bacteriuria. *Clin Infect Dis* **68**(10): e83–e110.

Sng CCA, Jap A, Chan YH, Chee SP (2008) Risk factors for endogenous Klebsiella endophthalmitis in patients with Klebsiella bacteraemia: a case-control study. *Br J Ophthalmol* **92**(5): 673–677.

20 Recurrent Urinary Tract Infection

Lee Pei Shan, Anupama Roy Chowdhury

Mrs R is a 78-year-old multiparous widow living with her son's family and a helper. Premorbidly, she is community ambulant, dually continent, and helping to look after her grandchildren. She has no drug allergies and is a lifelong non-smoker and non-drinker. She has no recent hospitalisations. She has been seeing her general practitioner over the past ten years for the problems of diabetes mellitus with Stage 3A chronic kidney disease and non-proliferative retinopathy for which pan-retinal photocoagulation was done last year. She also has hypertension, hyperlipidaemia, and osteoarthritis of both knees. Her medications include dapagliflozin 10 mg OM, metformin 850 mg BD, glipizide 15 mg BD, telmisartan 80 mg OM, atorvastatin 10 mg ON, and Anarex PRN for her osteoarthritis.

Mrs R was brought to the hospital for increasing confusion over the past week. She no longer recognises her grandchildren whom she usually cares for. She has also not been eating or drinking much in the past few days which got her family concerned. There are no sick contacts at home.

Question 1: What key aspects of corroborative history should be obtained?

Her helper noticed that she was having increased urinary frequency which started about a week ago but seemed to have resolved the day before. Mrs R had not complained of dysuria, haematuria, or abdominal/flank pain. Of note, she has long-standing incontinence attributed to uterine prolapse (she has had four normal vaginal deliveries). She has a vaginal pessary *in situ* which is changed monthly.

She typically has about two episodes of urinary tract infection (UTI) per year, each time presenting with dysuria. She was treated with co-amoxiclav for her last UTI six months ago. As such, she performs vaginal douching, taking care to clean her perineal region from front to back. She is not known to have renal calculi.

She does not have any other infective symptoms including respiratory symptoms, chills, or rigors. She is also not known to have any cognitive impairment prior to her current hospitalisation.

However, Mrs R is known to have a history of constipation. Her last stool screen was negative for occult blood and she does not exhibit other red flag symptoms for malignancy. Her helper noticed that she has not opened her bowels for the past four days.

On medication review, her caregiver reports that dapagliflozin was introduced about two weeks ago by her general practitioner for poorly controlled diabetes (HbA1c 9–11%), largely attributed to "dietary indiscretion". Mrs R had previously declined insulin but is otherwise compliant to her medications which are prepared by her helper. In the last general practitioner visit, Anarex was also prescribed for regular intake for an osteoarthritic flare.

She does not take any other traditional medicine, supplements, or over-the-counter drugs.

****

On examination, her vital signs were temperature 37.9°C, pulse rate 90/min, blood pressure 120/80 mmHg, and SpO_2 99% on room air. Mucous membranes were dry. She was confused and unable to comply with commands, though she could move all four limbs. Abbreviated mental test score was 6/10. Pupils were equal and reactive. Abdominal examination revealed a palpable bladder and no other masses. Cardiorespiratory examination was unremarkable.

Relevant investigations revealed white cell count 22 x 10^9/L (predominantly neutrophils), haemoglobin 13.2 g/dL, platelet count 300 x 10^9/L, urea 15 mmol/L, sodium 132 mmol/L, potassium 4 mmol/L, and bicarbonate 24 mmol/L, as well as creatinine 200 μmol/L and eGFR 22 mL/min/1.73 m^2 compared to results one month ago at the general practitioner (creatinine 100 μmol/L and eGFR 50 mL/min/1.73 m^2). HbA1c was 10.2% and albumin was 30 g/L; rest of liver panel was unremarkable.

800 mL cloudy urine was immediately drained upon inserting a urinary catheter. Urine microscopy showed RBC > 2,000, WBC > 2,000, epithelial cells 0, and microorganisms 3+. Urine dipstick showed glucose positive and ketones negative. Urine and blood cultures were sent off.

Ultrasound kidney, ureter, and bladder showed chronic renal parenchymal disease with no hydronephrosis, renal calculi, or perinephric stranding noted.

Question 2: What is your working diagnosis? List the medical issues including likely aetiology and complications.

In asymptomatic older adults, routine screening and treatment of pyuria or bacteriuria are ***not*** recommended. Changes in urine such as cloudiness without localised genitourinary symptoms or other symptoms to suggest an infection do not indicate

UTI! There exists a high prevalence of asymptomatic bacteriuria (from colonisation) in older adults above 70 years old: up to 19% in the community, up to 50% in long-term care facilities, and 100% in patients with in-dwelling urinary catheters. Asymptomatic bacteriuria does not increase the risk of mortality and treatment does not decrease the risk of symptomatic UTI and can, instead, potentially increase the risks of adverse events and antimicrobial resistance. Avoid sending urine cultures in an asymptomatic older adult!

In patients with symptomatic bacteriuria, the diagnosis of UTI depends on the presence or absence of an in-dwelling urinary catheter.

In a patient without an in-dwelling catheter or on intermittent catheterisation or condom catheter, one of the following features must be present:

(1) SPECIFIC GENITOURINARY TRACT PAIN (dysuria or inflammation of testes/epididymis/prostate).
(2) FEVER (oral temperature >37.8°C or 1.1°C above baseline), CHILLS, or LEUKOCYTOSIS + ≥1 of the signs in (3).
(3) ≥2 other urological signs of UTI viz. new/increased urinary urgency/frequency/incontinence, gross haematuria, new flank/costovertebral angle/suprapubic pain/tenderness.

In a patient with an in-dwelling catheter, the threshold for diagnosis is lower. at least one of the following features must be present:

(1) SPECIFIC GENITOURINARY TRACT PAIN (inflammation of testes/epididymis/prostate).
(2) FEVER (oral temperature >37.8°C or 1.1°C above baseline), CHILLS, or HYPOTENSION without alternate septic source.
(3) OBVIOUS SIGN — purulent discharge from/around the catheter.
(4) LEUKOCYTOSIS + SYSTEMIC NON-LOCALISING SIGN viz. acute change in mental status or acute functional decline.
(5) New flank/costovertebral angle/suprapubic pain/tenderness.

Foul-smelling or cloudy urine as reported by the patient or caregiver does not always signify a UTI especially in the absence of other symptoms of infection as detailed above. This may be related to diet, dehydration, medications, or personal hygiene.

Be mindful that patients with cognitive impairment may not be able to report symptoms. As such, delirium, unexplained instability and falls, incontinence, anorexia, or malaise may be the clinical manifestation of a UTI. However, an acute change in mental status, fatigue, poor appetite, or fall with unknown mechanism may also be contributed by pain, constipation, intravascular depletion, alternative causes of sepsis, electrolyte disturbances, depression, and medication changes. Hence, these causes must also be looked for and addressed concurrently if present.

Table 20.1 highlights the common risk factors for UTI in the elderly population:

Table 20.1. Pathophysiology of risk factors for UTI in the elderly.

Risk factors for UTI in the elderly	Possible mechanism(s)
Medical conditions (e.g., diabetes, cancer), use of immunosuppressive medication	Impaired cellular function; glycosuria from use of sodium-glucose cotransporter 2 inhibitors (SGLT2i) (e.g., empagliflozin, dapagliflozin, canagliflozin).
Comorbidities with concurrent cognitive impairment (e.g., dementia), stroke, Parkinson disease	Bladder and bowel incontinence, functional decline, immobility.
Oestrogen deficiency	Uterine/vaginal prolapse, vaginal atrophy, and urinary incontinence resulting in an ascending flow of bacteria into the sterile urinary tract; impaired protective action of bacterial colonisation of vagina.
Prostatic hypertrophy	Urinary retention with increased post-void residual urine and turbulent urinary flow may predispose to chronic prostatitis.
Other urological problems like voiding dysfunction (e.g., neurogenic bladder), urethral stricture	Increased risk of urinary retention, ascending flow of pathogens into the sterile urinary tract.
Long-term in-dwelling urinary catheterisation	Disruption of defence mechanisms, granting easier access of bacteria to the bladder. The catheter damages the protective uroepithelial mucosa, exposing new host cell binding receptors (which also attach to the catheter surface) for bacterial adhesins. These bacteria are more virulent and can create a biofilm by producing exopolysaccharides that entrap and protect replicating bacteria. Catheter encrustations may obstruct urine flow, promoting urine stagnation and bacterial replication.

(Continued)

Risk factors for UTI in the elderly	Possible mechanism(s)
Sexual activity	Risk factor in both men and women, especially in the elderly population. While the association is not as clear as in young women, it is believed that bacteria gain access to the urinary tract by colonising the periurethral mucosa and ascending to the bladder through the urethra.

****

Question 3: Outline your initial management plan for Mrs R.

The first step to treating UTI in the elderly is to ascertain if the UTI is complicated or not. Empirical antibiotics should be commenced (Table 20.2) and reviewed as soon as culture results are available.

Table 20.2. Antibiotic recommendations for uncomplicated female UTI.

Recommended treatment of uncomplicated UTI in females	Dose	Comments and caution
First-line		
Nitrofurantoin	50 mg QDS ($0.50 per tablet)	CrCl <30 mL/min: not recommended Only for treatment of lower UTI
Co-trimoxazole	960 mg BD ($0.10 per 480 mg tablet)	CrCl 15–30 mL/min: dose reduction CrCl <15 mL/min: not recommended
Fosfomycin	3 g oral granules ($11.86) single dose	Only for treatment of lower UTI
Amoxicillin	500 mg TDS ($0.12 per 250 mg capsule)	CrCl <50 mL/min: dose reduction Not for treatment of Klebsiella — consider combining with clavulanate instead
Cephalexin	250 mg QDS ($0.12 per capsule)	CrCl <50 mL/min: dose reduction (additional reduction if CrCl <15 mL/min)
Second-line		
Amoxicillin/clavulanate	1 g BD ($0.40 per tablet)	CrCl <30 mL/min: dose reduction
Ciprofloxacin	500 mg BD ($0.24 per tablet)	Avoid moxifloxacin as it does not concentrate in the urine and therefore is a poor option for UTI
Levofloxacin	500 mg OD ($0.83 per tablet)	

Treatment duration is typically seven days. A shorter duration of 5 days may be considered for an independent female living in the community. Complicated UTI such as pyelonephritis will require longer duration of therapy and a different choice of empirical antibiotics — it is out of the scope of this chapter. Note that all male UTIs are considered complicated UTIs.

In older patients with poor oral intake and/or delirium limiting consistent administration of oral antibiotics or vomiting, antibiotics may have to be administered via the intravenous route initially to ensure adequate therapeutic dosing. Once the patient is able to take and retain orally, they can be converted to oral antibiotics.

The complications associated with UTI in this elderly female should be concurrently managed. Acute urinary retention, acute kidney injury, and delirium are covered in other chapters.

Risk factor modification is necessary for secondary prevention of UTI. For her diabetes, a review with the dietician could help her gain an understanding on the need for dietary discretion and tailor a diet to her numerous comorbidities (including chronic kidney disease, hypertension, and hyperlipidaemia). Metformin needs to be held off in view of reduced creatinine clearance from the acute kidney injury. A potential alternative is a dipeptidyl peptidase-4 inhibitor such as linagliptin which is safe in renal impairment. Dapagliflozin also should be suspended during treatment of ongoing UTI, and the patient needs to counselled to monitor for UTI symptoms if it is to be restarted later. In this patient with poorly controlled diabetes on three oral drugs on optimal doses, insulin therapy would be an appropriate consideration. Mrs R and her caregiver should be counselled on the need for insulin therapy and appropriate caregiver training on insulin administration and glucose monitoring be arranged.

Tips for adding insulin in the elderly with type 2 diabetes:

— *The simplest strategy is to use a basal insulin analogue delivered in a pen injector device such as detemir (Levemir $14.53 for 300 U) or glargine (Lantus Solostar $30.46 for 300 U). There is little peaking effect and very low risk of hypoglycaemia. A cheaper alternative is isophane (Insulatard $8.35 for 300 U pen, $9 for 1,000 U by syringe and needle injection).*
— *10 U is a commonly prescribed starting dose.*
— *In elderly persons who live alone, be sure to assess their dexterity and eyesight when selecting an appropriate insulin.*
— *Treatment intensification to basal-bolus or biphasic insulin regimens should be performed judiciously; always "start low and go slow".*

The HBA1c target in the elderly must be individualised. Those with a life expectancy of more than ten years should aim for HBA1c <7.5%, while <8–8.5% is a reasonable target for the frail elderly with multiple medical comorbidities for which treatment is aimed more at protecting the quality of life and preventing hypoglycaemia.

Additionally for Mdm R, uro-gynaecological consult should be sought to manage the uterovaginal prolapse. Constipation can be managed with pharmacological and non-pharmacological measures as covered in another chapter. The association between vaginal douching and UTI is controversial and it is probably best avoided.

In patients with recurrent UTI (defined as a frequency of at least 3 UTIs per year or 2 UTIs in the last 6 months), low-dose prophylaxis for 3–6 months may be discussed in selected individuals, though this is not routinely practiced. Long-term antibiotics have risk of adverse effects including alteration of bowel flora and development of antimicrobial resistance which may outweigh the benefits. Options include nitrofurantoin, fosfomycin, or cephalexin. Current studies do not support cranberry products for UTI prophylaxis.

Hence, it is essential to try to identify underlying predisposing factors, such as urinary calculi, high residual volumes of urine, inadequate perineal hygiene, and inadequate water intake, and address these to try to prevent recurrent UTIs.

A good history and physical examination (especially the abdomen, per rectal, and per vaginal exam) will likely reveal some predisposing factors. Measurement of post-void residual urine volumes is easily done at the bedside with a bladder scan especially in continent patients as the scan can be done soon after the patient voids. A high post-void residual urine volume should trigger a hunt for an underlying cause (e.g., prolapse, constipation, pelvic mass) and the patient may have to be supported by intermittent catheterisation while the issue is being addressed. In our daily practice, we broadly accept a post-void residual urine volume of <150–200 mL.

A point to note is that the measurement of post-void residual urine with a bladder scan may not be accurate in patients with ascites or a pelvic mass. In such cases, a significant discrepancy is often observed between the measured volume with a bladder scan and the actual volume of urine drained.

Key messages

1. The diagnosis of UTI (complicated versus uncomplicated) should be established prior to empirical antibiotic therapy. Asymptomatic pyuria or bacteriuria does not require antibiotic treatment unless the older person is going for an invasive urological procedure involving instrumentation of the genitourinary tract.

2. An elderly person with UTI may present with non-specific symptoms such as delirium, anorexia, malaise, falls, or incontinence.
3. Careful assessment of precipitating/risk factors and complications associated with UTI is important as these issues should be addressed during management.

Answer key

1. Infective symptoms especially those of UTI (e.g., dysuria, haematuria, suprapubic pain, flank pain, incontinence, fever, chills, rigors);

   Precipitating factors for acute urinary retention and UTI;

   Medication review — changes or additions.
2. a. UTI with acute kidney injury (KIDGO Stage 2) secondary to poor oral intake and intravascular depletion;

   b. Acute urinary retention (contributing factors for urinary retention: constipation, anticholinergic effects of Anarex, uterine prolapse);

   c. Other predisposing factors for UTI would include vaginal douching, suboptimal diabetic control, and additional glycosuria from SGLT2i intake;

   d. Delirium secondary to UTI, AKI, ARU, constipation, and Anarex.
3. Treat the UTI, e.g., amoxicillin (tailor antibiotics based on culture results), fosfomycin if patient only has cystitis;

   Treat associated complications viz. urinary retention (leave in-dwelling urinary catheter for 2–3 days before trial off, check if vaginal pessary is *in situ*), acute kidney injury (intravenous hydration in view of poor oral intake, stop metformin and dapagliflozin, monitor renal function), delirium (frequent orientation, ensure sleep hygiene, stop Anarex, laxatives for constipation);

   Control risk factors viz. optimise glucose control with insulin while monitoring glucose levels.

References

Gupta K, Hooton TM, Naber KG, *et al.* (2011) International clinical practice guidelines for the treatment of acute uncomplicated cystitis and pyelonephritis in women: A 2010 update by the Infectious Diseases Society of America and the European Society for Microbiology and Infectious Diseases. *Clin Infect Dis* **52**(5): e103–e120.

Rodriguez-Mañas L (2020) Urinary tract infections in the elderly: a review of disease characteristics and current treatment options. *Drugs Context* **9**: 2020-4-13.

21 Acute Retention of Urine (Prostate)

Guo Weiwen, Shandy Wong Shan Li

Mr U is an 82-year-old gentleman who is premorbidly independent in his activities of daily living and ambulant in the community with a walking stick. His medical history includes diabetes mellitus, hyperlipidaemia, hypertension, and chronic obstructive lung disease. He does not smoke or drink. He is dually continent and stays with his wife and a helper.

His medications include bisoprolol 5 mg OM, simvastatin 20 mg OM, metformin 500 mg BD, tiotropium 2 inhalations of 18 mcg capsule a day, and salbutamol inhaler as needed. He has no drug allergy.

He is admitted to the ward for worsening right hip pain following a fall two weeks ago. The pain radiates to the knee and is worse on movement. His pain score is 8/10 and he has been unable to bear weight on his right lower limb. Since the fall, Mr U has not been able to ambulate and he has been largely bedbound, requiring assistance in his activities of daily living.

He visited a general practitioner who prescribed Anarex 2 tabs TDS and tramadol 50 mg TDS. The patient's wife also reported that he was suffering from constipation and has been more confused in the past two weeks. He does not have any fever, chest pain, shortness of breath, cough, or rhinorrhoea. His wife noted decreased urine output in the past one week.

Question 1: What additional pertinent history would you like to ask?

Mr U has no previous history of falls. This time, he slipped and fell while walking home on a rainy day. He landed on his buttocks and was unable to get up on his own following the fall. Since then, the right hip pain has been increasing and affecting the movement of his right leg. Analgesia from the general practitioner only provided temporary relief. He is compliant to all his medications. He has difficulty passing urine for the past two weeks but does not complain of any dysuria or gross haematuria. His wife noted that he has been increasingly confused in the last two weeks, becoming disoriented to place and time, and mixing up family members who came to visit. He spent most of his time sleeping on some days, while on other days, he had periods of agitation and was seen talking to himself.

On examination, Mr U opens eyes to calling and is not in distress. His vital signs are temperature 37°C, blood pressure 186/98 mmHg, heart rate 108/min, and respiratory rate 20/min with SpO_2 98% on room air. He is not oriented to time, place, or person. His oral mucous membranes are dry. Abdominal examination revealed suprapubic tenderness and a palpable bladder. Renal punch is negative. Per rectal examination revealed an empty rectum with intact anal tone and a smooth prostate at 4 finger breadths. His right lower limb is in a shortened and externally rotated resting position. His right hip range of movement is severely limited by pain. On neurological examination, his right lower limb power is 4/5 and examination is limited by pain. His distal pulses are intact. He scored 7/10 on the abbreviated mental test. His cardiopulmonary examination is unremarkable.

X-ray of the pelvis and right hip revealed a right neck of femur fracture.

Question 2: What is an appropriate immediate course of action?

This gentleman is in delirium. In an elderly patient with delirium, it is important to look for acute retention of urine as well as constipation as possible causes.

Obstruction is the most frequent cause of acute urinary retention, and the commonest cause in males is benign prostatic hyperplasia (BPH). Neurogenic bladder and decreased detrusor contractility in diabetes can also cause urinary retention.

Examination of the patient with acute retention of urine must include a digital rectal examination to look for enlarged prostate, masses, faecal impaction, perineal sensation, and anal tone. A female patient should undergo pelvic examination to look for tumour and pelvic organ prolapse. It is important to examine the abdomen for a palpable bladder. If available, a bladder scan can also be used to measure the urine volume in the bladder. A volume on ultrasound ≥400 mL is an indication for decompression.

If attempts to pass a catheter are unsuccessful, the patient should be referred to the urologist for bedside cystoscopy-guided catheter insertion. Note that urethral catheterisation is contraindicated in patients who have had recent urologic surgery and these patients should undergo suprapubic catheterisation instead.

Common complications of bladder decompression include transient haematuria, hypotension, and post-obstructive diuresis. Haematuria and hypotension usually resolve without intervention. Post-obstructive diuresis more commonly occurs with chronic retention of urine, so the fluid status of the patient should be monitored.

Bladder decompression decision-making algorithm based on urine volume from catheterisation

Initial urinary volume < 200 mL	• Removal of urinary catheter • Observe
Initial urinary volume > 400 mL	• Leave urinary catheter for initial urinary volume > 400 mL. • For urinary volume between 200-400 mL, the decision to remove or leave the urinary catheter should be based on the clinical scenario, underlying cause of urinary retention, and patient risk factors.
Voiding trial	• After 3 to 5 days, do a voiding trial if precipitating factor has been addressed. • Consider comorbidies, functional status, and ability to care for catheter and return to hospital when considering long-term catheterisation.

****

After insertion of an in-dwelling catheter, the initial volume drained was 600 mL of clear urine. Urinalysis showed no microscopic red or white blood cells. Mr U no longer complained of lower abdominal discomfort and was visibly more comfortable.

Question 3: What are the factors that contribute to the acute retention of urine in this patient? Select all relevant options.

a. Benign prostatic hyperplasia

b. Constipation

c. Immobility

d. Medications

e. Pain from hip fracture

f. Neurogenic bladder from diabetes

g. Urinary tract infection

Many pharmacologic agents are associated with urinary retention, including those with anticholinergic activity (e.g., antipsychotic drugs, antidepressant agents, anticholinergic respiratory agents), opioids and anaesthetics, benzodiazepines, α-adrenergic agonists, anti-arrhythmic drugs, anti-Parkinsonism drugs, non-steroidal anti-inflammatory drugs, hormonal agents, antihistamines, muscle relaxants, and even calcium channel antagonists.

Anticholinergic medication is the commonest contributing factor to acute retention of urine as it blocks the parasympathetic pathway and impairs the contraction of the detrusor muscle. Care should also be taken when prescribing opiate analgesics to the elderly — all opioids can cause urinary retention due to μ-opioid receptor agonism.

Polypharmacy is common in older patients as many of them have multiple medical conditions. It is important to review the medication list for drugs that may contribute to urinary retention. If a medication is no longer required or the dose can be reduced, they can be withdrawn to reduce pill burden for the patient and minimise side-effects.

****

Serum and urine investigations were done for Mr U.

Laboratory test	Baseline	Admission	Reference ranges
Sodium, mmol/L	140	130	136–146
Potassium, mmol/L	4.0	5.1	3.5–5.1
Chloride, mmol/L	100	98	98–107
Bicarbonate, mmol/L	24	23	19–29
Urea, mmol/L	5.0	10.2	2.7–6.9
Creatinine, μmol/L	100	155	59–104
eGFR, mL/min/1.73 m^2	60	35	
Calcium, mmol/L	2.14	2.2	2.09–2.46
Phosphate, mmol/L	1.25	1.3	0.94–1.5
Magnesium, mmol/L	0.80	0.78	0.75–1.07
Glucose, mmol/L	7.6	5.9	3.0–11.0
Albumin, g/L	35	36	40–51
Haemoglobin, g/dL	13.2	14	14–18
WBC count, $x10^9/L$	6.95	7.20	4–10
Platelets, $x10^9/L$	319	280	140–440
TSH, mIU/L		4.0	0.45–4.5
Free T4, pmol/L		12.0	10–20
HbA1c %	6.8	7.2	
Prostate specific antigen, μg/L		1.13	<4

Urine dipstick: RBC negative, leukocyte negative, nitrite negative, ketones negative, protein trace, glucose positive

Urinalysis: RBC 0, WBC 0, epithelial cell 7

Urine protein creatinine ratio: 0.2 g/g

Abdominal X- ray:

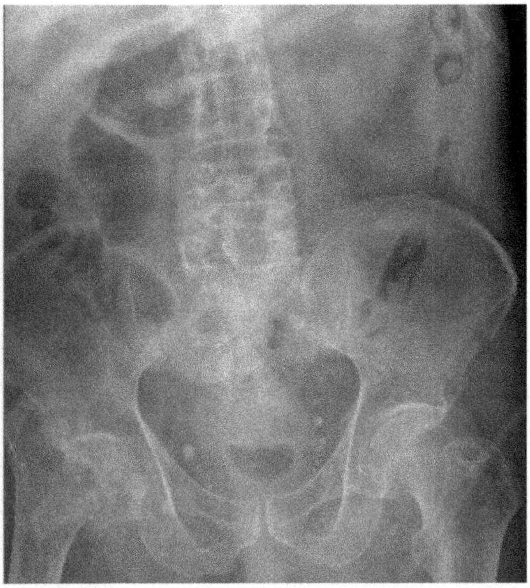

Question 4: Identify and explain the pertinent biochemical aberrations.

Question 5: Make three pertinent radiologic observations.

In all patients with acute or chronic urinary retention, recommended laboratory tests include full blood count (to look for infection), fasting glucose and HbA1c (to look for diabetes), electrolytes (to look for derangement as a complication of retention of urine), and thyroid function (to look for hypothyroidism, which may present as retention of urine or constipation). Urine dipstick or urinalysis are quick and effective screening tools for urinary tract infections. Serum creatinine should be screened to pick up acute kidney injury as a complication of urinary retention and dehydration.

Ultrasound of the kidneys, ureters, and bladder may be helpful to evaluate for urinary stones or strictures in the urinary tract, as well as to look for complications such as hydronephrosis.

If the aetiology for retention of urine is not found on initial evaluation, patients should be referred to a urologist for cystoscopy to look for strictures or structural abnormalities. Urodynamic studies can also be performed to look for functional bladder disorders.

A diagnosis of clinical BPH was made for Mr U as his prostatic enlargement has resulted in obstruction. BPH is caused by an increase in the total number of stromal and glandular epithelial cells within the transition zone of the prostate, resulting in its global enlargement.

Urinary symptoms of BPH typically include increased frequency of urination, nocturia, urgency, hesitancy, straining, intermittency, double voiding, weak urinary stream, and terminal dribbling. Pain and dysuria are usually not present. The International Prostate Symptom Score (IPSS) is a validated self-administered questionnaire (you can download an app called "Urology IPSS Prostate Score") that can provide information regarding the symptom burden to patients. A score of 1–7 indicates mild, 8–19 moderate, and 20–35 severe lower urinary tract symptoms.

Physical examination in a person with suspected BPH includes digital rectal examination to look for prostatic enlargement and nodules, faecal impaction, anal tone to look for the neurologic aetiology of retention of urine, and abdominal examination to look for palpable bladder and suprapubic tenderness.

Assessment of prostate size and morphology can be achieved by abdominal or transrectal ultrasonography, cystoscopy, computed tomography, or magnetic resonance imaging. Ultrasound can measure prostatic volume and intravesical prostatic protrusion (IPP). IPP correlates with the progression of BPH and predicts likelihood of successful trial without catheter.

Additional studies that may be used to confirm the diagnosis or evaluate the severity of BPH include post-void residual urine volume, uroflowmetry, and pressure flow studies. Urinalysis should be done to rule out infection. Prostate-specific antigen (PSA) may also be done for prostate cancer screening in appropriate patients aged more than 50 years with a life expectancy of more than 10 years. However, care should be taken in the timing of performing a PSA level as acute urinary retention, per rectal examination, and urinary catheterisation may also lead to spuriously elevated levels, amongst many other causes.

****

Mr U proceeded with an ultrasound of the kidney, ureters, and bladder which showed a partially distended urinary bladder after catheterisation. The urinary bladder wall is trabeculated, suggesting chronic urinary bladder outlet obstruction. The prostate gland is enlarged at 58.5 cm³.

His urine catheter drained 1,250 mL on the first day and 1,000 mL on the second day. On the third day, no urine output was noted.

Question 6: What is your plan of management?

In the event of decreased flow of urine or blocked urinary catheter, gentle pressure may be applied to the suprapubic region which may initiate urine flow.

Gentle irrigation through the end of the catheter using 10–20 mL sterile saline can be performed and should return the saline mixed with urine. If the saline is not returned, the catheter needs to be changed.

It is also important to assess the fluid status of the patient and ensure that the decreased urine output is not due to anuria or dehydration! A bladder scan or bedside ultrasound can be done and ≥200 mL suggests urinary retention.

In the elderly, a voiding trial is important as an in-dwelling catheter is in itself a risk factor for delirium. The duration of catheterisation depends on the aetiology of the acute retention of urine. If the underlying aetiology is treated and expected to resolve (such as infection), then a voiding trial should be done as soon as possible (usually around 3–5 days).

In a patient whose condition is expected not to resolve (such as neurogenic bladder from spinal injury or chronic urinary retention), trial without catheter may be attempted after 1–2 weeks. It is necessary to discuss with the patient and caregiver the options for long-term catheterisation (Table 21.1).

Table 21.1. Options for long-term urinary catheterisation.

Modality of long-term urinary catheterisation	Advantage(s)	Disadvantage(s)	Remark
Clean intermittent catheterisation	Less risk of urinary tract infections; Increased spontaneous voiding	Not suitable in cases of urinary obstruction (e.g., enlarged prostate, urethral stricture)	Patient and caregiver must be comfortable and competent
Suprapubic catheter	Prevents urethral trauma and stricture formation; Reduces the incidence of catheter-associated bacteriuria; Allows attempts at normal voiding without the need for re-catheterisation; Interferes less with sexual activity	Invasive and requires surgical procedure	
In-dwelling catheter	Easy to insert	Risk of urethral trauma and stricture; Increased risk of urinary tract infection; Interferes with sexual activity	Most common for short-term usage (<3 weeks)

Prior to discharge, patients and caregivers should be provided with adequate training on how to manage the catheter, empty the catheter bag, and monitor the urine output. In Singapore, follow-up with urology clinic or the Home Nursing Foundation should also be made for patients with a long-term in-dwelling catheter who may require catheter change.

The key long-term catheter care principles in the elderly are as follows:

A. Type of catheter

For most adults, a standard Foley catheter (double-lumen latex) is suitable. Single- or multiple-use straight catheters without a balloon are used for intermittent catheterisation. Silicone catheters are preferable when the patient requires prolonged catheterisation to decrease risk of urethral inflammation and strictures.

B. Preparation and cleanliness

Gloves should be worn whenever the catheter and drainage system are manipulated. Cleansing with soap and water around the catheter (periurethral, suprapubic) during daily bathing is adequate for ongoing maintenance.

C. Preventing backflow

Catheter and collecting tubing should be free from kinks and should be fixed to the patient's leg to prevent tugging or traumatic removal. The collection system must be positioned below the level of the bladder at all times.

D. Managing leakage

If leakage occurs around an established suprapubic catheter (>6 weeks after placement) or transurethral catheter, the catheter can be replaced with a new catheter that is larger by 2 to 4 F. Anti-muscarinic agents are often prescribed if catheter leakage is due to detrusor overactivity. However, care should be taken in the elderly as anti-muscarinic agents are a risk factor for delirium.

E. Replacement of catheters

Catheters with mechanical problems (poor drainage, encrusted) need to be replaced. Short-term indwelling catheters as a rule should not be replaced routinely. There is insufficient evidence to make a recommendation on long-term catheters.

F. Catheter removal

Remove urinary catheters as soon as possible once the indication for insertion is no longer present.

****

After gentle irrigation of the catheter, the flow was restored. Mr U was reviewed by orthopaedics for the right hip fracture and was offered a hip replacement. He was reviewed by the acute pain team for pain control but still required opioid medications. Per rectal bisacodyl suppository was given and he passed motion daily. Serum creatinine on day 3 has returned to baseline. He was diagnosed to have BPH and was counselled on treatment options.

Question 8: Mr U is planned for initiation of oral alfuzosin. How will you counsel the patient?

Lifestyle modifications are first-line treatment for all patients with urinary complaints. Patients should limit their intake of fluids prior to bed time and limit caffeine and alcohol intake — these can improve storage symptoms such as urgency and nocturia. Constipation should be avoided. Regular exercise and weight control are recommended. Behavioural interventions such as pelvic muscle exercises as well as voiding at timed intervals are also recommended.

Patients diagnosed to have BPH should be initiated on an α-1 adrenergic antagonist (Table 21.2) at the time of catheterisation for bladder decompression. α-1 adrenergic antagonists relax the smooth muscle at the bladder neck and prostatic capsule and have been found to increase success rate of trial without catheter. Treatment with alfuzosin delays the recurrence of acute retention of urine and the need for surgical treatment. Its effect is seen within days. Orthostatic hypotension should be observed for in the elderly on initiation of treatment. Patients with cataract surgery should avoid the initiation of α-blockers, especially tamsulosin until their cataract surgery is completed, to prevent intra-operative floppy iris syndrome (IFIS). Tamsulosin is uroselective, but it is also the most common cause of IFIS. One other point to note is that alfuzosin and tamsulosin need to be swallowed whole while terazosin can be crushed. This is of relevance to patients with dysphagia.

Table 21.2. Alpha-1 adrenergic antagonists for BPH.

α-1 adrenergic antagonist for BPH	**Dose**	**Side-effects (with estimated relative risks)**		
		Giddiness/ hypotension	**Rhinorrhoea (nasal congestion)**	**Ejaculatory dysfunction**
Second-generation Terazosin	1–10 mg daily	+++ (especially first dose syncope)	+	+ (0.3%)
Third-generation Alfuzosin	10 mg daily	+	+	++
Tamsulosin	0.4–0.8 mg daily	+	+	+++

5-α reductase inhibitors (e.g., finasteride 5 mg OM, $0.79 per pill; dutasteride 0.5 mg OM, $2.47 per pill — the latter may confer marginally greater clinical benefit in BPH and both carry a small risk of reducing libido) block the conversion of testosterone to dihydrotestosterone, causing prostatic epithelial atrophy and preventing prostate enlargement. Thus, they are used to prevent BPH progression rather than acute symptoms. They are indicated for patients with larger prostatic volumes (>30 g) and significant obstruction. However, treatment for more than one year is needed to prevent the retention of urine and reduce the need for surgery. 5-α reductase inhibitors reduce PSA levels by 50% and a baseline PSA should be checked before initiation of the drug.

Combination therapy with α-1 adrenergic antagonists and 5-α reductase blockers is recommended for patients who have prostate enlargement and moderate to severe symptoms of BPH or IPSS score >12, and for those with partial response to α-1 adrenergic antagonists.

It is recommended that patients have two trials without a catheter before considering surgical therapy. The first trial without catheter should be attempted in one to two weeks after catheter placement. For those who failed the initial trial without catheter, a second trial should be done after another two weeks. The second trial without catheter generally has a lower success rate than the initial attempt.

In patients with symptomatic BPH, transurethral resection of the prostate (TURP) reduces risk of acute retention of urine by 85 to 90%. Indications for surgery include moderate to severe voiding symptoms that are refractory to medical therapy, refractory urinary retention, recurrent urinary tract infections, recurrent gross haematuria, bladder stones, and hydronephrosis with renal function impairment.

Surgery is recommended to be done at least 30 days after an acute urinary retention episode to prevent operative complications, including bleeding and sepsis related to bacteriuria.

TURP complications include urinary tract infection, ejaculatory dysfunction, urethral strictures, urinary incontinence, failure (2.5% risk of requiring re-operation), and transurethral resection syndrome (dilutional hyponatraemia with the use of hypo-osmolar irrigation solution). Hyponatraemia in the older individual may precipitate delirium and in severe cases, the patient may develop seizures.

Key messages

1. Acute retention of urine is a urological emergency that requires immediate bladder decompression. The most common cause of acute retention of urine in elderly male patients is BPH.
2. Always exclude acute urinary retention in a patient presenting with delirium.

3. Many medications can contribute to acute retention of urine. It is important to review the medication list for all patients and minimise offending drugs.
4. In a patient with acute retention of urine, a trial without catheter should be attempted at 3–5 days if the underlying cause has been addressed, or 1–2 weeks in the case of BPH.
5. For patients with BPH, they should be initiated on an α-1 adrenergic antagonist at the time of catheterisation for bladder decompression.

Answer Key

1. ***Falls history*** — any pre-fall symptoms that predisposed to the fall? Mechanism of fall and presence of head injury and loss of consciousness? Any prolonged lie following fall that may predispose to rhabdomyolysis and acute kidney injury? Any decrease in food and water intake following the fall and immobility?

   Predisposing factors — any signs of infection, lower urinary tract symptoms, and delirium (orientation to time, place, and person)?

   Medication history — any new medications or increase in doses that can contribute to constipation, retention of urine, and confusion?
2. Acute retention of urine is a urological emergency which necessitates immediate decompression of the urinary bladder. This can be performed using either urethral or suprapubic catheterisation. Urine for microscopic analysis and culture should be sent during decompression to look for an infective cause of the urinary retention.
3. All except (g). Clinical history and urinalysis do not suggest infection (urinary tract infection, urethritis, or prostatitis).
4. Acute kidney injury (rise in serum creatinine to 1.5x baseline) from retention of urine contributed by dehydration, which is common in elderly patients with delirium as many of them develop poor oral intake. Hyponatraemia is a common complication following acute retention of urine, likely due to syndrome of inappropriate anti-diuretic hormone secretion (SIADH) triggered by bladder distension or pain.
5. Displaced right neck of femur fracture;

   Faecal matter in left hemi-colon;

   Absence of bowel dilatation, presence of phleboliths.
6. Check for a blocked or kinked catheter tube. Gentle irrigation can be attempted and if unsuccessful, change the urinary catheter.

7. Warn of side-effects such as dizziness, rhinorrhoea, and ejaculatory problems. Although the risk of hypotension is relatively low, it is still prudent to monitor blood pressure and observe for symptoms of postural giddiness when starting alfuzosin.

References

Elkabir JJ, Patel A, Vale JA, Witherow RO, Emberton M, Anson K (1999) Acute urinary retention in men. *BMJ* **319**(7215): 1004.

Ohn J, Asson HW, Eda OJR, Ruskewitz ECB, Ack J, Linson E, *et al.* (1995) A comparison of transurethral surgery with watchful waiting for moderate symptoms of benign prostatic hyperplasia. The Veterans Affairs Cooperative Study Group on Transurethral Resection of the Prostate. *N Engl J Med* **332**(2): 75–79.

Verhamme KMC, Sturkenboom MCJM, Stricker BHC, Bosch R (2008) Drug-induced urinary retention: incidence, management and prevention. *Drug Saf* **31**(5): 373–388.

22 Acute Kidney Injury

Teh Swee Ping, Anupama Roy Chowdhury

Mdm T is a 73-year-old female who presented with malaise and lethargy for a week, associated with loss of appetite and vomiting. Her medical history consists of atrial fibrillation, mitral stenosis with history of open valvulotomy in 1985, hypertension, hyperlipidaemia, and impaired glucose tolerance. Her usual medications are enalapril 10 mg BD, atorvastatin 10 mg ON, bisoprolol 2.5 mg BD, spironolactone 12.5 mg OM, furosemide 40 mg daily, and warfarin 2 mg daily.

A month ago, Mdm T saw her general practitioner for shoulder stiffness. She received an intramuscular injection of an anti-inflammatory agent as well as a one-week course of etoricoxib 90 mg daily with good control of her symptoms.

On arrival at the Emergency Department, her blood pressure was 95/60 mmHg, heart rate 105/min, and oxygen saturation 100% on room air.

Question 1A: What targeted physical examination should be performed expeditiously?

Physical examination must include an accurate assessment of her fluid status given the history of poor appetite and vomiting. For an older person with hypertension, her blood pressure is low and she is tachycardic, suggesting a hypovolemic state. Note, however, that it may be difficult to diagnose hypovolaemia in the elderly because the clinical signs of dehydration such as skin turgor and dry tongue (especially in mouth-breathers) may not be reliable. A malnourished patient with hypoalbuminaemia may be oedematous, which makes assessment more challenging.

****

Preliminary investigations showed:

WBC count	*13.0 x 10⁹/L*	*(4–10)*
Haemoglobin	*9 g/dL*	*(12–16)*
Platelet count	*110 x10⁹/L*	*(140–440)*

Urea	*30 mmol/L*	*(2.7–6.9)*
Sodium	*144 mmol/L*	*(136–146)*
Potassium	*5.0 mmol/L*	*(3.5–5.1)*
Chloride	*104 mmol/L*	*(98–107)*
Bicarbonate	*18.7 mmol/L*	*(19–29)*
Creatinine	*400 μmol/L*	*(45–84)*
Urinalysis	*RBC 135/UL, WBC 1360/UL, epithelial cells 18/UL, granular casts seen.*	

From the records, her creatinine result was 180 μmol/L three months ago.

Question 1B: What additional physical examination would you like to perform?

Question 2: Identify the contributing causes for Mdm T's current presentation.

Question 3: Propose an initial management plan for Mdm T.

An abdominal examination must be performed to identify presence of a suprapubic mass or dullness which would suggest urinary retention and a post-renal cause of acute kidney injury (AKI).

Bear in mind the need for urgent renal replacement in patients with uraemic complications — so check for pericardial rub, pulmonary oedema, Kussmaul breathing, uraemic flap and altered mental status.

Mdm T has acute kidney injury (AKI) based on creatinine increase >1.5× her baseline. Universal definition and staging of AKI are essential for standardisation of reporting of AKI in epidemiologic and outcome studies. We are using kidney disease: Improving Global Outcome (KDIGO) staging system (Table 22.1).

Table 22.1. Definition of AKI as per KDIGO guideline.

Stage	Serum creatinine	Urine output
I	↑ by **1.5**–1.9x from baseline (known or presumed to have occurred within prior 7 days) ↑ by ≥26.5 μmol/L (within 48 hours)	**≤0.5 mL/kg/hour ≥6**–12 hours
II	↑ by 2.0–2.9x from baseline	≤0.5 mL/kg/hour ≥12 hours
III	↑ >3.0x from baseline, or ≥353.6 μmol/L; or Requiring renal replacement therapy	≤0.3 mL/kg/hour ≥24 hours; or anuria ≥12 hours

Note: For staging purposes, patients should be staged according to the criteria that give them the highest stage.

The elderly with ageing kidneys usually have low kidney reserves. Any insult may precipitate a frank kidney injury. AKI in the elderly is ***often iatrogenic and multifactorial*** although the spectrum of the causes of AKI is similar to the general population. Mdm T is likely to have an inter-current illness with a urinary tract infection which resulted in poor oral intake and dehydration (pre-renal cause of AKI is common!). Moreover, she is also taking an ACE inhibitor, and two diuretics, with recent addition of a COX-2 inhibitor. Of note, risk factors for NSAID-induced AKI include chronic kidney disease (CKD), volume depletion from aggressive diuresis, and reduced effective arterial volume from heart failure or nephrotic syndrome.

It is also essential to entertain the possibility of a gastrointestinal (GI) bleed in this scenario: an elderly patient presenting with malaise and lethargy, hypotension, usage of anticoagulant (warfarin), recent exposure to NSAIDs/COX-2 inhibitor and anaemia (do not assume anaemia is from chronic illness!). GI bleed is a common medical and surgical emergency and is often treatable.

Risk factors of AKI in the elderly:

— *Diabetes mellitus*
— *Atherosclerotic cardiovascular disease*
— *Pre-existing CKD*
— *Renal hypoperfusion (sodium depletion, volume depletion, diuretic use, cirrhosis, congestive cardiac failure, hypotension)*
— *Drugs (NSAID, COX-2 inhibitor, ACE inhibitor, ARB, contrast etc.)*

It is very important to identify a change in a patient's routine prescription which may trigger an episode of acute kidney injury. Hence a thorough medication review is essential — this must include all prescription drugs (from public and private practitioners), over-the-counter medications, traditional medications and supplements. NSAIDs and COX-2 inhibitors are commonly prescribed in primary care for pain relief. When used alongside ACE inhibitors or angiotensin-II receptor blockers (ARB), the NSAID can induce a haemodynamically mediated AKI, the risk being highest within the first 30 days of therapy.

Prostaglandins (PG) play a significant role in modulating renal blood flow (RBF) and glomerular filtrate rate (GFR) by their vasodilatory effect. Increase in PG synthesis to preserve RBF is seen in subjects with CKD (eGFR < 60 ml/min), volume depletion (reduced effective arterial volume) and in the elderly. NSAIDs inhibit cyclooxygenase (COX) enzymes with subsequent reduction in PG synthesis. NSAID-induced inhibition of PG-mediated afferent vasodilation and reduction in peritubular blood flow may also increase the risk for ischaemic acute tubular necrosis (ATN) especially when used alongside other nephrotoxins such as aminoglycosides, amphotericin B and radiocontrast material. Furthermore, inhibition of PG results in sodium retention which exacerbates hypertension and causes peripheral oedema. It also reduces secretion of aldosterone producing a picture of Type 4 Renal Tubular Acidosis.

Hypotensive patients must be haemodynamically stabilised as soon as possible. If renal hypoperfusion is not reversed quickly, ATN sets in. Traditional urinary markers to differentiate pre-renal from intrinsic ATN may be difficult as they may reflect age-related disturbances in tubular handling of sodium and water as well as drug effects (diuretic). As a general guide, aim to keep mean arterial pressure above 65 mmHg. Antihypertensive medications should be suspended. Fluid resuscitation may predispose the elderly patient to inevitable complications of salt and water retention. Furthermore, in the elderly, fluid overload may set in more quickly and take longer time to resolve. Hence fluid status needs to be closely monitored — consider inserting an indwelling urinary catheter for strict input/output monitoring. Intravenous fluids should be withdrawn during stabilisation and de-escalation phases, while ensuring that urine output is adequate and there are no signs of hypoperfusion. Monitor renal function daily or more often as necessary.

Evaluate and ameliorate any reversible causes of the AKI. Appropriate antibiotic(s) should be started early (within one hour) upon recognition of sepsis. Urinary retention should be urgently relieved with catheterisation. Regular bowel clearance should be ensured if that may contributing to urinary retention. The indications and doses of possible nephrotoxic medications must be evaluated:

- Stop NSAIDs or COX-2 inhibitors
- Consider stopping diuretics
- Consider stopping metformin, SGLT-2 inhibitor (empagliflozin, dapagliflozin), ACE inhibitor, ARB during intercurrent illness
- Consider stopping extraneous potassium supplements
- Consider dose adjustment for antibiotics and anticoagulants
- Re-evaluate indication for use of radio-iodinated contrast and consider alternative imaging technique if possible

Life-threatening emergencies related to AKI should also be concurrently managed:

1. Hyperkalaemia. Patients with electrocardiographic changes should be placed on cardiac monitoring (consider admission to high-dependency unit) and treated with intravenous calcium gluconate 10% 10 ml slow bolus.
   a. Induce translocation of potassium:

i. Intravenous Actrapid 10 IU (in insulin syringe) with IV dextrose 50% 40 ml is generally recommended, but in the setting of AKI or CKD, consider attenuating the dose of Actrapid to 6–8 IU to reduce risk of hypoglycaemia. Monitor capillary blood glucose regularly. This "hyperkalaemia kit" may reduce serum potassium by approximately 1 mmol/L, but without excretion of potassium through the gastrointestinal route, renally or by dialysis, the serum potassium is likely to rebound.
ii. Intravenous sodium bicarbonate 8.4% 50–100 ml over 30–60 minutes may be considered as an adjunctive treatment especially in patients with metabolic acidosis.
iii. β2-adrenergic agonists e.g., salbutamol by metered dose inhalation 4 puffs stat may also be considered as an adjunctive treatment but be careful in the elderly as it can induce arrythmia/angina in susceptible individuals

b. Induce excretion of potassium:
i. PO sodium zirconium 10 g ($20 per sachet) stat and TDS. Mean reduction of 0.37 mmol/L of potassium level within four hours of administration is expected.
ii. PO Resonium® A 15 g (sodium polystyrene sulfonate 15/60 ml, $0.17 per ml) stat and QDS. An uncommon serious side-effect is bowel necrosis, hence nowadays zirconium is preferred.
iii. Supp Resonium® A 30 g (sodium polystyrene sulfonate 30 g/120 ml, $29.53 per enema) stat may also be considered for those who cannot take orally
iv. Loop diuretics e.g., furosemide can be useful in patients whose kidney function is not severely impaired.
v. Haemodialysis should be considered in refractory or rapidly rising hyperkalaemia.

2. Metabolic acidosis. The underlying cause must be evaluated so that it can be expeditiously treated. In an elderly patient with high anion gap metabolic acidosis, consider lactic acidosis in the setting of haemodynamic instability (type A) or association with metformin in the absence of haemodynamic instability (type B), ketoacidosis, and salicylate poisoning (in the presence of osmolal gap). Intermittent sodium bicarbonate infusions may be considered.

3. Fluid overload.

a. Ensure adequate dose of diuretic. In diuretic-naïve patients, consider intravenous furosemide 80 mg OD-BD to improve bioavailability, while patients who were on diuretic prior to the onset of AKI should receive a dose that is at least double of their usual dose. This can be escalated up to 600 mg per day as necessary (note: high dose of furosemide may result in sudden onset of sensorineural hearing loss which is usually reversible but can be permanent. Consider slow bolus when furosemide dose exceeds 80 mg).

b. Consider albumin with furosemide. Furosemide is bound to albumin for circulation. In hypoalbuminaemic states, there is reduced albumin bound furosemide to be delivered to the thick ascending loop of Henle. Salt-free albumin 20% is used in this setting.

Indications for urgent dialysis:

1. Hyperkaelaemia (K >6 mmol/L OR rapidly rising) despite medical treatment with or without ECG changes
2. Acidaemia (pH <7.15) with pure metabolic acidosis
3. Pulmonary oedema with severe hypoxaemia (FiO_2 >0.5, P/F ratio <300) refractory to medical treatment
4. Uraemic complications (altered mental state, pericardial rub) with serum urea >40 mmol/L
5. Certain alcohol and drug intoxications

Key messages

1. Multiple aetiologies are often operative in the development of AKI in the elderly, and certain causes of AKI are particularly common: post-renal obstructive disease especially in males with BPH, ischaemic ATN, and haemodynamically mediated AKI (NSAIDS, COX-2 inhibitor, ACEi/ARB).
2. Diagnostic and therapeutic issues in AKI are no different for the elderly patient as for the general population.
3. Unfortunately, the outlook for renal recovery is likely impaired in the elderly patient. Hence, prevention (judicious prescribing practices, risk factor control, good bowel clearance) is always prudent.

Answer key

1. A. Assessment of fluid status (vital signs, skin and tissue turgor, mucosal membranes; lung crackles).
1. B. Examine for palpable bladder (post-renal cause of AKI);

   Uraemic complications e.g., pericardial rub, altered mental state (need for urgent renal replacement therapy).

2. Pre-renal: poor oral intake and dehydration due to urinary tract infection and diuresis from furosemide and spironolactone. When used alongside diuretics, SGLT-ii inhibitors (empagliflozin/dapagliflozin) may result in pronounced hypovolaemia (note: they may also predispose to urinary tract infection).

   Renal: recent NSAID / COX-2 inhibitor intake; pre-existing chronic kidney disease.

3. Fluid resuscitation;

   Suspend enalapril, furosemide, spironolactone;

   BP and input/output monitoring with urinary catheterization;

   Daily renal panel monitoring;

   Electrocardiogram (hyperkalaemic changes include tall peaked T waves, short QTc, prolonged PR intervals, widened QRS complexes as well as ventricular tachyarrhymias);

   Treat urinary sepsis empirically with intravenous ceftriaxone (Mdm T's urine culture eventually returned as *Escherichia coli* sensitive to ampicillin, cefazolin, ceftriaxone, aztreonam, ertapenem, amikacin);

   Zirconium 10g TDS.

Reference

Anderson S, Eldadah B, Halter JB, *et al.* (2011) Acute kidney injury in older adults. *JASN* **22**: 28–38.

23 End-Stage Kidney Disease

Yeoh Lee Ying, Anupama Roy Chowdhury

Mr G is an 82-year-old man who was admitted for non-vertiginous giddiness. The giddiness had occurred on and off over the past week and is worse when getting up as well as on turning his head. He also felt tired easily and had reduced effort tolerance. Otherwise he had no chest pain, palpitations, fever, or acute respiratory symptoms. His appetite, which has generally been poor, was associated with nausea, constipation, and a sensation of abdominal bloating. He also had skin itch and insomnia.

His active medical problems are hypertension and moderate to severe aortic stenosis with preserved ventricular ejection fraction 61% for which he had opted for conservative management. He also has progressive chronic kidney disease (CKD) stage 5 likely secondary to hypertensive nephrosclerosis. Past medical history includes ischaemic stroke in 2011 with residual left ataxic hemiparesis and left hip intertrochanteric fracture after a fall with hip fixation in 2018.

His medications are amlodipine 2.5 mg OM, frusemide 40 mg OM, Sangobion (ferrous gluconate compound) 1 cap OM, aspirin 100 mg OM, omeprazole 20 mg OM, sodium bicarbonate 500 mg OM, calcium acetate 1334 mg TDS with meal, Senna (Sennosides) 2 tab ON, and SC Mircera [Epoeitin β-(methoxyl polyethylene glycol)] 100 mcg per month.

Mr G stays with his wife and daughter. He is independent in his basic activities of daily living, ambulating with a quad stick at home and using a wheelchair in the community.

On clinical examination, vital signs were supine blood pressure 174/85 mmHg, standing blood pressure 144/75, and heart rate 80/min, regular. He had mild pallor. There was no asterixis or pedal oedema. Jugular venous pressure was flat. An ejection systolic murmur was heard over the aortic region which radiated to the carotids. Lungs and abdominal examination was unremarkable. Neurological examination showed left upper motor neuron lesion of CN VII. No pronator drift was seen, but the muscle power for left lower limb was 4 (static since the stroke). No cerebellar signs were elicited.

Renal panel (comparing the results from the past few clinic visits).

Date	5/4/21	12/7/21	6/9/21	8/11/21
Urea (mmol/L)	*17.5*	*32.5*	*29*	*35.3*
Sodium (mmol/L)	*134*	*139*	*135*	*136*
Potassium (mmol/L)	*4.5*	*5.5*	*4.8*	*5.3*
Chloride (mmol/L)	*102*	*104*	*102*	*100*
Bicarbonate (mmol/L)	*22.4*	*22.1*	*20.9*	*21.3*
Creatinine (μmol/L)	*415*	*618*	*649*	*768*
CKD-EPI eGFR (mL/min)	*11*	*7*	*6*	*5*

Full blood count:

Hb 8.9 g/dL (12.0–16.0), MCV 96.4 fL (78.0–98.0), MCH 31.9 pg (27.0–32.0), MCHC 33.1 g/dL (32.0–36.0); WBC 4.3 x 10^9/L (4.00–10.00); platelet count 207 x 10^9/L (140–440).

Iron study:

Iron 10 μmol/L (8–32), ferritin 620 μg/L (13.0–150.0), Transferrin saturation 24% (≤50).

Bone mineral metabolism:

Corrected calcium 2.15 mmol/L (2.09–2.46), phosphate 2.15 mmol/L (0.94–1.50), serum albumin 31 g/L (40–51).

ECG: *Sinus rhythm, rate 60/min, left ventricular hypertrophy by voltage criteria.*
CXR: *Mild pulmonary venous congestion, mild blunting of left costophrenic angle.*
AXR: *Faecal loading in the colon.*

Question 1: What are the clinical benefits of kidney replacement therapy (KRT) for Mr G?

It is important to distinguish whether the symptoms that Mr G is experiencing are predominantly from:

(a) end-stage kidney disease (ESKD)
(b) ageing and frailty
(c) progression from the comorbidities (i.e., aortic stenosis)

Determine whether these symptoms are gradual or acute in onset. A more rapid GFR decline is associated with increasing symptom number and severity; always look for any reversible precipitating events. Conversely, most patients may adapt with gradual decline in GFR till ~6 to 8 mL/min/1.73 m^2 unless the patient has other concomitant illnesses such as congestive heart failure.

There are overlapping symptom burdens from ESKD and comorbidities in elderly patients. Recognising the kidney-specific versus general symptoms is crucial in order to address underlying issues as kidney replacement therapy alone will not reverse ageing or frailty and comorbidities. The interplay of aetiologic factors and Mr G's symptomatology is summarised in this diagram.

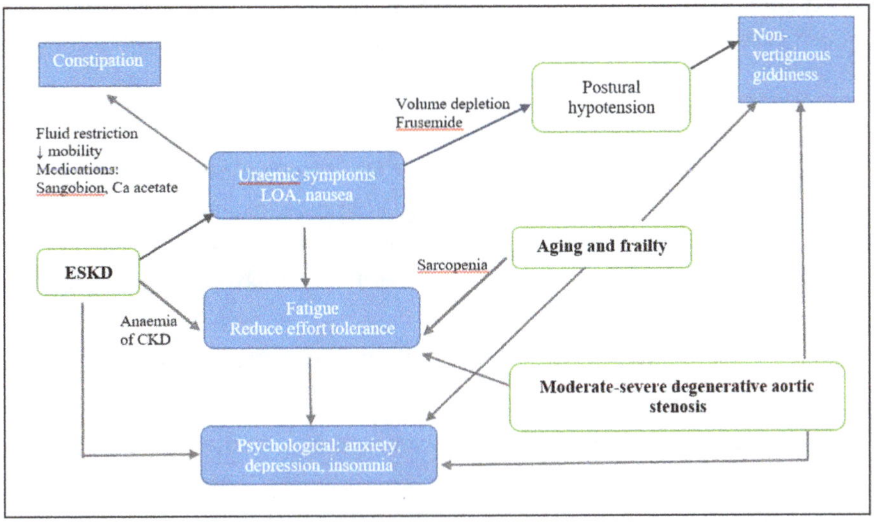

Kidney replacement therapy may ameliorate uraemic symptoms (e.g., poor appetite, nausea) and have some effect on other symptoms like fatigue and pruritus. However, the overall symptom burden is still substantial.

****

Question 2: What are your considerations when deciding on kidney replacement therapy (KRT) for Mr G?

Managing elderly ESKD patients and discussing treatment options (Table 23.1) is not just about dialysis or no dialysis. Debating the quantity or quality of life from the patient's perspective is of paramount importance. The decision can fluctuate from time to time depending on the patient's symptoms, experiences, encounters, and involvement of the family.

Table 23.1. Domains for Consideration of Kidney Replacement Therapy.

Objective	**Subjective**
Progressive versus reversible Extent of disease and comorbidities Complications from disease Cognitive and physical function Nutritional status Frailty	Emotional well-being Life style and coping Adherence to diet, medication, treatment Tolerable treatment burden or trade off
Treatment Options Pros and cons in each option Expected versus acceptable outcome Goals of care, preference and values	**Contextual** Home setting Family support versus dynamic Decisional congruence versus conflicts Care delivery

Most patients would like to know their life expectancy. Based on Singapore statistics in 2020, the life expectancy for males is 81.5 years and females is 86.1 years. A comparative analysis by Verberne WR, *et al.* in 2016 revealed that patients aged 80 and above or with multiple comorbidities did not have a survival advantage with dialysis compared to receiving supportive care.

Table 23.2 illustrates the common practical issues surrounding the options

Table 23.2. Kidney replacement options in end-stage kidney disease.

Long-term management options for end-stage kidney disease	**Haemodialysis (HD)**	**Peritoneal dialysis (PD)** **APD = automated peritoneal dialysis** **CAPD = continuous ambulatory peritoneal dialysis**	**Kidney supportive care**
Treatment			
Location	Dialysis centre	Home	Home
Manpower	Dialysis nurse	Family or caregiver	Palliative care or home hospice if life expectancy is less than 12 months
Schedule	Fixed	Flexible	According to the needs
Access	Tunneled dialysis catheter, arterio-venous fistula/graft	Peritoneal dialysis catheter	N/A

Table 23.2 *(Continued)*

Considerations in the elderly patient			
Physical	Mobility and travel to dialysis centre	Manual dexterity to perform the exchanges; Eyesight; Hearing — alarm from APD machine	N/A
Treatment burden	Sits on recliner for ~4 hours, 3x per week	Sleeps throughout night for APD ~8–10 hours/day; Perform 3 to 4 exchanges per day for CAPD; Storage space for dialysis solutions	Medication titration for symptom control
Dialysis-related complications			
Process	Hypotension on dialysis; Post-dialysis fatigue	Abdominal fullness from the dialysate; Metabolic effect, i.e., hyperglyceamia, hypertriglyceridaemia	N/A
Access site	Intervention for vascular access malfunction (stenosis, thrombosis); Access site-related infection	Intervention for PD catheter malfunction (block, migration); Peritonitis and exit site infection	

With the above considerations in mind, the managing physician should try to know Mr G as a ***person*** (Figure 23.3) so as to work through with him a plan that fits him the best:

1. What are the things that are important to him? [**Value**]
2. What are the expected versus acceptable outcomes? [**Preference**]
3. How much burden is Mr G willing to tolerate to achieve the goal versus what he wishes to avoid in pursuit of the goal? [**Goals**]
4. What are his worries or concerns at present and for the future?
5. What are the challenges for him and his family?

Should the patient opt for dialysis, it is important to explore a time- or event-limited trial of KRT weighing the treatment burden versus benefit.

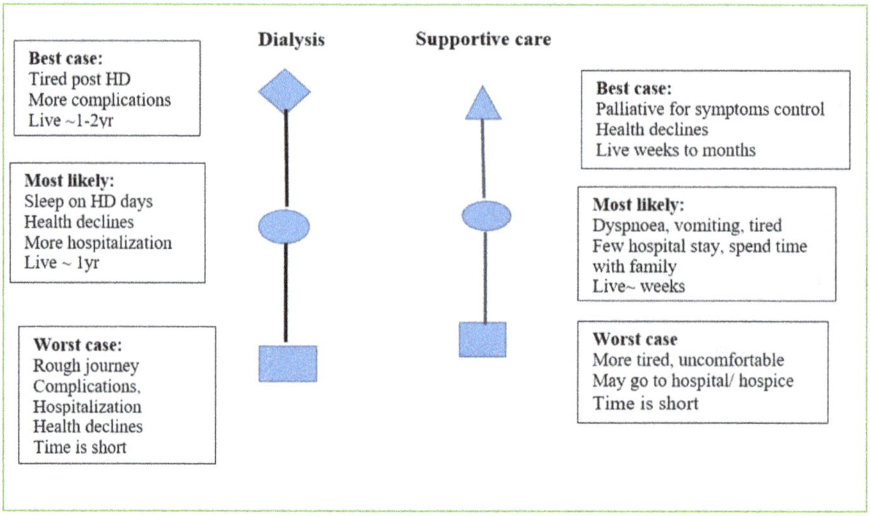

Fig. 23.3. Management Considerations in an Older Adult with End-stage Kidney Disease.

Advance care planning is important in order to elicit the patient's preferences as part of anticipatory care. These aspects are what he would consider in the event that he has serious complications with

(a) low chance of survival (e.g., 5 out of 100 patients will live)?
(b) loss of ability to move around or communicate (e.g., requiring 24-hour nursing care)?
(c) mental incapacity (e.g., he would never know who he is and require 24-hour nursing care)?

In such situations and in line with the patient's preferences, due consideration should be given for supportive care as the burden of KRT would likely outweigh its benefit.

****

After lengthy discussions with his family, Mr G decided to pursue conservative management for his ESKD. Of note, he was particularly irritated by the constant itch on his skin. Except for mild dryness, clinical examination failed to reveal any other primary dermatosis to account for the pruritus.

Question 3: Which of the following is the most appropriate management of his pruritus?

a. Calamine lotion TDS/PRN
b. Long warm bath soaks at bedtime
c. Oral hydroxyzine 10, 10, 25 mg
d. Topical betamethasone dipropionate 0.05% cream BD/PRN
e. Urea 10% cream BD

The essential principles of management of a patient who prefers kidney supportive therapy (non-dialysis) are as follows:

1. Identify and treat reversible causes. Address the biopsychosocial and spiritual perspectives.
2. Preserve kidney function (control risk factors, avoid nephrotoxic agents).
3. Consider non-pharmacological measures besides medication.
4. Modify medication regimens that require renal clearance. Start low, go slow, monitor treatment response, and be cautious with drug interactions and adverse effects.
5. Establish the acceptable and tolerable symptoms as symptoms can be relieved but **not** eradicated as kidney function declines.
6. Anticipatory care.

Table 23.4 shows some management tips for symptom control for Mr G

Table 23.4. Palliative management in end-stage kidney disease.

	Options		
Symptoms	**Non-pharmacological**	**Pharmacological**	**Considerations**
Reduced appetite, nausea	Treat constipation; Small, regular meals; Trial of ginger, lime/lemon/peppermint sweets; Avoid strong odours	Metoclopramide 10 mg TDS/PRN; Domperidone 10 mg TDS/PRN; Ondansetron 4–8 mg BD/PRN; Haloperidol 0.5–1.5 mg ON	Avoid prokinetic agents (metoclopramide, domperidone) if there is bowel obstruction.

(Continued)

(*Continued*)

Symptoms	**Options**		**Considerations**
	Non-pharmacological	**Pharmacological**	
Constipation	Allowable fluid and fibre intake; Physical activity (as tolerated)	Lactulose (max 60 mL/d); Sennosides 7.5 mg (max 4 tab BD); Bisacodyl (max 15 mg/d); Macrogol 4,000 oral powder BD; Sodium chloride enema (Centa enema) 20–40 mL PRN	Exclude bowel obstruction; Avoid sodium phosphate enema (fleet enema) (electrolyte derangement); Ispaghula husk (Fybogel) needs adequate fluid intake to work.
Pruritus	Cool environment; Keep skin hydrated (avoid hot baths/ excessive bathing); Adequate use of moisturisers (≥200 g/wk); Cold compresses PRN; Avoid skin irritants (harsh soaps, synthetic textiles like polyester or nylon clothing, keep finger nails short)	Topical: hydrocortisone 1% cream BD/PRN (mild), betamethasone ***valerate*** 0.1% cream BD/PRN (moderate); Gabapentin 100 mg ON (max 300 mg)/ pregabalin 25 mg ON (max 75 mg); Sertraline 25 mg ON/ mirtazapine 7.5–15 mg ON if concomitant depression	Look carefully for a primary dermatosis that may be reversible; Exclude allergic reactions; Avoid calamine lotions (as they can drying) and excessive prolonged use of topical corticosteroid; Consider dermatologist consult if there are underlying skin conditions; Be careful of older generation antihistamines such as hydroxyzine/ chlorpheniramine as they can often cause daytime drowsiness and may cause confusion and delirium particularly in the older patient due to their anticholinergic effect.

(*Continued*)

Symptoms	Options		Considerations
	Non-pharmacological	**Pharmacological**	
Fluid overload (oedema, dyspnoea)	Restrict salt and fluid; Sit upright ± lean forward (hands or forearms resting on thighs); Place fan (stationery or handheld) near face; ± oxygen supplementation for comfort; Endorphin-releasing techniques, e.g., massage, listening to music, meditation and controlled breathing exercises (mindful breathing or pursed-lips breathing)	Frusemide (up to 30 mg/hr, max 600 mg/d): IV bolus or infusion in inpatient setting OR PO frusemide (bioavailability 50%) ± PO metolazone 2.5–5 mg OM (up to 20 mg/d) IV/SC Fentanyl infusion (start at 5 mcg/hr and 10 mcg Q1H/PRN for breakthrough) if need titration for symptoms control. Once stable dose has been determined, consider transdermal fentanyl (patch formulations are 12 mcg/hr, 25 mcg/hr and 50 mcg/hr; can start at 6 mcg/hr) PO Lorazepam 0.5 mg ON (if there is anxiety)	Address dry mouth (oral care, avoid anticholinergic agent); Avoid high-dose morphine as the active metabolites accumulate in ESKD.

Key messages

1. Dialysis should not be the default treatment for elderly end-stage kidney disease (ESKD) patients.
2. Know the patient as a person from a medical perspective and align with the patient's preferences, values, and goals of care to derive an individualised treatment plan (shared decision-making).
3. Kidney supportive care is one of the treatment options for geriatric ESKD patients in order to maintain their quality of life and relieve their symptoms burden. The decision centres on balancing the benefits, risks, and trade-offs in the patients' care.

Answer key

1. KRT will help with his appetite loss and nausea, and possibly reduce fatigue and pruritus.
2. Before initiating KRT, it would be prudent to consider the following factors:
   - Biological age and life expectancy — At 82 years of age, Mr G has already surpassed his life expectancy (based on Singapore statistics in 2020). Furthermore, dialysis has not been shown to confer a survival advantage over conservative management for his age.
   - Cognitive, functional, emotional, and physical well-being — frequent travels to the dialysis centre may pose an inconvenience for him and his caregiver as he requires assistance. He also encounters the risk of hypotension during haemodialysis due to moderately severe aortic stenosis, as well as post-dialysis fatigue.
   - Concomitant morbidities and prognosis — dialysis has not been shown to confer a survival advantage over conservative management in view of his multiple comorbidities.
   - Nutritional status and frailty.
   - Patient's preferences and values.
   - Social support.
3. E.

References

Burns RB, *et al.* (2020) Management Options for an Older Adult With Advanced Chronic Kidney Disease and Dementia. *Ann Intern Med* **173**: 217–225.

Gelfand SM, *et al.* (2020) Kidney Supportive Care: Core Curriculum 2020. *Am J Kidney Dis* **75**: 793–806.

Verberne WR, *et al.* (2016) Comparative Survival among Older Adults with Advanced Kidney Disease Managed Conservatively Versus with Dialysis. *Clin J Am Soc Nephrol* **11**: 633–640.

24 Polyuric Syndrome

Cai Jiashen, Lalmalani Roshan Mahesh

Mr P is a 70-year-old man with a background of hypertension, hyperlipidemia, diabetes mellitus, and ischaemic cardiomyopathy presenting with an accidental fall. He had gotten up to urinate at night and encountered a wet floor in the toilet. He denies any head injury and was able to ambulate independently subsequently. He reports poor sleep with a two-year history of waking up to urinate, which is increasingly frequent from once to up to four times per night. He denies passing urine more often in the day and does not have any dysuria, haematuria, foul-smelling urine, or fever. He denies any involuntary leakage of urine or interruptions in urinary flow during micturition.

Question 1: What lower urinary tract symptom does the patient have?

The approach to a patient with lower urinary tract symptoms begins with correct identification of the problem (Table 24.1).

Table 24.1. Differentiating the lower urinary tract symptom.

Lower urinary tract symptom	Clinical presentation	Clinical interpretation
Hesitancy	Difficulty in initiating micturition resulting in a delay in the onset of voiding after the individual is ready to pass urine.	Bladder outlet obstruction, nervous system disorder (drug-induced or spinal/central), or psychological cause.
Incontinence (urinary)	Involuntary leakage of urine.	One or a mixture of: (1) Stress (increased intra-abdominal pressure). (2) Urge (see below).

(*Continued*)

(Continued)

Lower urinary tract symptom	Clinical presentation	Clinical interpretation
		(3) Overflow (chronic urinary retention due to reduced detrusor contractility and/or bladder outlet obstruction). (4) Functional (due to physical or mental impairment slowing down the process to micturate).
Intermittency	The situation when urinary flow stops and starts on one or more occasions during micturition.	Bladder outlet obstruction.
Nocturia	Waking at night to pass urine.	A wide variety of urologic and non-urologic causes.
Urgency	Sudden compelling desire to pass urine.	Overactive bladder due to detrusor overactivity (neurologic disorders, bladder structural or microbiota abnormalities) or poor detrusor compliance (post radiotherapy or prolonged catheterisation).

Nocturia is an extremely prevalent but under-reported condition, affecting 70–90% in the older population (≥70 years old). Although often neglected and often wrongly considered as part of normal ageing, nocturia warrants attention as it may be associated with serious underlying conditions and it affects patients' sleep, quality of life, mood, and fall risk amongst others.

When assessing a patient with nocturia, do take a history of falls and near falls. In addition, a complete falls risk assessment should be done with emphasis on:

- Vision (a patient with already compromised vision may suffer even more at night)

- Home environment (location of light switches, distance of room from bathroom, availability of urinals/commode, hazards such as kerbs, and home modifications such as grab bars and anti-slip mats)
- Footwear and walking aid assessment
- Postural blood pressure (some elderly people tend to stand up really fast to pass urine and their pre-existing postural hypotension is a recipe for a fall)
- Review of bone health (in particular due to risk of falls)

****

Further history revealed that Mr P takes around 4–5 cups of fluids a day. His systolic blood pressure at home ranges between 120 and 130 mmHg. His pre-breakfast capillary blood glucose level is 5–7 mmol/L. He reports poor sleep and wakes up to urinate 3 times per night, which is associated with increased day-time lethargy. He often dozes off while watching television. His partner has also noted episodes whereby he would stop breathing at times while asleep. His chronic medications include lisinopril 5 mg OM, bisoprolol 2.5 mg OM, simvastatin 20 mg ON, and furosemide 40 mg BD.

A bladder voiding diary was completed by Mr P as shown below:

Daytime		**Nighttime**	
Time	**Voided volume (mL)**	**Time**	**Voided volume (mL)**
Waking up 07:00 am	100	*Falling asleep* 10:30 pm	
09:30 am	150	00:30 am	150
12:00 am	100	02:00 am	200
03:30 pm	175	04:45 am	150
07:00 pm	100	Waking up 07:00 am	
10:00 pm	125		

Question 2: What is the MOST likely clinical syndrome?

It is important to distinguish between the three types of polyuric syndromes as they help in differential diagnosis (Table 24.2)

Table 24.2. Differentiating the polyuric syndrome.

Polyuric syndrome	Clinical definition	Clinical interpretation
Global polyuria	Increase in 24-hour urine volume of >40 mL/kg, representing excessive urine production during both the day and night.	Primary polydipsia, poorly controlled diabetes mellitus, diabetes insipidus or medications.
Nocturnal polyuria	Alteration in the usual day to night ratio of urine production, whereby >33% of total daily urine output occurs at night, although the total daily urine output remains normal.	Third-space fluid accumulation due to cardiac, renal, or hepatic causes, obstructive sleep apnea, loss of circadian control of urine output due to neurological impairment, or inappropriate timing of medications (especially ***diuretics***!).
Bladder storage disorders	Reduced voided volume, indicating a reduced capacity of the bladder to store urine, which may occur exclusively during the hours of sleep or globally.	Lower urinary tract pathology that affects the reservoir capacity of bladder storage such as bladder outflow obstruction (benign prostatic hyperplasia, neoplastic lesions), overactive bladder syndrome, cystitis, and neurogenic bladder dysfunction. Others may include medications with direct lower urinary tract effects.

The patient's medication list should be scrutinised as many drugs can potentially contribute to nocturia through one of three mechanisms:

A. Increased urine output

Diuretics
SSRIs
Calcium channel blockers
Tetracycline
Lithium

B. Insomnia and CNS effects

CNS stimulants (methylphenidate)
Antihypertensives (***α-blockers, β-blockers, methyldopa***)
Respiratory (albuterol, theophylline)

Decongestants (***phenylephrine***, ***pseudoephedrine***)
Hormones (corticosteroids, thyroxine)
Psychotropics (MAOIs, SSRIs, atypical antidepressants)
Dopaminergic agonists (carbidopa)
Anti-epileptics (phenytoin)

C. Direct lower urinary tract effects

Ketamine
Cyclophosphamide

It is not easy to get an accurate bladder diary from an elderly patient, especially from one with impaired cognition. A well-documented bladder diary is an invaluable resource in the assessment of urinary symptoms such as frequency, nocturia, and polyuria. Educating the caregivers and getting them to buy into the seriousness of the issue will result in better compliance and a more informative bladder diary. Ideally in addition to void timings and urinary volumes, the bladder diary should also include the timing and intake of fluids (and type of fluids) recorded over 48 hours if possible. Episodes of incontinence may additionally be documented.

****

Clinical examination revealed a grossly overweight (BMI 32.1 kg/m^2) man with mild lower limb oedema to the mid-shin. Cardiorespiratory examination revealed apex beat displaced to the 7th intercostal space 2 cm lateral to the midclavicular line, as well as very scant basal crepitations. There was no palpable bladder, and digital rectal examination revealed a one finger breadth smooth prostate. His vital signs showed blood pressure 130/70 mmHg, pulse rate 98/min, and oxygen saturation 95% on room air.

Investigations are as follows:

Haemoglobin	*18.6 g/dL*	*(14.0–18.0)*
WBC Count	*8.6 x10^9/L*	*(4.0–10.0)*
Platelet Count	*383 x10^9/L*	*(140–440)*
HbA1c	*6.6%*	*(4.6–6.4)*
Creatinine	*86 μmol/L*	*(60–104)*

Urine RBC 0/μL (0–4), WBC 0/μL (0–6), epithelial cell 2/μL (0–4)

Question 3: What are the most likely underlying causes of Mr P's symptoms?

Question 4: Propose an appropriate initial management plan for Mr P.

Mr P has predominant nocturia with no increase in daytime urinary frequency. The bladder diary reveals that this is actually nocturnal polyuria. He has risk factors to suggest obstructive sleep apnoea (OSA) viz. male gender, older age, obesity, hypertension, diabetes, daytime somnolence, and polycythemia. A useful screening tool for OSA is the STOP-BANG (Table 24.3) score which is also accessible via this link :

A STOP-BANG score of at least 5 points (age, gender, hypertension, apnoeic episodes, and daytime somnolence) suggests that the patient is at high risk of OSA and should be evaluated with a polysomnogram, the gold standard diagnostic investigation.

Third-space fluid accumulation due to congestive cardiac failure can lead to nocturnal polyuria due to a return of fluid to the intravascular compartment when in recumbent position. The evening time dose of diuretic can further contribute to this as well.

In this case, hypertension and diabetes mellitus are well controlled and unlikely to contribute to nocturia. Mr P also does not have a history of voiding or storage lower urinary tract symptoms to suggest benign prostatic hyperplasia or overactive bladder syndrome respectively, with an unremarkable prostate size on digital rectal examination. Note that chronic venous insufficiency is also associated with nocturnal polyuria, so this should be looked for in a physical examination.

Table 24.3. STOP-BANG scoring.

Snoring	Do you snore loudly (louder than talking or loud enough to be heard through closed doors)?
Tired	Do you often feel tired, fatigued, or sleepy during the daytime?
Observed	Has anyone observed you stop breathing during your sleep?
Blood **P**ressure	Are you being, or have been, treated for high blood pressure?
Body mass index	Is your body mass index >35 kg/m^2?
Age	Are you >50 years old?
Neck circumference	Is your neck circumference >40 cm?
Gender	Are you male?

Note: Score 1 point for each positive response. Low risk of OSA: <3. High risk of OSA: ≥ 5.

General non-pharmacological measures for managing nocturia include:

A. Reducing nocturnal urine output

- Reduction of overall fluid intake (especially if excessive) and specific reduction of evening intake
- Reduction in salt intake, particularly for those with congestive cardiac failure
- Reduction of evening consumption of diuretic fluids, including caffeine and alcohol
- Avoiding use of night-time diuretics (patients on twice-daily diuretics should consider moving night-time dose to mid-afternoon)
- Treatment of peripheral oedema by use of compression stockings or afternoon elevation of legs
- Avoidance of nocturnal hyperglycaemia in patients with diabetes
- Double voiding prior to bedtime in patients who feel that they have not completely emptied their bladder

B. Adjuncts

- Pelvic floor muscle exercise and urge-suppression strategies are useful in both women and men with nocturia
- Adopting good sleep hygiene can reduce episodes of night-time voiding
- Moderate daytime exercise has been associated with reduced episodes of nocturia

Medications or other interventions for nocturia include:

A. Addressing underlying medical causes viz.

- Congestive cardiac failure or peripheral edema — Optimisation of fluid status
- Poorly controlled diabetes mellitus — Optimisation of glycemic control
- OSA — Continuous positive airway pressure (CPAP) is the mainstay of therapy. It involves the maintenance of a positive pharyngeal transmural pressure so that the intraluminal pressure exceeds the surrounding pressure, thereby stabilising the upper airway. Oral appliances (e.g., mandibular advancement devices, tongue retaining devices) may be considered in patients who decline or fail to adhere to positive airway pressure therapy. Upper airway surgery can be considered when positive airway pressure or oral appliance is declined or ineffective after at least a three-month trial.

  Compliance with CPAP, however, is a continuous challenge in geriatric OSA patients. Additional measures such as weight loss, exercise, sleeping in a non-supine position, and alcohol avoidance may alleviate symptoms.

- Benign prostatic hyperplasia — Initial therapy with α-1-adrenergic antagonist to target the dynamic component of bladder outlet obstruction. Combination therapy with 5-α reductase inhibitor is superior to monotherapy, particularly in men with larger prostates.

B. Overactive bladder/detrusor hyperactivity: Bladder relaxant therapies including

i. Antimuscarinic agents
   - tolterodine 2 mg BD, $0.96 per pill, and can be reduced to 1 mg BD for maintenance — probably the most well tolerated of all;
   - solifenacin 5 mg OM, $0.53 per pill, can be increased to 10 mg OM but carries a higher rate of dry mouth;
   - oxybutynin 2.5 mg BD, $0.32 per pill, can be increased to 5 mg BD but may be limited by systemic side-effects; it also most easily crosses the blood-brain barrier.

   Antimuscarinics can cause side-effects such as dizziness, drowsiness, and cognitive impairment which may further increase fall risk. Agents such as oxybutynin may precipitate delirium. An agent that does not cross the blood brain barrier, such as trospium and darifenacin, may be useful in such cases. They are not widely available as yet.

ii. β-3 adrenergic agonists (mirabegron 25 mg OM, $3.09 per pill, can be increased to 50 mg OM if patient does not have severe renal disease or moderate liver impairment) may be a viable alternative for patients who cannot tolerate antimuscarinic agents. They reduce nocturia by increasing bladder capacity and decreasing urge-associated voids. Beware of the risk of urinary retention. Please check post-void residual urine while on treatment and avoid starting if there is significant post-void residual urine.

C. Others such as vaginal oestrogen therapy administered topically may be useful to reduce nocturia in postmenopausal women.

In patients with refractory nocturia despite the above-mentioned measures, desmopressin 0.1 mg taken prior to bedtime can reduce night-time free-water excretion due to its antidiuretic effect. Main contraindications relate to the risk of hyponatraemia and hence it is not commonly used in the older individual.

Key messages

1. Nocturia is a prevalent but under-recognised condition. It is important to elucidate the underlying aetiologies as they have serious effects on a patient's health and general well-being.
2. A bladder diary is an essential tool in differentiating various polyuric syndromes and aids in narrowing down the likely differentials.
3. Management of nocturia is often a multi-pronged approach involving initially lifestyle changes and addressing underlying medical conditions, followed by consideration of appropriate pharmacological measures.

Answer key

1. Nocturia
2. Based on the bladder diary, his 24-hr urine volume is 1,250 mL, with a nocturnal urine volume of 500 mL. The corresponding nocturnal polyuria index of 40% is consistent with nocturnal polyuria.
3. Obstructive sleep apnoea, congestive cardiac failure, medications.
4. Refer to respiratory physician for polysomnographic study to confirm OSA;

   Lifestyle changes including avoiding fluid intake at night, participating in moderate exercise, and elevating the legs in the afternoon;

   Pharmacologic adjustment — push timing of evening furosemide to mid-afternoon.

References

Gulur DM, Mevcha AM, Drake MJ (2011) Nocturia as a manifestation of systemic disease. *BJU Int* **107**(5): 702–713.

Hashim H, *et al.* (2019) International Continence Society (ICS) report on the terminology for nocturia and nocturnal lower urinary tract function. *Neurourol Urodyn* **38**(2): 499–508.

Kujubu DA, Aboseif SR (2008) An overview of nocturia and the syndrome of nocturnal polyuria in the elderly. *Nat Clin Pract Nephrol* **4**(8): 426–435.

Weiss JP, Everaert K (2019) Management of Nocturia and Nocturnal Polyuria. *Urology* **133S**: 24–33.

25 Chest Pain (Cardiogenic?)

Ibrahim Muhammad Hanif, Astrid Melani Suantio

Mdm C is a 78-year-old lady with a past medical history of hypertension, diabetes (HbA1c 6.7% two months ago), hyperlipidaemia, ischaemic heart disease (ejection fraction 60% three years ago), and chronic constipation. Her chronic medications are nifedipine-LA 30 mg OM, metformin 850 mg BD, atorvastatin 10 mg ON, aspirin 100 mg OM, and bisoprolol 1.25 mg OM. She presented to the Emergency Department for chest pain.

The chest pain could be localised to the left inframammary region and was described as stabbing in nature, with a pain score of 7 to 8 out of 10. It radiated to her left upper arm. The pain was unrelated to exertion or breathing. The pain was continuous over the last 24 to 36 hours with periods of waxing and waning. It was not relieved by paracetamol.

Her vital signs were blood pressure 138/88 mmHg, heart rate 78/min, respiratory rate 20/min, and SpO_2 99% on room air. Physical examination was unremarkable and pain was not reproducible on palpation or movement of the torso.

Question 1: What other clinical evaluation may be useful before ordering investigations?

In the elderly, the list of differential diagnoses of chest pain is wide. One approach is to think of the systems involved which may present as chest pain viz. cardiovascular, gastrointestinal, pulmonary, neurologic, or musculoskeletal systems. As the Singaporean population is very diverse in its ethnicity and language, obtaining a history from the patient may be best done in his/her best conversed language so as not to miss any significant history. It is also important to obtain a corroborative history from family members or caregivers who know the patient's condition best, especially in the setting of elderly with cognitive impairment. From this step, physical examination and targeted investigations help to rule out disorders which are immediately life-threatening, such as acute coronary syndrome, aortic dissection, pneumothorax, esophageal rupture, and pulmonary embolism.

Beware that the presentation of acute coronary syndrome (ACS) in the elderly may be unusual. Primary complaints of ACS in the elderly *without* chest pain include dyspnoea, diaphoresis, nausea and vomiting, syncope, weakness, and delirium. Furthermore, ACS may occur in the setting of a predominantly non-cardiac acute presentation such as exacerbation of chronic obstructive pulmonary disease, sepsis, pneumonia, or a fall! Eliciting a reproducible pain on palpation of the chest wall reduces the likelihood of ACS, but does not exclude it.

The elderly person with aortic dissection may not describe the classical "tearing" or "ripping" nature of chest pain — more often they report a "sharp" pain. In fact, they may sometimes present as migratory pain, syncope, or focal neurological deficits caused by a stroke from extension of the dissection into the carotid artery or by spinal cord ischaemia. Type A (involving ascending aorta) dissections are more likely to present with anterior chest pain while type B (involving descending aorta) dissections are more likely to present with back or abdominal pain.

The commonest symptom of pulmonary embolism is breathlessness at exertion and/or at rest. Pleuritic chest pain is less frequently reported in the elderly than in adults with pulmonary embolism and pneumothorax. In the elderly with decompensated chronic obstructive pulmonary disease or asthma, make sure pneumothorax is immediately ruled out!

Oesophageal rupture is rare but has high mortality and morbidity. The chest pain is abrupt, severe, ***worse with swallowing***, and often radiates to the neck, back, and shoulders. Vomiting and haematemesis may occur. Though frequently iatrogenic in origin, less common causes are spontaneous rupture (Boerhaave's syndrome — increased intra-abdominal pressure from vomiting), foreign body ingestion, and oesophageal tumours.

****

The ECG showed a normal sinus rhythm with no acute ischaemic changes. Chest radiograph did not show consolidation or free air under the diaphragm. The initial troponin level and at the six-hour mark were normal. The full blood count, liver, and renal panel were also normal.

Mdm C was admitted for monitoring. The pain intensity varied periodically over the night. The next day, the rounding team noted a few clusters of pustules on a red background over the left chest wall.

Question 2: What is an appropriate plan of management?

Preherpetic neuralgia is the prodromal stage of zoster which can last approximately three to five days. It can mimic a multitude of medical and surgical conditions depending on the location of the zoster reactivation and thus often poses a diagnostic challenge. For instance, it has been known to be mistaken for acute coronary syndrome (thoracic zoster), renal colic (lumbar zoster), and even migraine (cervical zoster).

****

Antiviral and analgesic treatment were commenced for Mdm C. Unfortunately, she fell while trying to go to the toilet that same night and sustained a pubic ramus fracture. The orthopaedics team recommended pain control and weight bearing as tolerated. The pain greatly limited her mobility, and she was planned for transfer to the community hospital for a period of inpatient rehabilitation with optimisation of pain control.

On the fifth day after the fall, Mdm C was noted to be persistently tachycardic. She also complained of vague chest discomfort at rest. Her vital signs were temperature 37.1°C, heart rate 110/min, blood pressure 125/80 mmHg, respiratory rate 18/min, and SpO_2 94% on room air.

Laboratory investigations were unremarkable for two sets of cardiac enzymes, full blood count, inflammatory markers, and renal panel with normal anion gap. Chest radiograph showed just minimal right-sided blunting of the costophrenic angle. Electrocardiogram showed sinus tachycardia with no other significant abnormality.

Arterial blood gas on room air is as follows:

pH	*7.50*	*(7.35–7.45)*
$PaCO_2$	*28 mmHg*	*(35–40)*
PaO_2	*90 mmHg*	*(80–100)*
HCO_3	*22 mEq/L*	*(22–26)*
SaO_2	*94%*	*(95–100)*

Question 3: What is your analysis and most appropriate immediate plan of action?

a. **Hospital-acquired chest infection; blood cultures and empirical broad-spectrum antibiotic**
b. **High-certainty pulmonary embolism; CT pulmonary angiogram and low-molecular weight heparin**
c. **Low-certainty pulmonary embolism; D-dimer level and Doppler ultrasound lower limb venous system**
d. **Myopericarditis; muscle enzymes and 2D-echocardiography**
e. **Occult sepsis; urinalysis and screen for pressure injury**

In elderly patients who are less mobile, it is good to always screen for complications of immobility syndrome (including chest/urine infections, constipation, retention of urine, pressure injuries on all pressure points [not just the sacral area], deep vein thrombosis, and pulmonary embolism) which can develop within a relatively short span of time.

If ordering a CT pulmonary angiogram (CTPA), ensure that the metformin is suspended and control the sugars with other oral agents or insulin. Monitor for the kidney function as the patient may already have underlying chronic kidney impairment with age which may worsen with contrast. Do discuss the contrast-induced nephrotoxicity (CIN) risk with the patient and family members prior to doing the CTPA. A useful free app for making this calculation is the CIN Risk Score Calculator developed by RenalGuard Solutions, Inc.

****

CT pulmonary angiogram was performed:

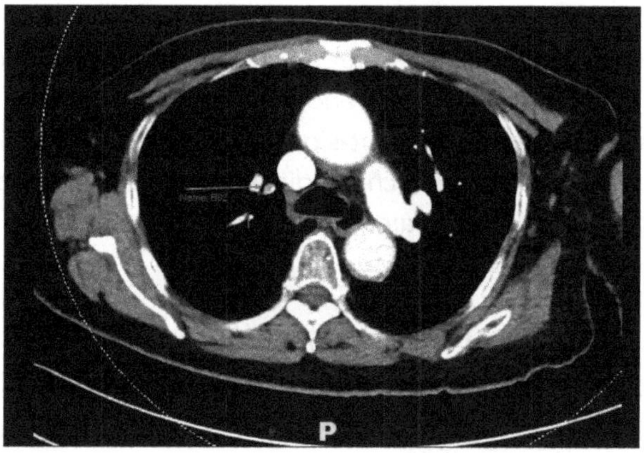

Green arrow indicating filling defects within pulmonary artery segmental branches of the right upper lobe.

The right calf measured 33 cm while the left calf measured 31.5 cm (at the level of 15 cm below the medial joint line of the knee). Doppler ultrasound scan confirmed above-knee deep vein thrombosis in the right lower limb.

Regular subcutaneous enoxaparin was commenced.

Three days later, Mdm C complained of epigastric and central chest pain, associated with vomiting of undigested food. Clinically she was alert but slightly disorientated to time. Vital signs were temperature 36.6°C, blood pressure 90/70 mmHg, heart rate 98/min, respiratory rate 18/min, and SpO_2 95% on room air. Cardiovascular system examination was unremarkable. The abdomen was soft with mild generalised tenderness. Per rectal examination revealed mixed brown and blackish stool.

Question 4: What is the most likely explanation of the chest pain now?

Question 5: Outline an appropriate management plan.

Although a cardiac cause of chest pain is a priority consideration, we still need to check for other causes of chest pain in this case viz. peptic ulcer disease, pancreatitis, gastroesophageal reflux disease, biliary tract causes, pneumonia, and surprisingly, urinary tract infection (many elderly patients present with vomiting and delirium and afterwards develop chest pain from the retching and vomiting). This case also highlights the importance of gastric protection in elderly patients even without history of peptic ulcer disease as stress ulceration can develop when they are ill and hospitalised.

Tips for Stress Ulcer Prophylaxis in Elderly

— *Identify patients at high risk of stress ulcers e.g., frail elderly with serious acute illness, chronic medical predisposing conditions (chronic renal failure, hypercalcaemia) and those on medications such as aspirin and NSAIDs.*
— *Choose an appropriate proton pump inhibitor (PPI) to be used and the route of administration.*
— *Review the duration of the PPI and cease once no longer deemed necessary.*

Key messages

1. Chest pain is a common symptom in the older patient with myriad causes. A detailed and comprehensive history from the patient and caregivers, thorough physical examination, and basic investigations often reveal the underlying cause.
2. It is crucial to identify life-threatening causes such as acute coronary syndrome, aortic dissection, pneumothorax, pulmonary embolism, and oesophageal rupture.
3. Atypical presentations are common in the older patient. Acute coronary syndrome may present as just a fall, delirium, or vomiting. Pulmonary embolism may present merely with a tachycardia with absence of classical symptoms, hence a high index of suspicion is required to identify these life-threatening conditions.

Answer key

1. History — ask for associated or atypical symptoms of acute coronary syndrome (e.g., breathlessness, diaphoresis, nausea) and pain after swallowing;

   Physical examination — check the blood pressure difference between the arms, as well as radioradial and radiofemoral delay.

2. Send blister fluid for varicella zoster virus DNA PCR (or Tzanck smear if the resource is available at the institution);

   Oral acyclovir 800 mg 5x/day or valacyclovir 1 g 3x/day (for better compliance);

   Topical antimicrobial agent (to prevent secondary bacterial infection);

   Gabapentin 300 mg ON and titrate gradually and according to pain and side-effects over next few days.

3. B. This patient has respiratory alkalosis with appropriate metabolic compensation. Oxygenation seems to be a potential problem. In view of the minimal abnormalities on the chest X-ray, pulmonary embolism should be considered even though the PaO_2 is still within normal limits. Given the context of age and immobility, this patient has a high pretest probability of pulmonary embolism, thus checking D-dimer is inappropriate. A stat dose of low molecular weight heparin, if no contraindication, should be administered while awaiting urgent CTPA.

4. Acute coronary syndrome precipitated by acute upper gastrointestinal bleeding due to recent anticoagulation.

5. Urgent investigations — laboratory viz. full blood count with reticulocyte count, urea and electrolytes, cardiac enzymes, liver function test, lipase, coagulation profile, group and cross match, electrocardiogram, and imaging viz. erect chest X-ray or abdominal X-ray (if intestinal obstruction is suspected);

   Keep nil by mouth;

   Fluid resuscitation and hourly parameters;

   Intravenous omeprazole infusion;

   Standby blood products;

   Urgent referral to gastroenterology and preparation for oesophagoduodenoscopy.

Reference

Gupta R, Munoz R (2016) Evaluation and Management of Chest Pain in the Elderly. *Emerg Med Clin North Am* **34**(3): 523–542.

26 Breathlessness I (Cardiogenic)

Peh Wee Ming, Jessica Chen Weizhen

Mr S is an 85-year-old Chinese man, a nursing home resident, who was transferred to the general hospital following a recent accidental fall and functional decline. He used to be ambulant with a walking frame and required minimal assistance in his activities of daily living. His medical history includes type 2 diabetes mellitus, chronic hypertension, and mixed Alzheimer's dementia with stroke disease.

History from the patient is limited apart from complaints of mild pain over his lower back. The nursing home staff, however, are concerned that he appears to be breathing rapidly and heavily at multiple times of the day.

Question 1: What is your diagnostic framework for evaluating shortness of breath in the elderly?

Shortness of breath (SOB) is a common presentation of the elderly at the acute hospital. It is also a strong predictor of mortality in elderly individuals! Adopt a comprehensive approach while being mindful of the SOB unmasking underlying medical issues specific to the elderly. Never assume that a complaint of SOB is simply because of "getting old"!

As you take a history about breathlessness, it is known that the elderly patient is less likely to report that the breathing problem stopped him or her from doing most activities. Hence, you may need to be direct and ask two questions to evaluate this:

1. What are your daily activities?
2. Have you stopped doing any activities because of breathing discomfort?

Cardiovascular system

A few conditions common to the elderly present as non-specific presentations of SOB viz. ischaemic heart disease, heart failure with preserved ejection fraction (HFpEF), cardiac arrhythmias, and valvular heart disease. Heart failure with reduced ejection fraction (HFrEF) is usually caused by ischaemic heart disease. What is less frequently recognised is that heart failure with preserved ejection fraction (HpEF) is ***significantly more common*** than HFrEF in the elderly as chronic hypertension leads to diastolic dysfunction.

Conduction system diseases are more prevalent in the elderly manifesting as atrial fibrillation and bradyarrhythmia. Age is the most important risk factor for the development of atrial fibrillation due to age-related dilation and remodelling of the left atrium. Elevated left atrial pressure, especially in the presence of stress, can lead to SOB secondary to reduced effort tolerance and pulmonary oedema. Ageing is also associated with an increase in the prevalence of sinus node dysfunction, atrioventricular nodal block, and bundle branch block.

Valvular heart disease such as aortic stenosis and mitral regurgitation is a frequently encountered problem in the older person. Aortic stenosis, for instance, is more than ten-fold higher in prevalence in the elderly compared to young adults! Echocardiography is an indispensable tool for assessing the severity of valve lesions.

Respiratory system

First, one should recognise that the respiratory system undergoes changes in ageing such as a decreased vital capacity, reduced elastic recoil of the lung, and decreased respiratory strength. Work of breathing increases and gas exchange becomes less efficient.

In addition, chronic lung diseases such as chronic obstructive pulmonary disease and interstitial lung disease are more prevalent. A number of lifestyle choices, such as chronic smoking and occupational exposure to pollutants, can contribute to their development.

Venous thromboembolism increases with age with an incidence rate of 1% per year in the elderly. Common presentations include SOB and even syncope. Venous thromboembolism is also associated with immobility and underlying malignancy of which the incidence is higher in the elderly.

Pneumonia is the most common infection in the elderly. A special consideration in the evaluation of pneumonia is swallowing dysfunction causing aspiration. Other predisposing factors include age-related immune dysregulation and underlying chronic lung disease. Silent aspiration may not be easily diagnosed and might be missed. Hence, in a patient with risk factors for dysphagia, recurrent pneumonia, or consolidation in the right lower zone, a swallowing assessment must be undertaken to identify aspiration as a potential cause. In some instances, cervical osteophytes may indent the pharyngeal wall and also cause dysphagia.

Anaemia

There is an increased incidence of anaemia in the elderly. While there are many causes, the more important ones are iron deficiency anaemia (e.g., gastrointestinal bleeding), vitamin B12 deficiency (e.g., vegan diet adopted by the elderly), and underlying bone marrow dysfunction (e.g., multiple myeloma and myelodysplastic syndrome).

Sarcopenia and cachexia

With ageing, there is the involuntary generalised accelerated loss of skeletal muscle mass, strength, performance, and function called sarcopenia. Muscle mass declines about 5% per decade after 30 years of age, and the decline is more significant after 60 years of age. Decline in muscle mass is also related to increases in fat mass with changes in body composition. Sarcopenia predicts poor outcomes for older people including falls, functional decline, loss of independence, morbidity, and mortality.

The underlying mechanism of the development of sarcopenia is complex and includes comorbidity, chronic illness, protein malnourishment, and inactivity. The main muscle groups associated with breathing are the intercostal muscles and diaphragmatic muscle. The condition of muscle fibre atrophy and weakness that occurs in respiratory muscles along with systemic skeletal muscle with age is known as respiratory sarcopenia. This may be perceived by the elderly as a reduced effort tolerance and SOB.

What can aggravate and accelerate this process is deconditioning which is brought on by inactivity or bed rest (especially upon hospitalisation, the elderly patient is often labelled with "fall precautions" which translates into minimal supervised ambulation during the inpatient stay, often spending most of the day and night in bed). In the elderly, deconditioning begins within hours of lying on a trolley or a bed. Without early intervention, the constellation of weakness, fatigue, reduced food intake, weight loss, and depression rapidly cascades into dependency.

Psychological

The elderly with mood issues have more physical symptoms than young adults due to increases in the prevalence of medical comorbities with ageing. The older individual has a tendency to convert one's psychological stress into somatic symptoms like SOB.

Anxiety and depression are prevalent among the elderly. This may be due to multiple physical comorbidities, but conversely older persons with anxiety disorders and depression commonly complain about physical symptoms like SOB and chest tightness. Evaluation of SOB in the elderly should preferably include an objective measure of anxiety and depressive symptoms. However, it is challenging to evaluate somatic symptoms of anxiety from symptoms of medical conditions. Sometimes these can even co-exist.

In short, the evaluation of shortness of breath in the elderly should be comprehensive with an index of suspicion of elderly-specific causes. Unfortunately, it can also be challenging to differentiate between SOB that is associated with a reduction in physiological reserves and SOB as an atypical manifestation of sarcopenia and psychological conditions.

****

Mr S was afebrile and his vital signs were blood pressure 190/95 mmHg, heart rate 80/min regular, respiratory rate 26/min, and oxygen saturation 95% on room air. A small haematoma was noted over his occipital scalp. Clubbing and conjunctival pallor were absent. Mild lumbar spinal tenderness was elicited, but there was no spinal deformity. Bilateral leg oedema was present up to the mid-shin level. Multiple blisters were seen over his left leg. Jugular venous pressure was elevated at 5 cm with no giant "v" waves. The apex beat was undisplaced, and there was no palpable P2 or parasternal heave. An ejection systolic murmur was heard over the left lower sternal edge which radiated to the carotids. Bibasal crepitations with reduced air entry were heard. There was no prolonged expiration or wheeze. Liver and spleen were not palpable.

Laboratory investigations showed:

WBC count	*6 x 10^9/L*	*(4–10)*
Haemoglobin	*12 g/dL*	*(14–18)*
MCV	*87 fL*	*(78–98)*
MCH	*30 pg*	*(27–32)*
RDW	*15%*	*(11–16)*
Platelet count	*250 x 10^9/L*	*(140–440)*
Blood urea	*8 mmol/L*	*(2.7–6.9)*
Sodium	*132 mmol/L*	*(136–146)*
Potassium	*4 mmol/L*	*(3.5–5.1)*
Bicarbonate	*25 mmol/L*	*(19–29)*
Chloride	*103 mmol/L*	*(98–107)*
Serum creatinine	*90 μmol/L*	*(62–106)*

CKMB	*2 µg/L*	*(1–5)*
Trop-T	*10 ng/L*	*(<29)*
ProBNP	*2,500 pg/mL*	*(<149)*
Lactate	*1 mmol/L*	*(0.5–2)*
C-reactive protein	*10 mg/L*	*(<4.9)*
Serum procalcitonin	*<0.49 mcg/L*	*(<0.49)*
Total protein	*60 g/L*	*(68–85)*
Serum albumin	*35 g/L*	*(40–51)*
Total bilirubin	*20 µmol/L*	*(7–32)*
Serum ALT	*50 U/L*	*(6–66)*
Serum AST	*30 U/L*	*(12–42)*
Serum ALP	*40 U/L*	*(39–99)*
Gamma-GT	*35 U/L*	*(6–42)*
Serum TSH	*2 mIU/L*	*(0.7–4.28)*
Free T4	*15 pmol/L*	*(12.7–20.3)*
Folate	*80 nmol/L*	*(10.4–78.9)*
Vit B12	*200 pmol/L*	*(145–569)*

His chest X-ray is as follows:

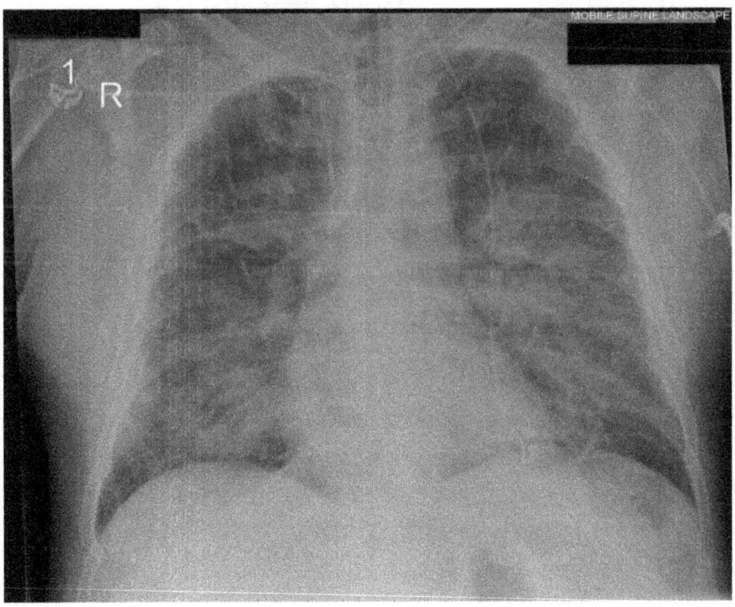

His ECG is as follows:

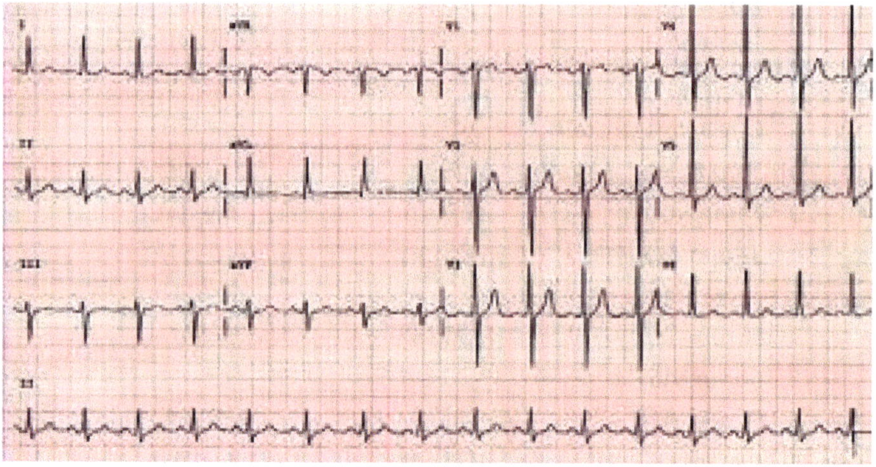

Question 2: What is the most likely explanation for the patient's acute deterioration?

a. **Acute pulmonary oedema secondary to hypertensive urgency**
b. **Acute right heart failure due to severe aortic stenosis**
c. **Fulminant bronchopneumonia**
d. **High-output heart failure secondary to anaemia**
e. **Right heart failure due to rapid atrial fibrillation**

****

Over the next three days, intravenous frusemide 40 mg BD was administered. His usual enalapril 5 mg BD was continued while amlodipine 10 mg OM was added. Mr S achieved a negative balance of 1–2 L of urine per day with improvement of bilateral lower limb oedema and bibasal crepitations. The patient was able to wean off oxygen.

On the seventh day of admission, Mr S developed fever and cough. He required 2 L of oxygen and saturations maintained at 95%. His blood pressure was 100/80 mmHg and he appeared to be slightly lethargic. The nurse observed that he was coughing while eating. The family was concerned that he appeared as breathless as at admission time. His daughter offered more history that he has had difficulty with swallowing and hence had a reduced oral intake which might have accounted for his weight loss of 5 kg over 6 months.

Repeat laboratory investigations showed:

WBC count	*15 x 10^9/L*	*(4–10)*
Haemoglobin	*16 g/dL*	*(14–18)*
Platelet count	*150 x 10^9/L*	*(140–440)*
Blood urea	*15 mmol/L*	*(2.7–6.9)*
Sodium	*149 mmol/L*	*(136–146)*
Potassium	*3.2 mmol/L*	*(3.5–5.1)*
Bicarbonate	*32 mmol/L*	*(19–29)*
Chloride	*90 mmol/L*	*(98–107)*
Serum creatinine	*160 µmol/L*	*(62–106)*
CKMB	*4 µg/L*	*(1–5)*
Trop-T	*<29 ng/L*	*(<29)*
Lactate	*5 mmol/L*	*(0.5–2)*
Serum procalcitonin	*7 mcg/L*	*(<0.49)*

Repeat ECG did not show any acute changes.

Repeat chest X-ray showed:

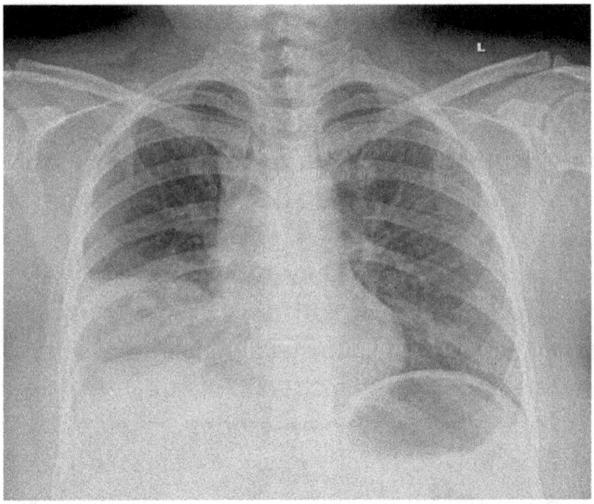

Question 3: What are some possible explanations for his hypotension?

It is not uncommon for the physician to be aggressive in diuresis in a patient who presents with pulmonary oedema and an eagerness to normalise the blood pressure with higher than usual doses of antihypertensives. Diuresis in patients

Tips and precautions on using diuretics in the elderly:

— *The combination of small doses of diuretics with a conventional antihypertensive agent has an important place in the treatment of the elderly hypertensive person.*
— *Diuretics are more likely to cause*

(a) prerenal uraemia due to their diminished renal reserve
(b) hearing impairment (esp. high doses of loop diuretics)
(c) greater impact on carbohydrate metabolism (overt diabetes)
(d) incontinence complicating care and quality of life (esp. those with limited mobility and overactive bladders); hence timing the diuretics so as to avoid night time diuresis is useful
(e) uraemia and hyponatraemia (esp. if receiving concomitant potassium-sparing agents)

— *Giving potassium supplements or potassium-sparing agents does not obliterate the need to monitor the electrolytes.*
— *It may be useful to separate the administration of a diuretic from an ACE-inhibitor by several hours as the reduction in systemic blood pressure or influence on glomerular haemodynamics may reduce the effect of the diuretic.*
— *The use of NSAIDs is an important cause of apparent diuretic resistance due to interference with prostaglandin synthesis (prostaglandin E2 antagonises the antidiuretic effect of vasopressin in the collecting tubule, resulting in sodium and water retention).*

who are diuretic-naive can lead to relative hypovolaemia which is compounded by antihypertensive treatment.

A new fever during admission associated with coughing in a patient with moderate to severe dementia should raise the suspicion of aspiration pneumonia or nosocomial pneumonia. An increase in oxygen requirement would be compatible with this too.

Development of acute kidney injury in the patient is likely prerenal and due to sepsis. Metabolic acidosis from acute kidney injury can manifest as dyspnoea as there is an increased need for ventilation leading to increased respiratory workload.

In the elderly, it is important to moderate the treatment approach as they are more susceptible to side-effects and complications of therapy due to reduced physiological reserves. Close monitoring by physical examination as well as laboratory investigations helps to guide treatment and prevent complications. The diuresis was held off and a renal-adjusted dose of piperacillin-tazobactam was initiated.

****

A transthoracic echocardiogram was ordered to evaluate cardiac function as well as to determine the significance of the aortic murmur. It showed severe aortic stenosis with diastolic dysfunction of the heart. The left ventricular ejection fraction was 25%.

Question 4: What are the therapeutic implications of this finding for Mr S?

The commonest valvular lesion in people over 75 is aortic stenosis, and it is severe in about a quarter of them. In Mr S, both chronic hypertension and severe aortic stenosis increase afterload. This combination is likely responsible for the development of diastolic dysfunction.

Aggressive diuresis can decrease preload to the extent of reducing left ventricular end-diastolic volume causing hypotension. On the other hand, the stenotic aortic valve leads to increased pressure work by the heart leading to concentric hypertrophy. The subsequent reduction in left-ventricular end-diastolic volume and increase in left-ventricular end-diastolic pressure results in impaired pulmonary venous return leading to pulmonary congestion. This is often triggered by aggressive fluid resuscitation. During the fluid challenge, great care was taken not to precipitate another episode of acute pulmonary oedema.

The only treatment that has been demonstrated to improve quality of life and increase survival in patients with severe aortic stenosis is replacement of the valve. For the one-third of the elderly who are not considered surgical candidates, transcatheter aortic valve replacement options can be considered. Aortic valves can be inserted percutaneously (i.e., transcatheter aortic valve implantation or TAVI) and they can be balloon-expandable or self-expanding. Transcatheter aortic valves appear to be non-inferior to surgical intervention with regards to outcomes of mortality and short-term and long-term outcomes with faster in-hospital recovery.

Mr S was referred to cardiology who recommended TAVI.

Key messages

1. Shortness of breath in the elderly requires a systemic approach and workup to consider a wide range of differentials. The most important areas to consider are the cardiovascular system, respiratory system, anaemia, psychological aspects, and sarcopenia. Metabolic acidosis may also cause dyspnoea in a select group of patients.
2. Beware of premature closure after you identify a primary cause of the breathlessness in the elderly. They often have other contributory causes too.
3. The reduced physiological reserves of the elderly put them at high risk of complications to treatment.
4. Do not miss aortic stenosis in the elderly as it is common and is an important cause of diastolic dysfunction.
5. TAVI can be considered a semi-invasive intervention for frail elderly in critical aortic stenosis.

Answer key

1. There is no model answer for such a question as different physicians will have their own diagnostic frameworks. Your preferred approach should be sensible and immediately practical, but the most important thing is that it should always work for you. Our thought process for SOB in the elderly is:

	Common causes of SOB in the elderly^	
First rule out organic causes	Cardiovascular system*	• HFpEF > HFrEF • AF • Valvular disease
	Respiratory system*	• Obvious: COPD,bronchiectasis, pneumonia • Subtle: VTE,pulmonary hypertension
	Anaemia*	• Deficiencies: Fe, Vit B12 • Haematological malignancy e.g., MDS
Next consider functional cause	Psychological	• Anxiety • Depression
And don't forget frailty syndrome	Sarcopenia	• Respiratory muscle atrophy, weakness and dysfunction • Impact of deconditioning

^Influenced by inaccurate history, compliance issues and challenging social circumstances.

*Background of age-related reduced cardiorespiratory reserve.

2. A.
3. Hypovolaemia due to poor intake and aggressive diuresis;
   Sepsis due to hospital-acquired pneumonia;
   Antihypertensive medications.
4. A balance need to be made between sufficient diuresis: severe hypovolaemia → ↓preload → ↓left-ventricular end-diastolic volume → hypotension;
   versus fluid resuscitation of hypotension: liberal fluids → ↑left-ventricular end-diastolic pressure (left ventricle unable to accommodate the extra fluid) → flash pulmonary oedema.

References

Lindman BR, Alexander KP, O'Gara PT, Afilalo J (2014) Futility, benefit, and transcatheter aortic valve replacement. *JACC Cardiovasc Interv* **7**(7): 707–716.

Mahler DA (2017) Evaluation of dyspnea in the elderly. *Clin Geriatr Med* **33**: 503–521.

Otto CM (2013) Medical management of symptomatic aortic stenosis. In: UpToDate, Basow DS (Ed.), UpToDate. Waltham, MA.

Upadhya B, Taffet GE, Cheng CP, Kitzman DW (2015) Heart failure with preserved ejection fraction in the elderly: scope of the problem. *J Mol Cell Cardiol* **83**: 73–87.

27 Breathlessness II (Aspiration)

Jonathan Goh Teow Koon, Anupama Roy Chowdhury

Mr A is an 86-year-old Chinese male who was admitted to the general ward from the Emergency Department. He has a notable past medical history of Parkinson disease, hypertension, hyperlipidaemia, ischaemic stroke, and dementia. At baseline, he is assisted in his activities of daily living by his live-in helper. He is a non-smoker.

His current medications include aspirin 100 mg OM, nifedipine LA 30 mg OM, Madopar (levodopa/benserazide) 250 mg TDS, and simvastatin 10 mg ON. He also takes zolpidem 10 mg ON regularly for insomnia.

History was taken from his helper as the patient's bradykinaesia and dysarthria made it difficult for him to speak. The presenting complaint was fever for three days. On the day of presentation to the Emergency Department, he had also started to become more breathless. He has had a chronic cough for many years with intermittent sputum production. He had difficulty swallowing his saliva resulting in some drooling, and had also been noted to choke and cough after taking solid foods. However, his helper noted that his cough had worsened over the past week with increasing mucopurulent greenish phlegm.

On examination, his vital signs are temperature 38.7°C, blood pressure 100/60 mmHg, pulse rate 110/min, and respiratory rate 26/min with SpO_2 90% on room air. Mr A is visibly distressed with use of accessory muscles of respiration. There is a paucity of facial expressions and a resting tremor in both hands. Chest examination was remarkable for right-sided dullness to percussion and basal coarse crepitations. Dental hygiene was satisfactory.

Pertinent laboratory investigations are as follows:

Haemoglobin	*12.5 g/dL*	*(12–16)*
WBC count	*19.2 x 10^9/L*	*(4–10) predominantly neutrophilic*
Platelet count	*200 x 10^9/L*	*(140–400)*
Urea	*8 mmol/L*	*(2.7–6.9)*
Creatinine	*94 µmol/L*	*(45–84)*

Bicarbonate	*18 mmol/L*	*(19–29)*
Sodium	*130 mmol/L*	*(136–146)*
Potassium	*3.6 mmol/L*	*(3.5–5.1)*
Chloride	*100 mmol/L*	*(98–107)*
C-reactive protein	*120 nmol/L*	*(0.2–9.1)*

Blood cultures are pending.

This is the chest X-ray:

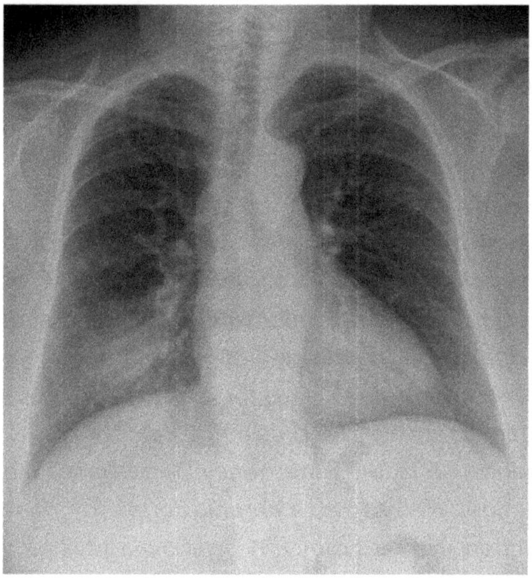

A diagnosis of pneumonia likely due to aspiration is made.

Question 1: What are the risk factors for aspiration pneumonia in Mr A?

Question 2: What empirical antibiotic(s) will you commence Mr A on?

Aspiration of oropharyngeal secretions in small amounts occur during sleep. A healthy adult with an intact cough reflex and active ciliary transport together with a normal immune system is able to clear the low levels of virulent bacteria.

However, if any of these protective mechanisms is impaired (Table 27.1) or if the aspiration is large enough to overwhelm these protective mechanisms, then aspiration pneumonia will result. The responsible pathogens can come from a previously colonised oropharynx or upper gastrointestinal content.

The diagnosis of aspiration pneumonia is made if there are characteristic clinical features of pneumonia with risk factors for aspiration and compatible findings

Table 27.1. Risk Factors for Macro-aspiration.

Impaired swallowing • tumours in the head and neck • oesophageal diseases (cancer or strictures) • motility disorders such as achalasia, gastro-oesophageal reflux disease (GERD) • neurological diseases such as seizures, stroke, degenerative diseases (e.g., multiple sclerosis, Parkinson disease, dementia) • frequently seen after liberation from mechanical ventilation	**Impaired cough reflex** • degenerative neurological diseases, stroke, and any cause of impaired consciousness
Impaired consciousness • neurological diseases such as stroke • medications that induce drowsiness such as hypnotics, antidepressants, antipsychotics, general anaesthesia, and alcohol • frequently seen post cardiac arrest	**Increased chance of gastric contents reaching the lung** • GERD • tube feeding (due to loss of anatomical integrity of the upper and lower oesophageal sphincter)

on a chest radiograph. A history of witnessed macro-aspiration will further support the diagnosis.

Compatible chest radiograph findings include infiltrates in the gravity-dependent areas of the lung segments which in turn depend on the patient's position:

- If the patient is upright, these are the basal segments of the lower lobe.
- If the patient is supine, these are the superior segment of the lower lobe and/or the posterior segment of the upper lobe.

Note that in early aspiration pneumonia, chest radiographs may appear normal.

Historically, the microorganisms that cause aspiration pneumonia were predominantly anaerobes especially oral flora. However, numerous studies in recent years, even amongst elderly patients, have seen a shift towards bacteria more commonly seen in the community (*Streptococcus pneumoniae, Staphylococcus aureus, Haemophilus influenzae,* and Enterobacteriaceae) or in the hospital (predominantly gram-negative organisms viz. *Pseudomonas aeruginosa, Klebsiella pneumonia, Escherichia coli,* and *Enterobacter* spp.).

Hence, the selection of antibiotics will depend on whether there are risk factors for infection with multi-drug-resistant organisms (treatment with broad-spectrum antibiotics in the past 90 days or hospitalisation for 5 days).

For community cases, treatment as per community-acquired pneumonia is sufficient (ceftriaxone and azithromycin). For patients who are critically ill or have risk factors for multi-drug-resistant organisms, piperacillin/tazobactam (Tazocin) should be considered. If MRSA is suspected, then vancomycin should be added.

If there are risk factors for anaerobes such as poor oral dentition or lung abscesses, anaerobic cover with clindamycin can be added in favour of metronidazole which has been shown to have a higher treatment failure rate. Amoxicillin/clavulanate has also been used in place of ceftriaxone for its additional anaerobic cover.

Duration of treatment should be 5–7 days depending on clinical response and if there are no complications of pneumonia such as necrotising pneumonia, lung abscess, or empyema.

On the other hand, chemical pneumonitis is a non-infectious inflammatory response of the airways and pulmonary parenchyma to acidic gastric content or bile acids. Chemical pneumonitis does not require antibiotics if it is mild to moderately severe, although in severe cases, empirical antibiotics should be started and clinical progression monitored. If subsequently there is lesser concern of pneumonia and the patient improves, antibiotics may be discontinued.

****

A speech therapist assessed Mr A's swallowing and concluded that he has mild to moderate oropharyngeal dysphagia.

Question 3: Which of the following is probably the most useful long-term intervention to lower the chance of another episode of aspiration pneumonia in Mr A?

a. Assisted hand feeding by his helper

b. Feeding via nasogastric feeding tube

c. Feeding via percutaneous endoscopic gastrostomy tube

d. Reduce the dose of Madopar as tolerated

e. Swallowing retraining strategies by a speech therapist

The goals in management of elderly patients with dysphagia is to optimise the safety, efficiency, and effectiveness of the oropharyngeal swallow to maintain adequate nutrition and hydration.

A full speech and swallowing assessment should be conducted for all patients at risk of aspiration by a qualified speech therapist. A clinical assessment can first be carried out and, if required, a video-fluoroscopic swallow assessment should be performed.

Once dysphagia has been established, compensatory strategies may be taught to the patient or the patient's caregiver to allow a safer or more efficient swallow. Examples of such techniques are:

- Postural changes, e.g., raising the head of bed by 30° for bed-bound patients, chin tuck, head rotation — may be tricky in patients with cervical spine problems.
- Swallowing manoeuvers, e.g., supraglottic swallow (hold breath → double swallow → forceful expiration which ensures the vocal folds close before and during swallow) — can be problematic in persons with dementia and those with cardiovascular problems.

The consistency of solid and liquid food may have to be modified. Soft diet with thickened liquids is usually preferred over pureed and thin liquids in reducing the risk of aspiration. However, the consistency of the patient's food should be individualised. Modification of consistency must be taught to the caregiver preparing the food, and their competency and understanding must be checked. In reality, many older patients dislike the modified consistency and hence may be non-compliant to the modifications suggested. In such cases, patients and families may need to make a conscious decision to prioritise the patient's wishes over the risks of aspiration.

Slow and careful hand feeding by the patient's caregiver may be required to control the rate of ingestion as some patients, particularly those with cognitive impairment, may impulsively feed themselves rapidly without allowing for adequate time to swallow and subsequently end up choking. Vary the placement of food in the patient's mouth according to the type of deficit — for example, the food should be placed on the side of the mouth opposite to that of the facial weakness. ***Patients with dysphagia who are receiving assisted hand feeding encounter fewer episodes of aspiration than those who are tube-fed!*** The personal participation of a loved one in this activity, preferably in a calm and peaceful environment, may also promote food intake.

If a patient is on enteral feeding, this should be done with the head elevated rather than in a supine position, with the head-up position being maintained for a minimum of half to one hour after feeding. This allows for a period of gastric emptying.

The effectiveness of a nasogastric tube in preventing aspiration pneumonia is uncertain with studies showing that the rate of aspiration events did not decrease. Neither did inserting a nasogastric tube improve survival in patients with advanced dementia. Similarly, there is no data to suggest that patients with gastrostomy tubes (though more comfortable for the patient) have a lower incidence of pneumonia compared to those with nasogastric tubes. In patients with advanced dementia with severe dysphagia, insertion of a nasogastric tube may nevertheless be considered for short-term tube feeding ***where there is an expectation that the patient's dysphagia will improve***.

Care should be taken to maintain good oral hygiene. A soft toothbrush or electric toothbrush is recommended for brushing. For edentulous patients, brush the gums gently using a soft paediatric toothbrush. Dentures should be well-fitting and regularly cleaned. Regular oral toilet daily with a chlorhexidine swab can help keep the oral cavity clean in patients who are unable to brush their teeth or gargle.

Pharmacological precautions in elderly patients with dysphagia are as follows:

- Medications that have sedating effects should be avoided if possible.
- As medications that raise gastric pH such as H2-blockers or proton-pump inhibitors may increase the risk of pneumonia, their indications must be reviewed on a regular basis with cessation of these drugs if they are no longer required.
- In stroke patients, there is some evidence that angiotensin converting enzyme inhibitor, L-dopa and amantadine may be helpful to improve swallowing and reduce the risk of aspiration pneumonia. However, the older patient needs to be closely monitored for the side-effects of these drugs.

As elucidated in the points above, reducing the risk of an aspiration pneumonia requires a multi-pronged approach.

Key messages

1. Risk factors for aspiration pneumonia are impaired swallowing, impaired consciousness, increased chance of gastric contents reaching the lung, and impaired cough reflex.
2. Choice of empirical antibiotics follows that of community or hospital-acquired pneumonia. Anaerobic cover should be added only if there is high clinical suspicion.
3. The goal in the management of elderly patients with dysphagia is to optimise the safety, efficiency, and effectiveness of the oropharyngeal swallow to maintain adequate nutrition and hydration. Nasogastric tubes have ***not*** been shown to reduce the risk of aspiration pneumonia.

Answer key

1. Parkinson disease, stroke, dementia, sedating medication (zolpidem).

2. In line with our hospital antibiotic guidelines, ceftriaxone + azithromycin is appropriate for this patient with community-acquired pneumonia with low risk of anaerobic infection.
3. A.

References

DiBardino DM, Wunderink RG (2014) Aspiration pneumonia: a review of modern trends. *J Crit Care* **30**: 40–48.

Luk JKH, Chan DKY (2014) Preventing aspiration pneumonia in older people: do we have the "know-how"? *Hong Kong Med J* **20**: 421–427.

Mandell L, Niederman MS (2019) Aspiration pneumonia. *N Engl J Med* **380**: 651–663.

Wirth R, Dziewas R, Beck AM, *et al.* (2016) Oropharyngeal dysphagia in older persons — from pathophysiology to adequate intervention: a review and summary of an international expert meeting. *Clin Interv Aging* **11**: 189–208.

28 Breathlessness III (Chronic Obstructive Pulmonary Disease)

Kenneth Koh Hsien Hui, Lalmalani Roshan Mahesh

Mr A is an 80-year-old man who was diagnosed with chronic obstructive pulmonary disease (COPD) ten years ago but is not on regular follow-up. His other medical conditions include ischaemic heart disease with previous percutaneous coronary intervention, hypertension, and diabetes mellitus. He has no personal or family history of asthma.

He has a 60 pack-year smoking history and is still smoking 20 sticks of cigarettes daily. He gets breathless on walking a few steps and hardly leaves his HDB flat. He only uses inhaled salbutamol whenever he gets breathless. He has had 6 hospitalised COPD exacerbations in the past year. He relies on his daughter-in-law for assistance in his activities of daily living.

Question 1: Which of the following features can be used to diagnose COPD?

I. **Clinical features of progressive exertional dyspnoea, chronic cough, and chronic sputum production.**
II. **Chest X-ray/CT thorax findings**
III. **Spirometry**
IV. **Exposure to risk factors**

Options

a. **I, II, and III**
b. **I, III, and IV**
c. **I, II, and IV**
d. **All of the above**

Evidence of expiratory airflow limitation on spirometry is required to confirm a diagnosis of COPD in a symptomatic patient with exposure to known risk factors for COPD. Symptoms of COPD include persistent exertional dyspnoea, chronic cough, and chronic sputum production. Unrecognised heart failure may be found in elderly patients with stable COPD. It is therefore important to correlate symptoms with the presence of airflow obstruction.

Spirometry is a physiologic test that measures the maximal volume of gas inhaled and exhaled by an individual with maximal effort. The forced vital capacity (FVC) is the volume of gas that is maximally exhaled from full inspiration. The volume of exhaled gas in the first second of a FVC manoeuvre is the FEV1. Decrease in the FEV1 is the factor most associated with deterioration in the quality of life in elderly COPD patients. The FEV1 and FVC values are measured during spirometry and the FEV1/FVC ratio is calculated.

The FVC manoeuvre has multiple steps that require a rapid transition between maximal inhalation and maximal exhalation without hesitation. This can be challenging to perform in elderly patients. A prolonged expiratory breath-hold is required in an FVC manoeuvre, but this may lead to syncope in elderly patients. There are other stringent acceptability criteria for spirometry which include no mouthpiece obstruction and no leak. Ill-fitting dentures may occlude the mouthpiece, but an edentulous geriatric patient may not be able to produce a good seal. A good seal around the mouthpiece is needed to prevent a leak. Meeting the repeatability criteria for spirometry indicates maximal effort by the patient but can be limited by fatigue in the elderly patient. Having an experienced lung function technician who is able to keep instructions simple, patiently demonstrate acceptable technique for each step of the FVC manoeuvre, and provide encouragement and useful feedback to the elderly patient is crucial in obtaining acceptable and reproducible spirometry results.

The Global Initiative for Chronic Obstructive Lung Disease (GOLD) guidelines use a post-bronchodilator FEV1/FVC ratio of less than 0.7 to diagnose expiratory airflow limitation. However, this may lead to an over-diagnosis of COPD in elderly patients. There are spirometry reference equations derived from different populations. These equations are affected by the ethnicity, gender, and height of the patient. The **lower limit of normal (LLN)** of these spirometry reference equations is used as a cut-off for the FEV1/FVC ratio in the diagnosis of COPD. Using the LLN as the cut-off improves the diagnostic accuracy of COPD in the elderly.

Impulse oscillometry is a physiologic test that measures respiratory impedance during tidal breathing by the application of pressure oscillations at the mouth. It requires less effort and patient cooperation but has greater day-to-day variability compared to spirometry. It has the potential to be used as an alternative technique to measure airflow resistance in patients suspected to have COPD but who are unable to perform spirometry. This promising tool is currently limited by its availability, but it will likely be a more practical option for measuring airflow obstruction in elderly patients.

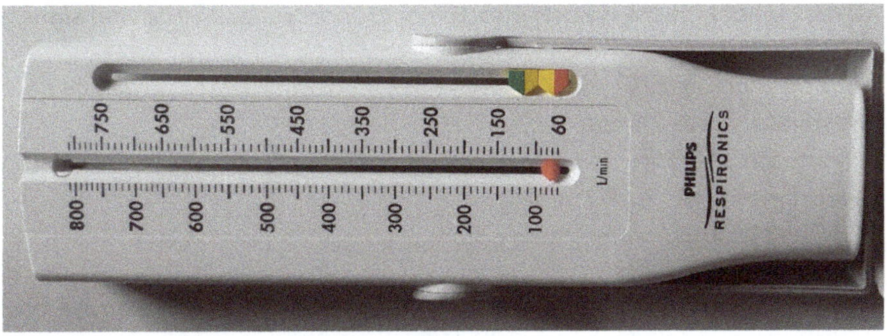

Fig. 28.1. Handheld peak flow meter. A decrease in PEF is an indicator of declining health in the elderly in terms of functional ability and physical activity.

The use of questionnaires and handheld devices (Fig 28.1) such as peak expiratory flow (PEF) to diagnose COPD has a lower specificity compared to spirometry and is not recommended for use in the diagnosis of COPD. The sensitivity of radiology in diagnosing COPD is limited by inter-observer variability and disease heterogeneity. In one study, chest radiographs were found to have only a sensitivity of 35% in diagnosing COPD. The relationship between lung function and radiology findings is inconsistent across different disease morphologies on CT thorax.

A confirmatory diagnosis of COPD by way of a spirometry is challenging in older adults. With a significant proportion of the geriatric population having some degree of cognitive impairment, they may not be able to follow the precise instructions required for a spirometry. Hence choosing patients who can understand and cooperate is important when ordering a lung function test. More often than not, a diagnosis of "presumptive COPD" is made based on symptoms, risk factors, and/or imaging findings. A trial of treatment, however, should not be delayed while awaiting spirometry.

****

Mr A's spirometry result from 10 years ago is as follows:

FEV1/FVC ratio: 0.67 and less than LLN
FEV1: 1.28 L (55% predicted)
FVC: 1.90 L (65% predicted)

Mr A now presents at the emergency department with acute worsening of breathlessness in the past one day. He had fever, sore throat, and worsening cough with increased sputum production for the past three days. His sputum was green.

On examination, he was able to speak in short phrases. His vital signs were:

Temperature 36.8°C
Respiratory rate 24/min
Heart rate 110/min
Blood pressure 170/90 mmHg
SpO_2 92% on 2 L intranasal oxygen

He was using his accessory muscles of respiration. Jugular venous pressure was not raised. Heart sounds were dual with no added heart sounds. Symmetrical breath sounds with wheeze were heard bilaterally. There were no crackles. Calves were supple with no pedal oedema.

A chest X-ray revealed bilateral hyperinflated lung fields with no focal consolidation and no pneumothorax.

Arterial blood gas done on 2 L intranasal oxygen: pH 7.35, $PaCO_2$ 52 mmHg, PaO_2 70 mmHg, bicarbonate 23 mmol/L

Full blood count: Hb 11.8 g/dL, WBC 12,000/L (neutrophils 73%), platelets 180,000/L

Renal panel: Urea 5.8 mmol/L, Na 132 mmol/L, K 4.1 mmol/L, C^- 97 mmol/L, Cr 39 umol/L

Troponin <13 ng/L

Electrocardiogram: Sinus rhythm. No acute ischaemic changes.

He was diagnosed as having an acute exacerbation of COPD precipitated by infection. He received intravenous hydrocortisone, multiple doses of inhaled bronchodilators, and intravenous amoxicillin-clavulanate.

At the ward, he produced a bag of medicine. It contained multiple inhalers of various drug classes — inhaled corticosteroid (ICS), combination long-acting antimuscarinic and long-acting β2-agonist (LAMA-LABA), combination long-acting β2-agonist and inhaled corticosteroid (LABA-ICS), long-acting antimuscarinic monotherapy (LAMA), short-acting antimuscarinic (SAMA), and short-acting β2-agonist (SABA).

Question 2: What inhalers would you prescribe for Mr A now?

a. Ipratropium, salbutamol with LAMA-LABA

b. Ipratropium, salbutamol with LABA-ICS

c. Ipratropium, salbutamol with LAMA

d. Ipratropium, salbutamol with LAMA-LABA-ICS

During an acute exacerbation of COPD, a short course of corticosteroids and short-acting bronchodilators, such as inhaled salbutamol and ipratropium, are prescribed in addition to maintenance therapy for COPD. The use of antibiotics in treating acute exacerbations of COPD is controversial. A meta-analysis suggested a reduction in treatment failures and mortality in those patients who were admitted to the intensive care unit, while the benefit in other patients was less clear. Nevertheless, the GOLD guidelines 2023[2] recommend the use of antibiotics in patients with exacerbations of COPD in the following situations:

I. Increased sputum purulence + increased dyspnoea and/or increased sputum volume; **OR**
II. Requires mechanical ventilation.

The risk of potential adverse effects must be considered when prescribing antibiotics in the elderly.

The prescription and titration of inhalers in COPD patients is guided by the presence of symptoms and a history of exacerbations (Fig 28.2):

- The COPD assessment tool can be used to assess symptomatology. Alternatively, the MMRC dyspnea score is easier to administer and can be used to grade the severity of symptoms. You can assess these tools from the free app "COPD pocket consultant guide".
- Inhaled salbutamol 2 puffs PRN for wheeze or breathlessness (maximum 16 puffs/day) is prescribed to all COPD patients.
- For the stable COPD patient with few symptoms and few exacerbations, inhaled ipratropium 2 puffs TDS may be added.
- For patients with multiple exacerbations or who have more symptoms, dual bronchodilator (LAMA-LABA) is preferred. Options include inhaled tiotropium/olodaterol (Spiolto Respimat) 2 inh OM and inhaled umeclidinium/vilanterol (Anoro Ellipta) 1 Inh OM.

ICSs such as inhaled budesonide 2 puffs BD or inhaled fluticasone propionate 2 puffs BD may be added on for patients who continue to have exacerbations in spite of being on dual bronchodilator therapy.

Despite his multiple hospitalised exacerbations for COPD, Mr A remained non-adherent to his maintenance therapy. He was thus kept on LAMA-LABA. Although the addition of ICS to LAMA-LABA has been shown to reduce the risk of exacerbations and improve lung function, the use of ICS in COPD is associated with a higher prevalence of oral thrush and pneumonia. Other side-effects of

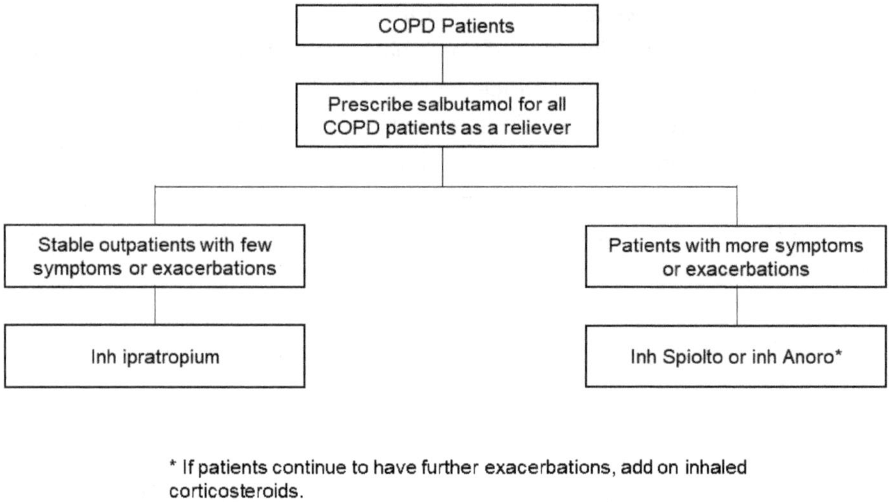

Fig. 28.2. Suggested treatment algorithm for COPD patients.

osteoporosis, cataracts, and diabetes mellitus are more commonly associated with patients receiving systemic corticosteroids for prolonged periods of time. Therefore, maintenance inhaler therapy needs to be optimised in COPD patients to reduce exacerbations and thus reduce exposure to systemic corticosteroids. There is no role for prolonged courses of oral steroids in a COPD patient.

Inhalers come in different designs. There are three main classes of inhalers: metered-dose inhaler (MDI), soft mist inhaler (SMI), and dry powder inhaler (DPI). All three classes require a coordination of inspiratory effort with dose actuation. MDIs and SMIs require dexterity during dose actuation and a slow, deep inhalation of three to five seconds followed by a breath hold of five to ten seconds. A space-chamber may be prescribed with MDIs to improve drug delivery. Drug particles generated in SMIs are finer and there is increased deposition of the drug in the smaller airways compared to MDIs. DPIs require a higher inspiratory flow compared to MDIs and SMIs but require less dexterity to administer. The choice of inhaler device should be individualised to the elderly patient.

The inhaled route of drug delivery is associated with less systemic side-effects compared to oral drugs. Oral theophylline has a modest bronchodilator effect but a narrow therapeutic index. If used in the elderly, especially those on polypharmacy, dose adjustments must be made in view of reduced drug clearance and the possibility of drug–drug interactions. Most of the drugs used in COPD treatment are therefore administered via the inhaled route. Having good inhaler technique with strict compliance to maintenance therapy is key to optimal control of COPD.

Older adults may have reduced dexterity. As a result, they may not be able to handle inhalers as well as younger people for a variety of reasons including upper limb weakness from previous strokes, sarcopenia and cervical myelopathy, upper limb apraxia secondary to underlying neurodegenerative conditions, and tremors secondary to movement disorders. Furthermore, other difficulties including poor vision and impaired cognition can result in improper use of inhalers.

Therefore, attention must be paid to selecting an appropriate delivery device, using the help of a spacer when indicated and ensuring proper usage by training both the patient and the caregiver on the relevant techniques. Furthermore, inhaler technique must be regularly reviewed by the physician at clinic visits especially when previously well controlled disease has worsened. If found to be inadequate, a switch to an inhaler which can be administered via a spacer device would be prudent.

Mr A was experiencing **polypharmacy**. Polypharmacy increases the risk of adverse drug reactions and impacts on adherence. Therefore, it is important to simplify drug prescription in the elderly. A single inhaler with once-daily dosing for maintenance therapy is preferable in the elderly. Mr A continued to improve and completed a five-day course of corticosteroid and antibiotics. He was kept on a LAMA-LABA and Inh salbutamol 2 puffs as needed for dyspnoea or wheeze, up to a maximum of 16 puffs per day.

Smoking cessation improves survival and slows down lung function decline in COPD patients. A combination of behavioural counselling and pharmacologic therapy showed greater efficacy in smoking cessation compared to either treatment on its own. Unfortunately, smoking cessation in the elderly is easier said than done. There are a wide variety of challenges: smoking cessation clinics face high dropout rates, healthcare providers encounter language barriers, and many elderly patients harbour longstanding behavioural habits and deep-seated misconceptions about smoking. In practice, knowledge about counselling and smoking cessation techniques is often limited to psychologists and pharmacists.

Nicotine replacement therapy comes in many forms such as patches, gums, and lozenges. However, success rate is low and it may affect glycemic control in diabetics. Since the recall of varenicline, bupropion, an atypical antidepressant used to treat geriatric depression, is presently the only alternative to nicotine replacement therapy in the market which may help in the early stages of smoking cessation by attenuating the effects of nicotine withdrawal.

Our recommendation would be to involve a loved one in the smoking cessation journey. This will encourage compliance and potentially reduce clinic dropout rates. In addition, smoking cessation treatment is best begun in the inpatient setting as this is when the motivation would be at its peak, especially when the admission is due to COPD. The primary physician should be proactively and actively involved in the process.

Finally, pneumococcal vaccination and annual influenza vaccination reduce the risk of COPD exacerbations. Having a case manager to monitor and support the COPD patient reduces hospital re-admissions and improves health-related quality of life.

****

Mr A was referred to the smoking cessation service and was started on nicotine replacement therapy. He had completed his pneumococcal vaccine regimen in the past and last received his influenza vaccine ten months ago. He was referred to a case manager. He was coached on the appropriate use of his inhaled medications and proper inhaler technique and was deemed competent in the administration of his medications.

Although Mr A was no longer wheezing, he still had breathlessness on exertion with a drop in his SpO_2 to 85% on mild exertion. A repeat arterial blood gas on room air at rest showed pH 7.37, $PaCO_2$ 48 mmHg, PaO_2 54 mmHg, and bicarbonate 24 mmol/L.

Question 3: What is the next most appropriate course of management?

a. **Arrange for long-term home oxygen therapy**
b. **Evaluate for other causes of breathlessness**
c. **Refer for pulmonary rehabilitation**
d. **Start him on opioid drugs for symptomatic relief**

Mr A underwent a computed tomographic pulmonary angiogram which did not show any pulmonary embolism, infection, or pneumothorax. A transthoracic echocardiogram showed normal biventricular function, no significant valvular heart disease, and no regional wall motion abnormalities. He was subsequently discharged on supplemental oxygen and referred for pulmonary rehabilitation.

He will need to be reassessed in the outpatient setting for severe chronic hypoxaemia (i.e., **$SpO_2 \leq 88\%$** or **$PaO_2 \leq 55$ mmHg**), which is an indication for long term oxygen therapy. The prescription of long-term oxygen therapy in COPD patients with severe chronic resting hypoxaemia has been shown to reduce mortality.

Pulmonary rehabilitation is a comprehensive intervention based on a thorough patient assessment followed by patient-tailored therapies that include, but are not limited to, exercise training, education, and behaviour change designed to improve the physical and psychological condition of people with chronic respiratory disease and to promote the long-term adherence to health-enhancing behaviours. Pulmonary rehabilitation has been shown to improve exercise capacity and the quality of life of patients following a recent COPD exacerbation. Participation in group activities allows the elderly patient to socialise and is useful in helping the elderly patient come to terms with the disease and adjust to it. The COPD Association (Singapore) helps to raise awareness of the condition and provides activities for patients and their caregivers.

Mr A had a body mass index of 19.2 kg/m^2/BSA and was seen by the dietitian and started on dietary supplements. COPD patients who are malnourished should be referred to the dietitian to devise a diet plan to ensure that they get an adequate daily caloric and protein intake. A more caloric dense oral nutritional supplement such as Ensure Plus (1.5 kcal/mL) or Fresubin (2 kcal/mL) may be more appropriate in this setting.

The decision regarding the use of an opioid-based treatment for the management of dyspnoea in elderly patients with advanced COPD should take into account the risk of adverse effects from opioid use, such as dizziness that can lead to falls, respiratory depression, constipation, and urinary retention. The American Thoracic Society guidelines on the pharmacologic management of COPD 2020 advocated a personalised decision-making process regarding the use of opioid-based therapy in advanced COPD patients with refractory dyspnoea in spite of optimal medical therapy.

If breathlessness persists despite optimising inhalers and non-pharmacological techniques, we can start oral morphine mixture 2.5 mg Q4H/PRN in patients with CrCl >15 mL/min/1.73 m^2. In patients with CrCl <15 mL/min/1.73 m^2 or if the patient remains distressed by the symptom despite PRN oral morphine mixture, consider a referral to the hospital's palliative care team for further titration of medication. Lower doses, longer dosing intervals, or use of safer alternatives like fentanyl patches may also be considered in such situations.

"The hand that writes the opioid prescription should write the laxative prescription."

— Cicely Saunders

> Managing dyspnea in terminally ill patients is complex. While opioids are the pharmacological mainstay, there is a lot more we can do for them:
>
> — Breathing techniques, energy conservation techniques, and accommodation techniques (change in living arrangements, allowing more frequent rests)
> — Supplemental oxygen
> — Fan blowing cool air on face
> — Looking for and treating any concomitant mood/anxiety disorders

In opioid-induced constipation, stimulant laxatives (senna, bisacodyl) are the laxatives of choice. Bulk laxatives are best avoided as they may worsen the constipation if these patients are unable to maintain adequate fluid intake.

****

Mr A was reviewed in the outpatient clinic in eight weeks. His symptoms have improved but he remained hypoxaemic on room air. He was maintained on long-term oxygen therapy. Advance care planning (ACP) was initiated.

Question 4: Which of the following statements best describes advance care planning?

a. **A legal document signed by the patient that allows the doctor to suspend extraordinary life-sustaining treatment when the patient is terminally ill and has no decision-making capacity.**
b. **A legal document allowing the patient to appoint a substitute decision-maker to make financial or personal welfare decisions on the patient's behalf when the patient loses their decision-making capacity.**
c. **A series of conversations about a patient's wishes for care and treatment in event that the patient loses their decision-making capacity.**
d. **A series of conversations about the disposition of a patient's assets following their demise.**

ACP is a series of conversations about a patient's wishes for care and treatment in the event that the patient loses their decision-making capacity. Members of the healthcare team can be advocates or facilitators to help patients reflect and decide on their future healthcare treatment.

There are different stages of advanced care planning:

(1) General ACP discussion — for healthy adults or those with early chronic disease
(2) Disease-specific ACP — for patients with progressive life-limiting illness and declining function suffering from frequent complications
(3) Preferred plan of care (PPC) — for patients with less than 12 months' prognosis

A disease-specific ACP was worked out for Mr A. In the event of critical illness, Mr A has decided to prioritise symptom control and was not keen for aggressive resuscitation measures.

Key messages

1. Exclude mimics of COPD in the geriatric patient.
2. Prioritise ease of use of inhaler devices and once-daily dosing of inhalers in selecting treatment for the geriatric patient.
3. Non-pharmacologic aspects like vaccination, smoking cessation, pulmonary rehabilitation, and nutrition are important in holistic care of the geriatric COPD patient.
4. Establish goals of care early.

Answer key

1. B.
2. A.
3. B.
4. C.

References

Graham BL, Steenbruggen I, Miller MR, Barjaktarevic IZ, Cooper BG, *et al.* (2019) Standardization of spirometry 2019 update: an official American Thoracic Society and European Respiratory Society technical statement. *Am J Respir Crit Care Med* **200**(8): e70–e88.

Global Strategy for Prevention, Diagnosis and Management of Chronic Obstructive Pulmonary Disease: 2023 Report.

Spruit MA, Singh SJ, Garvey C, ZuWallack R, Nici L, *et al.* (2013) ATS/ERS Task Force on Pulmonary Rehabilitation. An official American Thoracic Society/European Respiratory Society statement: key concepts and advances in pulmonary rehabilitation. *Am J Respir Crit Care Med* **188**: e13–e64.

Yang IA, Clarke MS, Sim EH, Fong KM (2012) Inhaled corticosteroids for stable chronic obstructive pulmonary disease. *Cochrane Database Syst Rev.* **2012**(7): CD002991.

29 Drowsiness (Hypoglycaemia)

Lim Kai Xiong, Melvin Chua Peng Wei

Mr O is an 82-year-old gentleman was admitted to general medicine for pneumonia. He had presented with purulent cough, fever, and poor oral intake over the past three days. His past medical history includes hypertension, hyperlipidaemia, and type 2 diabetes mellitus (latest HbA1c 7.1%) complicated by stage 3a chronic kidney disease. His chronic medications are metformin 500 mg BD, NovoMIX 30 Flexipen (insulin aspart 30%, insulin aspart protamine 70%) 16 units pre breakfast/10 units pre dinner, atorvastatin 20 mg ON, and lisinopril 5 mg OM. He is now receiving intravenous ceftriaxone for his chest infection. He is served a low-salt, low-fat, low-carbohydrate diet for meals.

On day two of admission, a staff nurse informs the junior doctor in the ward that Mr O was found to be drowsy and poorly responsive. His Glasgow Coma Scale was E3V3M4. A capillary blood glucose (CBG) performed stat showed a reading of 2.4 mmol/L.

Question 1: What is your immediate plan of action?

a. **Give a bolus of 40 ml of dextrose 50% (D50%)**
b. **Order intramuscular glucagon 1 mg**
c. **Serve the patient a dextrose drink**
d. **Serve the patient a hot chocolate drink**
e. **Start intravenous dextrose 5% infusion of 2 L over 24 hours**

Question 2: Postulate an explanation (or explanations) for the development of hypoglycaemia in Mr O.

Mr O would not have been able to take a dextrose drink safely as he was drowsy, unable to follow commands, and did not have an enteral feeding tube. Hence, the hypoglycaemia was corrected by the administration of 40 mls of D50% as a bolus.

In the event that intravenous access cannot be obtained, intramuscular glucagon 1 mg could have been considered as an alternative.

Should the patient be able to take orally safely, the hypoglycaemia could be corrected as follows:

- For CBG of **2.8–3.9 mmol/L**, administer 1 sachet of dextrose (anhydrous) oral powder with half a cup of water or 15 g of fast-acting carbohydrates
- For CBG <***2.8 mmol/L***, administer 2 sachets of dextrose (anhydrous) oral powder with half a cup of water or 30 g of fast-acting carbohydrates

It is essential to recheck CBG ***15 minutes*** after treatment to ensure the resolution of hypoglycaemia. Repeated treatment may be required if the patient remains hypoglycaemic.

After the patient's hypoglycaemia has been corrected, it is important to review the underlying reasons for hypoglycaemia so that the necessary interventions are performed. The ultimate aim is to obliterate the recurrence of further potentially preventable hypoglycaemic episodes. Prolonged and unrecognised hypoglycaemia may result in irreversible cognitive impairment due to neuroglycopenia. Repeated hypoglycaemic episodes contribute to depression and lower quality of life.

On review of Mr O's medical records, it was noted that his renal function had deteriorated over time with progression of diabetic kidney disease over the last few years. Reduced renal clearance of insulin prolongs the half-life of insulin which led to a progressive improvement of his HbA1c. Hence, seemingly better glycaemic control may in fact be due to ominous worsening of renal function in the older patient. On further history taking, it was noted that the patient was already having symptoms suggestive of hypoglycaemia at home.

The other significant contribution to hypoglycaemia is poor oral intake. In the elderly, this is often associated with inter-current illness, nausea, poor dentition, dementia, depression, and unfamiliar/modified hospital diets.

Elderly individuals are at increased risk of hypoglycaemia:

— *impaired cognitive function making it difficult to adhere to complex medication regimes, diet, and glucose monitoring*
— *reduced renal clearance of insulin*
— *poor eyesight and/or reduced dexterity of fingers due to arthritis of the joints of the hands resulting in insulin injection errors*
— *limited hypoglycaemia awareness*
— *blunted glucagon and epinephrine response in hypoglycaemia*
— *inconsistent oral intake*
— *polypharmacy (especially ≥5 medication classes)*

Table 29.1. Common Medications Interacting with Antidiabetic Medications in the Elderly to Potentially Cause Clinically Significant Hypoglycaemia.

Medication	Likely mechanism	Remarks
Antibiotics: ***Clarithromycin*** ***Fluoroquinolones*** Cotrimoxazole	 Inhibits P-glycoprotein and CYP enzymes Stimulates insulin release	 Especially sulphonylurea
Ethanol	Inhibits gluconeogenesis	Especially sulphonylurea
Pantoprazole	Reduced renal excretion of sitagliptin via transporter OAT3	Sitagliptin
Colchicine		DPP4-inhibitor (sitaglitpin, linagliptin, etc).
Acetaminophen		DPP4-inhibitor (sitaglitpin, linagliptin, etc).
Common herbal preparations in Singapore: Ginseng Lycium (Goji berries)	 Stimulates insulin secretion Improves glucose transport and insulin signaling	

It is imperative to review all patients' medications on admission (Table 29.1) and continue to do so throughout the hospitalisation and on discharge. As Mr O was at increased risk of hypoglycaemia for the reasons mentioned above, adjustments to his diabetic medication could have been made earlier to prevent the hypoglycaemic episode.

Thus, during routine outpatient reviews, it is imperative to review not just the older patient's blood sugars and HbA1c but also take into account renal function, eating habits, and other factors that may have affected their his/her oral intake.

****

After correcting the hypoglycaemia with dextrose 50%, Mr O was started on a maintenance dextrose 5% drip and his diabetic medications were adjusted accordingly. His oral intake and CBG trend were closely monitored over the next few days. Proactive titration of medications ensured that further hypoglycaemic episodes did not occur. The dextrose drip was subsequently stopped when he began eating well.

A plan was tailored after reviewing his medical condition, social setup, and caregiver requirements. It was later revealed that he was not competent with insulin injections due to deteriorating vision contributed by diabetic retinopathy which resulted in errors in the units of insulin injected. In addition, his caregivers were unable to help with the twice-daily injections as they had to go to work.

As such, his NovoMIX injections were stopped and he was started on once-daily basal insulin injection. This allowed Mr O's caregivers to assist with the injection before going to work. The simplified regime and caregiver involvement should improve compliance, and reduce errors and risk of hypoglycaemia.

Whilst inpatient, appropriate caregiver training was given. Insulin injection technique and rotation of injection sites to avoid lipodystrophy were reinforced. Mr O and his caregivers were also educated on CBG monitoring, as well as how to recognise and correct hypoglycaemia.

On discharge, Mr O was given an appointment to follow up on his diabetic control and to review for any further episodes of hypoglycaemia.

Question 3: What would be an appropriate HBA1c target for Mr O?

a. **5%**
b. **6%**
c. **7%**
d. **8%**
e. **9%**

The HbA1c target of each patient needs to be individualised. A less stringent HbA1c target can be considered in ***elderly and frail*** patients, especially if the diabetes duration is long and the patient is at high risk of hypoglycaemia and has shorter life expectancy and multiple comorbidities.

Mr O fits all the criteria for a less stringent HbA1c! In other patients with limited life expectancy, the focus should not be on a HbA1c target. Instead, avoidance of hypoglycaemia and symptomatic hyperglycaemia should be the main goals of diabetes management. During follow-ups, the CBG diary should be reviewed paying close attention to the fasting CBG — levels <4 mmol/L are a big NO!

On the websites of many local healthcare institutions, you can find helpful practical advice for patients and caregivers on how to quickly identify and appropriately act on hypoglycaemia. One handy resource is found in the free Healthhub app → "A–Z" → search for "diabetes" → "Diabetes: Management of Hypoglycaemia and Hyperglycaemic Crisis".

Key messages

1. It is important to recognise symptoms of hypoglycaemia — neurogenic and neuroglycopaenic — promptly. CBG is a critical point of care test for drowsiness.
2. Hypoglycaemia should be corrected expeditiously:
   a. Quick-acting carbohydrates if the patient is able to take orally
   b. Intravenous dextrose 50% if the patient is unable to take orally or has severe symptoms
   c. Intramuscular glucagon 1 mg if venous access is not available

   Check CBG 15 minutes later!
3. Review the underlying reasons for hypoglycaemia. If the underlying causes are not rectified, hypoglycaemia will recur.
4. The elderly are more prone to hypoglycaemia. Review the patient's diabetic history, including medications and baseline control. Make the necessary adjustments to medications before hypoglycaemia occurs.
5. HbA1c target needs to be individualised for each patient.
6. A tailored plan is required for each elderly diabetic patient, taking into consideration the medical condition, social setup, and caregiver requirements. Patient education and getting the caregiver on board in caring for the elderly with diabetes and other chronic diseases help to improve compliance and reduce potential complications.

Answer key

1. A.
2. Poor appetite, tightly controlled HbA1c, chronic (and worsening) renal impairment.
3. D. Age, comorbidities, long duration of disease, and risk of hypoglycaemia are reasons for his less stringent HbA1c target.

References

American Diabetes Association Professional Practice Committee (2022) 13. Older Adults: Standards of Medical Care in Diabetes — 2022. *Diabetes Care* **45**(Suppl 1): S195–S207.

Freeman J (2019) Management of hypoglycemia in older adults with type 2 diabetes. *Postgrad Med* **131**(4): 241–250.

Kalra S, Sharma SK (2018) Diabetes in the elderly. *Diabetes Ther* **9**(2): 493–500.

Mohissi E (2013) Management of Type 2 Diabetes Mellitus in Older Patients: Current and Emerging Treatment Options. *Diabetes Ther* **4**: 239–256.

30 Bradycardia (Hypothyroidism)

Tan Zaw Oo, Anupama Roy Chowdhury

Mdm B is a 72-year-old lady who was referred from the general practitioner for the evaluation of bradycardia. She had a history of type 2 diabetes mellitus, and her chronic medications are metformin 850 mg BD, glipizide 5 mg BD, and calcium 450 mg/vitamin D 200U supplement 2 tabs daily. Her general practitioner was checking her parameters and was concerned about her regular heart rate of 45/min.

Mdm B revealed that in the past three months, she has been feeling easily tired throughout the day and night. She was increasingly forgetful and unable to concentrate on daily tasks like cooking and cleaning the house. Her mood was low. However, she did not have any fever or infectious symptoms. She slept on one pillow at night and did not have chest pain or exertional breathlessness. She is single and does not have any close relatives.

Question 1: Excluding cardiogenic and infectious causes, which other systems would you pay attention to when obtaining further history concerning her lethargy?

In elderly patients, lethargy is a common presenting complaint. Albeit a non-specific symptom, it could represent an insidious manifestation of an underlying serious medical condition. Top differential diagnoses should always include infectious, metabolic/endocrine, and neoplastic causes as well as possible side-effects of medications (e.g., antidepressants, sedating antihistamines). Moreover, a depressive illness needs to be ruled out in elderly patients.

Bear in mind that hypothyroidism is commoner in older people, especially females, likely due to the increasing prevalence and incidence of autoimmune thyroiditis. In addition, the clinical presentations of hypothyroidism in the elderly differ from younger adults in that they have less complaints of cold intolerance, weight gain, and muscle cramps, but more of them present with neurological symptoms and signs like impaired hearing, ataxia, and hypogeusia. Fatigue and exertional dyspnoea are also more common in older hypothyroid individuals.

Evaluating sinus bradycardia in the elderly can be challenging as sinus rates below 50/min are often in keeping with age-related physiology. Symptomatic sinus bradycardia can have many differential diagnoses. All kinds of sinus node dysfunction are commoner in the elderly, especially those with diabetes, and hypothyroidism can both cause it or mimic its symptoms of lethargy, fatigue, and weakness. All kinds of atrioventricular blocks are also more common in the elderly. Slow ventricular response atrial fibrillation can appear to be sinus in nature, caused by hypothermia from hypothyroidism. Diabetic dysautonomia can rarely cause bradycardia, apart from orthostatic dizziness.

****

On a systems review, Mdm B related recent and increasing difficulty in passing motion. She did not have cold or heat intolerance, cold sweat, giddiness, tremor, or feelings of hunger. Her intake was as per normal (meal delivery service), but she was steadily gaining weight and her legs were swelling. She denied osmotic symptoms such as polydipsia and polyuria. Although she did not monitor her glucose levels, she took her medications regularly and was told by her general practitioner that her diabetes was well controlled.

Additionally, Mdm B has been sleeping earlier and waking up later in the last few months. She did not find enjoyment in her usual hobbies and had lost interest in watching television. She has no neurological complaint. She has no history of cancer or surgery. She denied taking traditional medication. Her geriatric depression score was 9, indicative of moderate depression.

On examination, her vital signs were as follows: temperature 36.1°C, heart rate 49/min, and blood pressure 140/80 mmHg. Her BMI was 29 kg/m^2. Her abbreviated mental test score was 7/10 — she failed to answer her age, give the Prime Minister's name, and recall the memory phrase.

She was not pale but appeared to have dry skin. There was non-pitting oedema over the lower limbs to mid-shin level. There was no mass or tenderness of the neck. Neurological and other systemic examinations were grossly normal.

The thyroid panel showed:

Thyroid stimulating hormone (TSH)	*27.4 mIU/L*	*(0.701–4.280)*
Free thyroxine (T4)	*8 pmol/L*	*(12.7–20.3)*

Question 2: Outline an appropriate management plan for Mdm B.

One must have an index of suspicion for thyroid disorder when an elderly patient presents with generalised and non-specific symptoms despite only having a few dysthyroid symptoms. As the hypothyroidism also contributes to the low mood in most elderly patients, it is essential to be investigated.

Although TSH is the most important test and can adequately detect overt primary hypothyroidism in the elderly, assessing free T4 is also crucial for management as it helps to differentiate between overt and subclinical hypothyroidism, and it can predict and affect TSH level inversely. While there are some discrepancies in the definitions of subclinical hypothyroidism, it is widely accepted as having a raised TSH level with normal free T4 and without positive antibodies in the serum. Hence in general, it is advisable to check both TSH and free T4 for a better interpretation and to expedite further management.

It is a known fact that the levels of TSH and free T4 change with ageing with a mild increase in TSH as the patient ages. Older patients also tend to have non-thyroidal illnesses causing derangements of their thyroid function. Several studies on treating mild thyroid hypofunction in the elderly have shown mixed results. While there is no consensus for treating elderly patients based on high TSH levels alone (5–10 mIU/L), most practices accept a slightly higher TSH threshold before instituting thyroxine replacement

Hypothyroidism impacts multiple systems, and the severity depends on the chronicity and degree of hypothyroidism. Mdm B's basic laboratory works revealed mild hyponatraemia (Na 130 mmol/L), mild anaemia (Hb 11 g/dL), and creatinine kinase level 277 U/L (44–201). Liver profiles were normal. Lipid panel showed high total cholesterol, low-density lipoprotein, and triglycerides. In addition, her thyroid peroxidase (TPO) antibody level was 61.4 IU/ML [<9.0 IU/ML]. ECG showed sinus bradycardia with no evidence of old infarcts.

Mdm B was diagnosed with hypothyroidism secondary to Hashimoto's thyroiditis. Note that unlike younger adults, elderly patients with autoimmune thyroiditis are more likely to present with the atrophic form of the disorder (i.e., without goitre).

The medical team decided to start levothyroxine (L-thyroxine). The goal of therapy is the euthyroid state with improvement of symptoms and TSH in the long term towards a level considered acceptable for the age of the patient. Early identification and treatment of hypothyroidism is particularly important in the elderly as they are more prone to developing severe medical complications such as myxoedema coma and peri-operative and intra-operative complications.

Subclinical hypothyroidism is also a common biochemical abnormality seen in the older patient where the TSH is elevated with normal free T4. These patients may have sought medical attention for other complaints. For such patients, it would be reasonable to start thyroxine if TSH >10 mIU/L or TPO antibodies are positive and monitor their response 6–8 weeks later.

In older patients (age >60 years) or those with coronary artery disease, L-thyroxine should be started at a lower dose (0.25 to 0.5 mcg/kg/day) and increased gradually in 4–6 weeks. For practical purposes, a starting dose of 12.5 to 25 mcg/day may be considered.

Atorvastatin was started because of significant dyslipidaemia. Mdm B was then discharged once medically fit and given a follow-up in the outpatient clinic.

****

Six weeks after the discharge, during the follow-up clinic consultation, Mdm B expressed that she felt better yet not her usual self. Her geriatric depression score was 4 which showed some improvement. While her leg swelling had improved, her weight was still the same.

The thyroid panel showed:

TSH	*23.2 mIU/L*	*(0.701–4.280)*
Free T4	*9.1 pmol/L*	*(12.7–20.3)*

The lipid panel showed improvement. She claimed compliance to her medications and had not taken any traditional medication. She was able to tell the correct dose of thyroxine prescribed.

Question 3: What do you think could be happening?

In compliant patients with under-achieving treatment goals, consider the impact of pharmacokinetic interactions. Thyroxine absorption is significantly reduced with meals and other minerals, especially iron and calcium, as gastric pH appears to influence the absorption. In postmenopausal women with primary hypothyroidism, oestrogen replacement therapy can lead to higher thyroxine dose requirements due to the increased production of thyroid-binding globulin.

When caring for the elderly patient, it is paramount to educate the patient as well as the family or caregivers on the medication timings, dosages, and how to monitor for side-effects.

****

Upon further clarification, the patient took thyroxine with other medications and breakfast. She was counselled on the correct way of taking thyroxine, which is supposed to be at least 1 hour away from meals or food and other medication so as to achieve better absorption. She was given further follow-up in the clinic.

Key messages

1. Although there are multiple causes of lethargy in the elderly, it is essential to rule out infections, metabolic disorders, and malignancy. Even though the most common cause of hypothyroidism in all ages is autoimmune (Hashimoto's) thyroiditis, thorough assessment is needed to exclude other causes such as medications (e.g., lithium, amiodarone) and iatrogenic causes (e.g., surgery, radiotherapy).
2. Conduct the thyroid function test (TSH and free T4) in the older patient with non-specific symptoms and a suspicion for hypothyroidism.
3. The antibodies tests are not strictly recommended once the hypothyroidism is diagnosed, but it is helpful for confirmation of the diagnosis. It is also useful in determining the need for treatment in subclinical hypothyroidism. Metabolic and liver profiles may show hyponatraemia, dyslipidaemia, and raised transaminase levels. Hypothyroidism is known to be associated with anaemia and increased creatinine kinase. Imaging will be needed for further evaluation if there is nodular thyroid or compression symptoms.
4. Exercise caution when starting thyroxine replacement as elderly patients may have underlying undiagnosed coronary artery disease or risk factors which increase its risk.
5. Thyroxine absorption is significantly reduced with meals and other minerals, especially iron and calcium.

Answer key

1. Metabolic disorders, especially glucose control and thyroid symptoms; malignancy and psychiatric illness (depression).
2. Renal panel, liver panel, full blood count, creatinine kinase;

   Fasting lipid profile;

   Thyroid antibodies tests viz. anti-thyroid peroxidase (anti-TPO) and anti-thyroglobulin (anti-Tg);

   ECG;

   L-thyroxine starting dose 25 mcg daily (12.5 mcg daily if she has electrocardiographic changes of coronary artery disease with gradual increase in dose).

3. Check if the patient has been taking thyroxine together with meals and other medications/supplements.

Reference

Barbesino G (2019) Thyroid Function Changes in the Elderly and Their Relationship to Cardiovascular Health: A Mini-Review. *Gerontology* **65**: 1–8.

Bensenor IM, Olmos RD, Lotufo PA (2012) Hypothyroidism in the elderly: diagnosis and management. *Clin Interv Aging* **7**: 97–111.

Colucci P, Yue CS, Ducharme M, Benvenga S (2013) A Review of the Pharmacokinetics of Levothyroxine for the Treatment of Hypothyroidism. *Eur Endocrinol* **9**(1): 40–47.

31 Itch

Derrick Aw Chen Wee, Melvin Chua Peng Wei

A 80-year-old man with Parkinson disease was admitted with dehydration and consequent acute kidney impairment. He also complained of itchy rash on his legs for one month.

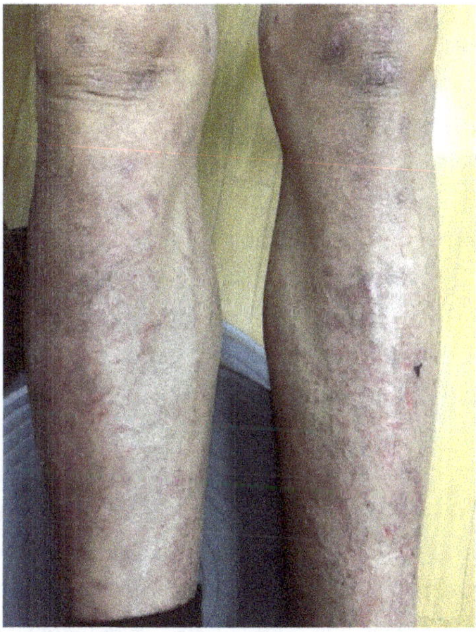

Question 1: What is the most likely diagnosis?

a. **Asteatotic eczema**
b. **Contact dermatitis**
c. **Renal pruritus**
d. **Stasis eczema**
e. **Tinea corporis**

The first priority in approaching an elderly with itch is to determine if the itch is due to a dermatologic condition or not. The latter refers to ***primary pruritus***, which means that the itch occurs on normal-looking intact skin. We can group the known causes into four categories:

(1) Systemic, e.g., chronic kidney disease (even if on haemodialysis), chronic liver disease, hyperthyroidism, paraneoplastic.
(2) Neuropathic, e.g., post-herpetic, diabetes (due to small-fibre polyneuropathy), radiculopathy (brachioradial pruritus which typically affects the upper limbs, and notalgia paraesthetica which typically affects the interscapular region on one side).
(3) Psychogenic, e.g., depression and anxiety disorders, delusional parasitosis.
(4) Adverse drug reaction, e.g., calcium channel blockers, thiazides, angiotensin-converting enzyme inhibitors, codeine. Polypharmacy renders the elderly particularly at risk.

If none of the above is evident, then we may offer a diagnosis of exclusion of "senile pruritus". Clinically, you may see secondary skin lesions such as scratch marks, but otherwise the skin looks normal.

This patient, however, has a primary dermatosis to account for his itch. The presence of scaling and redness suggest a dermatitis (interchangeable with "eczema") while its ***crazy-paving pattern*** is classical of asteatotic eczema. Tinea often exhibits an annular pattern of peripheral scaling and central clearing. While it is a rule of thumb to always consider the possibility of contact dermatitis in any adult with new-onset dermatitis, the morphology in this case and the absence of a contactant history rule this out.

Xerotic eczema is an overarching entity of dermatitis due to skin dryness (xerosis), and asteatotic eczema with the characteristic haphazard pattern of scaly erythema is a subset of it. More than half of elderly people have xerosis, and most of them experience itch and inflammation as a consequence.

Elderly people are prone to developing xerosis because of an age-related increase in epidermal surface pH which reduces the activity of lipid-forming enzymes, decreases the production of natural moisturizing factor, and impairs the activity of ceramide-forming enzymes in the stratum corneum. Additionally, the expression of Aquaporin 3 (AQP3; a protein that facilitates the transport of water and glycerol through the cell membrane to maintain epidermal hydration) is reduced in elderly skin.

Elderly people are prone to developing itch in their skin because the increase in skin alkalinity enhances the activity of serine proteases that activate protease-activated receptor 2 (PAR2) receptor signaling which induces itch. Xerosis itself may further reduce the itch threshold to other stimuli. An acquired abnormality in keratinisation in the elderly has also been suggested.

Note that an elderly person may have xerosis and not have eczema, yet. If the xerosis remains unmanaged, there is a high likelihood that eczema will eventually occur. Interestingly, the characteristic pattern of asteatotic eczema almost always shows up only on the shins. The legs in the elderly are a site that is prone to another form of eczema: ***stasis eczema*** (Fig 31.1). Many elderly patients have oedema on their legs due to heart failure and chronic venous insufficiency.

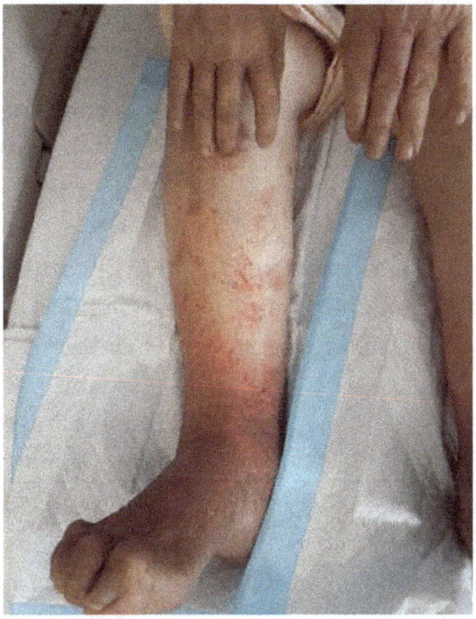

Fig. 31.1. Patient with dual stasis and asteaotosic eczema.

****

Question 2: Which of the following topical anti-inflammatory agents is the most appropriate for this patient?

a. Betamethasone dipropionate 0.05% cream BD

b. Betamethasone dipropionate 0.05% ointment BD

c. Betamethasone valerate 0.05% cream BD

d. Betamethasone valerate 0.05% ointment BD

e. Clobetasol propionate 0.05% cream BD

Presently, there are two types of topical anti-inflammatory therapies for eczema: topical corticosteroids (TCS) and topical calcineurin inhibitors. The topical calcineurin inhibitor that is more commonly used by dermatologists for elderly patients is topical tacroliumus 0.1% ointment, and we often reserve this expensive product (about S$60 for a 10 g tube) for limited-extent eczema on the sites of very thin skin such as the eyelids and where steroid atrophy is present. Patients should be warned of the risk of a transient burning sensation after application which decreases with repeated use. It is clearly inappropriate for use in this situation.

This table gives the potency rankings of the common TCS (alone or in combination) used in local institutions:

Potency	Example of TCS (generic versions available for all)	Example of fixed-dose combination of TCS and antimicrobial
Mildly potent	Hydrocortisone cream/ointment Betamethasone valerate 0.025% cream/ointment Desonide 0.05% lotion/cream	Hydrocortisone et clioquinol cream Hydrocortisone et fusidic acid cream Hydrocortisone et miconazole cream Betamethasone valerate 0.025% et clioquinol cream
Moderately potent	Betamethasone valerate 0.05% cream/ointment Betamethasone valerate 0.1% lotion/cream	Betamethasone valerate 0.05% et clioquinol cream Betamethasone valerate 0.05% et clioquinol cream
Potent	Betamethasone valerate 0.1% ointment Mometasone furoate 0.1% lotion/cream/ointment Betamethasone dipropionate 0.05% cream/ointment	Betamethasone dipropionate 0.05% et fusidic acid cream/ointment Betamethasone dipropionate 0.05% et gentamicin cream Betamethasone dipropionate 0.064% et clotrimazole and gentamicin cream
Very potent	Clobetasol propionate 0.05% lotion/cream/ointment	

Many factors come into consideration before we make a judgement call on the most appropriate TCS for a patient's eczema.

A. Disease-related

Determine if the eczema is ***acute or chronic***. An acute eczema is likely to comprise mainly of papules, discharge, blistering, oedema, and pain. A chronic eczema is likely to look like thickened, possibly lichenified plaques. Lower potency TCS and a cream formulation are preferred for acute stage. You may elect to use a TCS combined with an antiseptic like clioquinol as flares of eczema are often provoked by an abundance of *Staphylococcus aureus* on the skin. TCS-containing antibiotics like fusidic acid and gentamicin would be suitable for eczema with secondary impetiginisation (exemplified by the presence of honey golden crusting). Fusidic acid-containing topicals are generally reserved for outpatient use and for short periods of use to prevent the development of resistance. Chronic eczemas respond better to higher potency TCS and an ointment formulation that is more occlusive in texture. A subacute eczema will exhibit features of both acute and chronic eczema, and the potency and formulation of TCS depends on which type is predominant.

Look at the extent of the eczema. Creams and lotions are easier to apply and spread than ointments for application over large areas.

B. Site-related

Certain parts of the body are physiologically thin and thus very vulnerable to developing steroid atrophy viz. ***eyelids, flexural areas*** (antecubital fossae, popliteal fossae, neck), and external genitalia. For other areas of the body where the skin is fragile and easily wrinkled with purpura, a lower potency TCS is preferred.

Eczema over hairy areas such as the scalp, pubic areas, and moustache is best treated with a TCS in lotion formulation.

C. Drug-related

Some TCS are less atrophogenic than others, so these may be better choices for a patient with eczema over atrophied skin or sensitive sites. Mometasone furoate 0.1% cream and lotion only needs to be applied once instead of twice daily. Desonide 0.05% cream/lotion ($20 for a 60 ml bottle) is slightly more potent yet gentler than hydrocortisone cream.

D. Patient-related

Information from the patient's past experience may be helpful. For instance, if you think a strong TCS like betamethasone dipropionate 0.05% ointment is needed to manage a patient's lichen simplex chronicus, but the patient has expressed that he had previously had excellent response with a weaker TCS such as betamethasone valerate 0.1% ointment, you can elect to persist with it instead of escalating the potency.

Most TCS are available in generic versions so with few exceptions, affordability is not a major concern today.

After you have decided on a most appropriate TCS for the patient and counseled on proper use (rub the TCS into the rash until you don't see the white of a cream, or feel the greasiness of an ointment), the next important aspect of prescribing is the quantity. Very often, a patient's rash needlessly flares due to insufficient amounts of TCS given to last till the clinic review. As a rule of thumb, ***one*** 15 g tube of TCS applied twice daily should suffice for a rash whose body surface area covers ***one*** palm, for ***one*** month.

Advise the patient to continue using the TCS regularly to complete skin clearance. Complete skin clearance is observed when the rash is no longer palpable, not itchy, and not red (though it may look brownish due to post-inflammatory hyperpigmentation). When that happens, the TCS can be applied to the same areas twice weekly for two months to prolong remission. A common mistake is to completely stop the TCS the moment complete skin clearance is achieved!

****

Question 3: How many 15 g tubes of TCS would you prescribe for this patient before he goes home? His outpatient appointment with dermatology is in three months.

a. One

b. Two

c. Three

d. Four

e. Five

Question 4: A typical restructured hospital in Singapore has the following moisturising items in its formulary: aqueous cream, urea 10% cream, emulsifying ointment, white soft paraffin, white soft paraffin-liquid paraffin (3:2) ointment (Table 31.2). Which and how would you prescribe for this patient?

This patient definitely needs a moisturising skincare regime as the underlying problem is xerosis (age-related).

Table 31.2. Moisturizers in formularies of restructured hospitals in Singapore.

Formulary moisturiser	Aqueous cream (sodium lauryl sulphate-free)	Urea 10% cream	White soft paraffin	White soft paraffin-liquid paraffin (3:2) ointment
Active ingredient(s)	White soft paraffin, liquid paraffin	Urea 10%, white soft paraffin	Petrolatum	Petrolatum plus mineral oil in 3:2 ratio
Characteristic(s) of note	Occlusive	Humectant > Occlusive	Occlusive; very greasy and not so easy to spread	Occlusive; greasy but easier to spread
Cost	$3 for a 100 g tube	$5 for a 100 g tube	$3 for a 100 g jar	$4.15 for a 100 g jar

You may select any of these moisturisers for your patient, though the following considerations may influence the choice presently or at a later time:

- Urea cream confers a theoretical advantage over the others by conferring an additional humectant (attracting water into the stratum corneum) property
- Urea cream confers an additional weak (10% only) keratolytic effect, so it may be particularly beneficial when there is significant scaling on the skin
- Aqueous cream and urea cream contain emulsifiers which may cause sensitivity reactions in certain individuals
- The petrolatum-based products are less likely to irritate skins with significant amounts of excoriation
- The greasiness of the petrolatum-based products may significantly affect adherence

You may also have heard of "therapeutic moisturisers" available in retail. These purportedly confer additional benefits (e.g., directly replenishing defective or deficient molecules in the skin barrier such as natural moisturising factor and ceramides, providing an antibacterial property, reducing skin inflammation, reducing itch) on top of just occlusion and water attraction. While much more expensive than the formulary moisturisers, their superior textures generally allow the product to glide and absorb more easily in the skin, hence enhancing adherence. Adherence is key to ensuring successful therapeutic outcomes in dermatology.

Moisturisers must be applied to the entire body at least ***twice*** daily, preferably after a shower and at bedtime. This must be re-enforced to the patient if he is applying the moisturiser himself, as many of the elderly are non-compliant with the frequency of application. In the event that the patient is unable to do the application himself in view of impaired dexterity of fingers or the presence of cognitive impairment, caregivers must be educated on the optimal frequency of application. To ensure optimal bioavailabilities, moisturisers and TCS should be applied at separate times, preferably spaced thirty minutes apart.

Whichever moisturiser you select, you need to ensure that adequate quantities are dispensed. An average-sized adult should require a minimum of ***200 g*** of moisturizer for the ***entire body per week***.

Emulsifying ointment that is petrolatum-based may be prescribed as a soap substitute. However, it is very greasy and contains a small amount of sodium lauryl sulphate which can cause irritation to hyper-sensitive skin. We usually prescribe this as adjunctive skincare for people with *very* dry skin. In the elderly, excessive greasiness of the skin may predispose to falls!

In the event that multiple creams or formulations have been prescribed for different parts of the body, it would be prudent to write the instructions in an easy-to-understand format for the patient and caregiver to follow.

Key messages

1. The approach to an elderly with itch (with "eczema") can be summarised in three steps:
   a. Distinguish between primary and secondary pruritus (as investigations and management differ).
   b. Make sure you are dealing with a dermatitis (not urticaria, for instance, which may portend pemphigoid!).
   c. Consider the likely causes of the dermatitis. The commonest cause of itch in the elderly is xerosis, and the commonest cause of an itchy rash in the elderly is xerotic eczema.
2. Dermatitis needs a three-pronged management:
   a. Treat the cause if it is treatable (e.g., chronic venous insufficiency, heart failure, contact with external irritants).
   b. Treat the inflammation. A topical corticosteroid is the usual treatment. When used in the proper way (twice daily for most TCS, rub into the rash until you don't see the white of the cream or don't feel the greasiness of the ointment), side-effects are uncommon.
   c. Treat the skin barrier. Prescribe at least 200 g/week of a moisturiser for application to the entire body at least twice daily at separate times of the TCS.

Answer key

1. A.
2. C.
3. C. *The body surface area covered by the rash on both legs adds up to about one palm only.*
4. There are many prescription possibilities of moisturiser for this patient. A reasonable one would be urea 10% cream BD. The patient should be advised to apply the cream all over the body even if the rash is currently confined to the legs, because xerosis affects everywhere and it is a matter of time that inflammation occurs outside the legs. Hence, if you can convince the patient (and the caregiver), the ideal quantity to dispense is 200 g per week.

Reference

Aw DCW (2021) My Dance with Eczema: And 80 lessons for the patient and the doctor. Singapore: Partridge Publishing.

32 Blistering Disorder

Phoon Yee Wei, Foo Swee Sen

An 85-year-old female who is a resident of a nursing home was admitted following a recent fall associated with functional decline. She used to be ambulant with a walking frame and required some assistance in her activities of daily living. Her pre-existing medical problems are type 2 diabetes mellitus, hypertension, ischaemic cardiomyopathy, old strokes, and mixed dementia with recurrent falls.

History from the patient is limited apart from complaints of mild pain over her lower back. Vital signs are blood pressure 140/85 mmHg, heart rate 80/min regular, oxygen saturation 95% on room air, and afebrile. Physical examination revealed a small

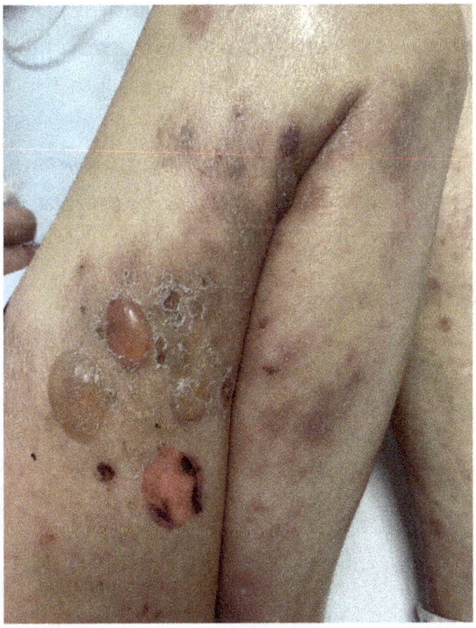

Fig. 32.1. Tense bullae and erosions on an urticarial background and overall dry scaly skin.

haematoma over her occipital scalp and mild lumbar spinal tenderness, otherwise no spinal deformity was noted. Of note, blisters were noted over her left leg (Fig 32.1).

Question 1: What other targeted physical examinations and diagnostic investigations would you perform?

Blistering dermatoses can be broadly classified in this way:

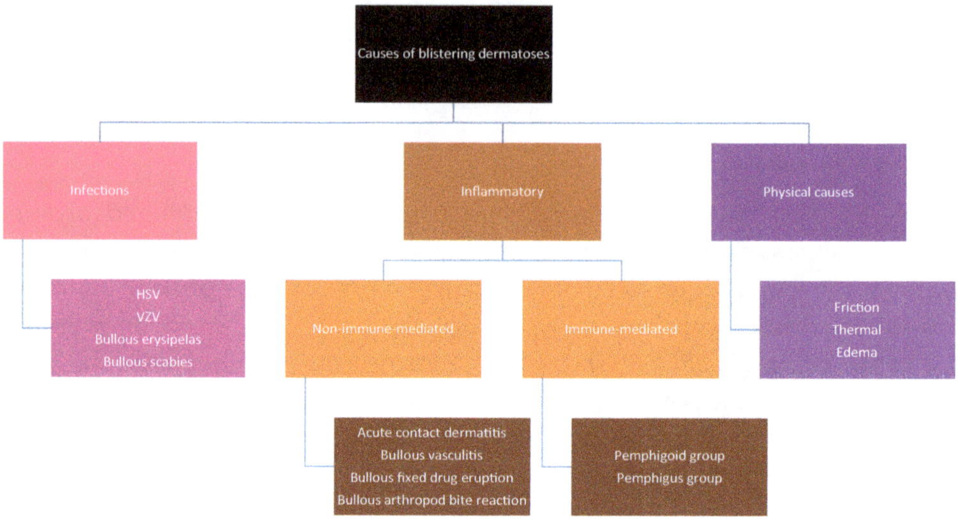

The presence of blisters on one limb should always prompt one to look for the same on the contralateral and other limbs, as blisters confined to a single limb may suggest herpes zoster infection (Fig 32.2) especially if the blisters are distributed in a dermatomal pattern.

Also, the evaluation of blistering dermatoses must include meticulous inspection of the mucosal surfaces: oral, conjunctiva, and genitalia. Several

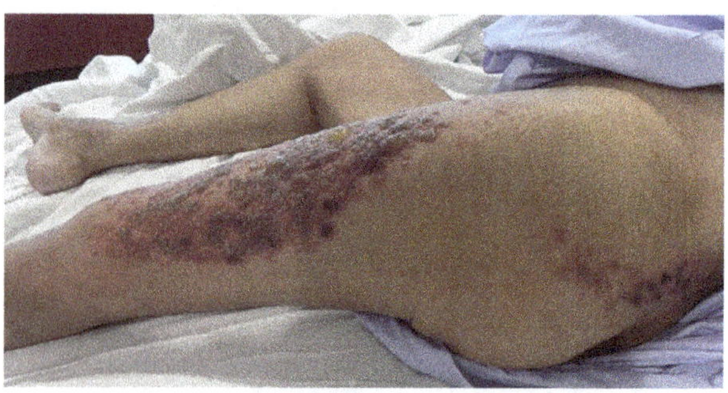

Fig. 32.2. Shingles: clusters of haemorrhagic vesiculobullae on an erythematous base with characteristically scalloped edges over the L3 and L4 dermatomes. The right leg is conspicuously spared.

autoimmune-mediated blistering diseases, especially the pemphigus group, have concomitant mucosal involvement. Similarly, up to 50% of patients with bullous pemphigoid (BP) may have buccal erosions too! These can be an important cause of poor feeding amongst elderly patients with BP and will be missed without examination of the oral cavity.

Bullous scabies has been reported to mimic autoimmune blistering diseases such as bullous pemphigoid both clinically as well as immunologically. This should be considered as a differential especially in the appropriate clinical setting: patients from community care facilities, other residents or caregivers reporting similar signs and symptoms, and lack of improvement expected with anti-inflammatory treatment.

In the work up for sub-epithelial autoimmune blistering diseases, most commonly BP, we send serum samples for enzyme-linked immunosorbent assay: BP 180 (or BPAG2), BP 230 (or BPAG1) antigens. BP 180 is almost always positive in BP and its titre has been shown to correlate with BP disease activity. Another test that substantiates a diagnosis of BP is indirect immunofluorescence which uses a serum sample and 1 molar salt split skin as substrate. A "roof pattern" is seen in BP.

****

Over the next few days, new blisters appeared over her hands, arms, feet, and trunk.

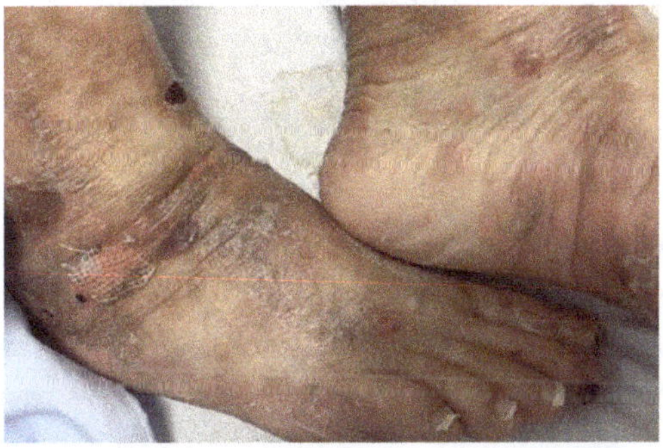

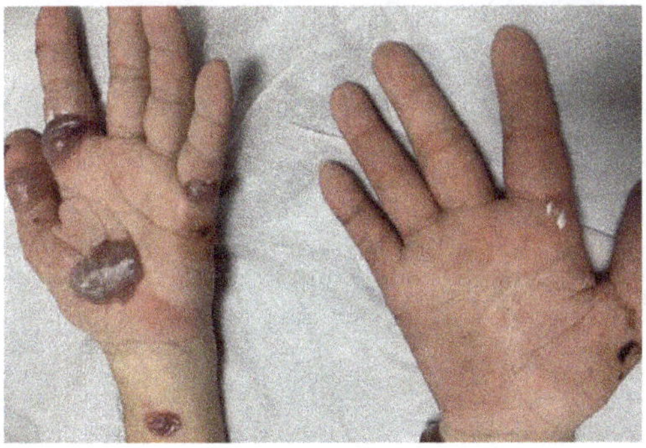

Question 2: What is the most likely diagnosis?

a. **Bullous contact dermatitis**
b. **Bullous pemphigoid**
c. **Bullous scabies**
d. **Pemphigus vulgaris**
e. **Varicella zoster infection**

Progression of the blistering rash in a generalised symmetrical distribution renders zoster and contact dermatitis unlikely. The blistering eruption in this case may be too florid for bullous scabies which typically presents with a polymorphous eruption alongside characteristic scabetic lesions such as crusted plaques over the palms and soles or papules, nodules, pustules, linear burrows, and eczematous plaques located over sites of predilection such as the finger or toe-web spaces, peri-areolar area, axillary, groin, or genitalia. The lack of oral or mucosal involvement and the predominance of tense bullae as opposed to flaccid bullae or crusted plaques makes pemphigus vulgaris (PV) less likely. Moreover, PV usually affects younger age groups compared to BP.

Bullous pemphigoid is the most common autoimmune-mediated blistering disease amongst those aged above 70. The prevalence of neuropsychiatric disorders such as dementia, Parkinson's disease, stroke, epilepsy, and depression has been reported to be 10-fold higher in BP patients. Typically, these disorders precede the development of BP. During the pre-bullous phase, BP can present with gyrate urticarial plaques or eczematous lesions. These give rise to tense clear or haemorrhagic bullae during the bullous phase. Sites of predilection include the palms and soles, flexural sites of the trunk, and proximal limbs. Remember that up to 50% of BP patients may have involvement in mucosal sites.

BP is characterised by the presence of circulating auto-antibodies to the basement membrane hemi-desmosomal antigens BP 230 and BP 180. Proteolytic cleavage as a result of binding of these auto-antibodies results in the formation of tense bullae.

****

A diagnostic skin punch biopsy (for histological examination and direct immunofluorescence, or DIF) was considered.

Question 3: Which of the positions (A, B, or C) should the punch biopsy be performed over for

1. **Histology?**
2. **DIF?**

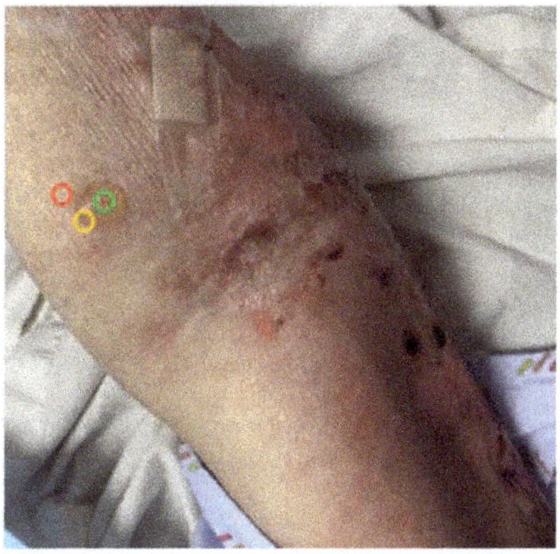

Skin biopsy, if performed for blistering dermatoses, should be done over the edge of the blister as this would allow for delineation of the level of the split. Of course if the blister is small enough, then the entire blister can be punched out.

Characteristic histological features in BP are a sub-epidermal split and an inflammatory infiltrate comprising of predominantly eosinophils and lymphocytes. When sending specimens taken for DIF in blistering dermatoses, care should be taken to obtain samples from the peri-lesional skin as opposed to that from blister skin as we will need an intact epidermis for adequate visualisation.

****

Question 4: Which of the following is the most appropriate management?

a. Start medium-potency topical corticosteroid (e.g., betamethasone 0.1% valerate cream) to rash + wound care

b. Start oral prednisolone at 0.5 mg/kg/day and very high-potency topical corticosteroid (e.g., clobetasol propionate 0.05% cream) to rash + wound care

c. Start potent topical corticosteroid (e.g., clobetasol propionate 0.05% cream) to rash + wound care

d. Start oral anti-Staphylococcal antibiotics (e.g., cephalexin) and medium-potency topical corticosteroid combined with anti-septic (e.g., betamethasone valerate 0.1% et clioquinol cream) to rash

e. Only wound care is required

Corticosteroids form the cornerstone therapy of BP.

Topical corticosteroids can be used as monotherapy in mild or localised BP — body surface area (BSA) involved <10%.

Systemic corticosteroids are first line therapy for moderate to severe BP (BSA involved >10%). Suggested starting doses of systemic corticosteroid are:

Moderate disease: oral prednisolone 0.5 mg/kg/day
Severe disease: oral prednisolone 0.75–1 mg/kg/day

Once disease control is achieved (no new blisters forming or erosions and existing lesions beginning to heal), the dose of oral prednisolone can be gradually tapered.

Potent topical corticosteroids are used in the treatment of BP and can be applied to areas of blisters and erosions or even the whole body when used as monotherapy. Oral tetracyclines (e.g., doxycycline at doses of 100–200 mg/day) are often used as an immunomodulatory agent in combination with oral prednisolone or potent topical corticosteroids in the treatment of BP. Erythromycin at a dose of 1,000 mg/day may be used if reflux esophagitis or peptic ulcer disease is a concern. Steroid-sparing agents (e.g., mycophenolate mofetil and rituximab) may be considered in refractory cases with frequent relapses or patients requiring protracted periods of high-dose (>1 mg/kg/day) oral prednisolone.

Oral antibiotics are not indicated in most cases of BP unless there are clear clinical signs of infection. Blisters occur as part of the clinical manifestation of BP.

Wound care in BP comprises of non-adhesive dressings (e.g., paraffin-impregnated tulle gras) to areas of erosion. Dressings are preferably secured with crepe or tubular bandages instead of direct application of adhesive tape to the skin. Large tense blisters can be pricked and drained with a sterile needle. Take care not to de-roof these blisters as their roof acts as a natural barrier to infections.

****

After 3 weeks of starting oral prednisolone, her glycaemic trend was noted to be high, ranging between 14 and 20 mmol/L.

Her medications are aspirin 100 mg OM, amlodipine 5 mg OM, calcium/vitamin D 2 tablets OM, glipizide 5 mg BD, linagliptin 5 mg OM, omeprazole 20 mg OM, and spironolactone 12.5 mg OM.

Question 5: Which of the following changes to her medications would you make?

a. Increase linagliptin dose to 10 mg daily

b. Increase linagliptin dose to 10 mg daily and glipizide dose to 10 mg twice daily

c. Increase linagliptin dose to 10 mg daily and replace glipizide with a subcutaneous intermediate-acting insulin injection

d. Stop linagliptin and add a subcutaneous intermediate-acting insulin injection

e. Stop linagliptin and increase glipizide dose to 10 mg twice daily

There are two themes to this question — dipeptidyl-peptidase-4 inhibitor (DPP-4i)-associated BP and steroid-induced hyperglycaemia.

To date, more than 60 drugs have been reported to induce BP including loop diuretics (e.g., furosemide), certain antibiotics, and more recently immune checkpoint inhibitors against programmed death-1 (anti-PD-1) and programmed death ligand 1 (anti-PD-L1). There is growing epidemiological evidence of DPP-4i-associated BP which is strongest for vildagliptin but also emerging reports to linagliptin and sitagliptin.

The mechanism of DPP-4i-associated BP is unclear, though hypotheses have indicated possible immunological and structural alterations to the basement membrane zone. The DPP-4/CD 26 protein is ubiquitously expressed in many cells, including T lymphocytes, and is upregulated in several skin diseases including BP. Inhibition of DPP-4 has been shown in murine models to increase infiltration of eosinophils into the skin. The suppression of DPP-4 has also been postulated to be associated with the development of epitopes for DPP-4i-BP auto-antibodies via the epitope-spreading phenomena.

Reported clinical and immunological characteristics of DPP-4i-associated BP include: male, elderly over 80 years, less florid or severe compared to typical BP, negative or low titre for anti-BP 180 auto-antibodies, and quick and sustained remission following discontinuation of DPP4-i. The latency period between commencement of DPP4-i and onset of BP is variable, ranging from 1 month up to 3 years — the long latency period suggesting that this may be a drug-aggravated rather than a true drug-induced skin disease.

The incidence of hyperglycaemic complications has been reported in almost 40% of patients following the diagnosis of BP which is likely due to the widespread prescription of systemic glucocorticoids in the treatment of BP. Hyperglycaemic complications include newly diagnosed diabetes, worsening glycaemic control leading to up-titration of diabetic medications, hospitalisation, or hyperglycaemic crisis. The risk of glucocorticoid-induced hyperglycaemia more often occurs post-prandially and its risk is highest during the first few weeks of glucocorticoid initiation. As such, a regimen with an ***intermediate to long-acting basal insulin coupled with an additional hypoglycaemic agent*** for post-prandial glycemic control is preferred. Another management challenge includes the risk of hypoglycemia on tapering of glucocorticoids as control of BP improves.

In addition, treatment with glucocorticoids introduces a risk of infectious complications amongst BP patients, which is further compounded by the burden of multi-morbidity and poor functional status.

Close vigilance for the development of delirium is important when treating elderly BP patients with high-dose glucocorticoids especially in the presence of pre-existing neurological problems such as dementia and previous strokes.

****

As part of evaluation for her fall, the following investigations were sent off:

Bone mineral density (T-score):
Lumbar Spine: –2.0
Neck of Femur: –1.5
Serum vitamin D Level: 8 ng/mL (30–100)
Serum iPTH level: 20 pg/mL (normal)

Question 6: Outline an appropriate management plan.

The use of glucocorticoids increases the risk of fragility fractures by more than two-fold. Glucocorticoid-induced osteoporosis occurs early, within 3 months of initiation of treatment and its incidence increases in a dose- and duration-dependent manner. The mechanism of glucocorticoid-induced osteoporosis occurs primarily through the upregulation of osteoclasts and increased apoptosis of osteoblasts, leading to increased bone resorption and decreased bone formation. Bone quality is also affected due to decreased function and increased apoptosis of existing osteocytes. Therefore, the increase in fracture risk is not fully assessed by bone mineral density (BMD) measurements as it is also contributed by degradation in bone quality and increased risk of falls.

BMD T-score < –2.5 indicates osteoporosis while a T-score between –1 and –2.5 indicates osteopenia. Thus, T-score < –2.5 will be an indication for treatment but a higher threshold (< –1.5) has been proposed for patients on chronic glucocorticoid treatment.

The WHO fracture risk assessment (FRAX) algorithm has been developed to estimate the 10-year risk of hip and other major fractures based on clinical risk factors, with or without BMD. The risk factors included in FRAX are age, sex, body mass index, personal history of fracture, smoking, alcohol intake, glucocorticoid use, rheumatoid arthritis, and other causes of secondary osteoporosis. FRAX cannot be used in premenopausal women, in men aged <40 years, and in subjects previously treated with anti-osteoporotic drugs.

The American College of Rheumatology guidelines recommend treatment in older adults at moderate or high risk of osteoporotic fractures. This include patients with a history of osteoporotic fracture, men ≥50 years, postmenopausal women with a BMD T-score ≤2.5 at the hip or spine, FRAX (glucocorticoid-adjusted) 10-year risk for major osteoporotic fracture ≥10% OR FRAX (glucocorticoid-adjusted) 10-year risk for hip fracture >1% and very high-dose glucococorticoids (prednisolone ≥30 mg/day and a cumulative dose of >5 g in the past year).

The risk of major osteoporotic fracture calculated with the FRAX tool should be multiplied by 1.15 and risk of hip fracture by 1.2 if the prednisolone dose is >7.5 mg/day.

This elderly woman with osteopenia is exposed to very high doses of glucocorticoids, and with a history of recurrent falls, she will benefit from bisphosphonate therapy.

One of the rare side-effects of bisphosphonate treatment is osteonecrosis of the jaw. Hence, it would be prudent to have prior dental clearance and completion of dental work before starting treatment.

As the patient is also severely deficient in vitamin D, aggressive replacement can more quickly achieve optimal levels before commencing bisphosphonate therapy (a reasonable dosing of cholecalciferol is 50,000 IU/week for 8 weeks) and subsequent re-checking of levels would be appropriate.

Finally, a fall risk assessment is also important for this lady to address the reversible factors that are contributing to her fall.

Key messages

1. BP is the most common autoimmune-blistering disorder amongst the elderly characterised by the appearance of urticarial or eczematous plaques and tense bullae. ***If an elderly person recurrently develops "urticaria" over the flexural sites, beware that it may be pemphigoid waiting to manifest!***
2. An association of BP and neuropsychiatric disorders is commonly reported. ***Beware of bullous scabies in the appropriate clinical context: an institutionalised elderly patient who is mentally and physically disabled!***
3. Anti-BP 180 antibodies are almost always elevated in BP and titres correlate with BP disease activity.
4. Drug-induced BP has been reported to DPP4-inhibitors, loop diuretics, and anti-PD1 inhibitors.
5. Glucocorticoids remain the mainstay treatment of BP. However, hyperglycaemic, infectious complications, and steroid-induced delirium are therapeutic considerations especially in the elderly.
6. A lower threshold for bisphosphonate treatment should be adopted especially in postmenopausal women with the presence of other risk factors such as glucocorticoid use and propensity for falls.

Answer key

1. Look for blisters in the other limbs and oral erosions. Perform skin scrapings for scabies microscopy. Send serum samples for enzyme-linked immunosorbent assay: BP 180, BP 230 antigens, as well as indirect immunofluorescence.
2. B.
3. 1 – B, 2 – A.
4. B.
5. D.
6. Calculate the patient's FRAX score;

   Consider starting oral bisphosphonates (e.g., alendronate 70 mg per week) after dental clearance;

   High-dose oral cholecalciferol 50,000 IU weekly for 8 weeks;

   Fall risk assessment.

References

Buckely L, Guyatt G, Fink HA, *et al.* (2017) 2017 American Colleage of Rheumatology guideline for the prevention and treatment of glucocorticoid-induced osteoporosis. *Arthritis Rheumatol* **69**(8): 1521–1537.

Chai ZT, Tan C, Liau MM, *et al.* (2020) Diabetes mellitus and hyperglycemic complications in bullous pemphigoid. *J Am Acad Dermatol* **82**(5): 1234–1237.

Montagnon C, Tolkachjov S, Murrell D, *et al.* (2021) Subepithelial autoimmune blistering dermatoses: Clinical features and diagnosis. *J Am Acad Dermatol* **85**: 1–14.

Phoon YW, Fook-Chong S, Koh HY, *et al.* (2015) Infectious complications in bullous pemphigoid: an analysis of risk factors. *J Am Acad Dermatol* **72(**5): 834–839.

Sim B, Fook-Chong S, Phoon YW, *et al.* (2017) Multimorbidity in bullous pemphigoid: a case-control analysis of BP patients with age- and gender-matched controls. *J Eur Acad Dermatol Venereol* **31**(10): 1709–1714.

33 Pressure Injury

Sivagame D/O Maniya, Derrick Aw Chen Wee,
Anupama Roy Chowdhury

Mdm K is an 82-year-old lady who was admitted for urinary sepsis. She has a past medical history of cortical stroke, hyperlipidaemia, hypertension, type 2 diabetes (HbA1c 9%), and advanced dementia. She is bed-bound, incontinent, and dependent on her caregiver for her activities of daily living. Nutrition was provided by a liquid formulation through percutaneous endoscopic gastrotomy tube three times daily.

On admission, she was found to have a chronic wound over her sacrum (Fig. 33.1). The helper has been applying gauze packing and changing it twice daily to absorb a modest amount of discharge. When the base of the ulcer was probed, the finger encountered a hard surface. Mdm K neither winced nor reacted during the examination of the ulcer.

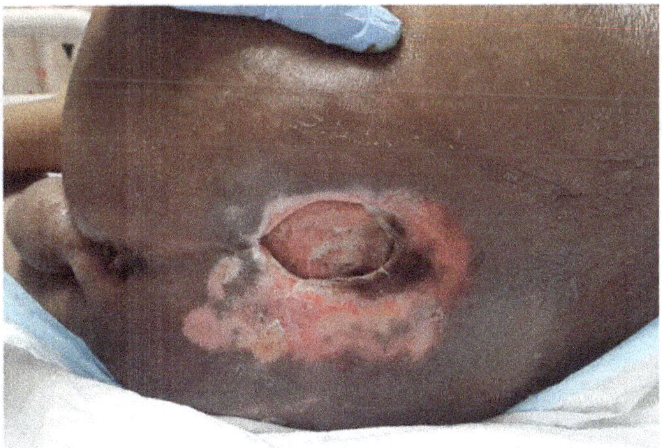

Fig. 33.1. Buttock ulcer of Mdm K.

Question 1: What is the stage of this pressure injury?

a. 2
b. 3
c. 4
d. Unstageable
e. Deep tissue injury

Staging pressure injuries can be challenging as assessment of tissue involvement can be equivocal. Nevertheless, clinicians should strive to determine the stage as accurately as possible as it has a direct influence on the development of a pressure injury prevention plan and selection of an appropriate treatment. It also allows communication between healthcare professionals.

Pressure injuries are classified according to the amount of actual and potential tissue damage using the National Pressure Injury Advisory Panel classification system (Table 33.2).

Table 33.2. Pressure injury staging.

Stage	Appearance	Important to note	Illustrative examples
1: Non-blanchable erythema of intact skin	Localised area of persistent redness.	Often under-detected in individuals with darkly pigmented skin — shining a light is helpful to visualise the redness.	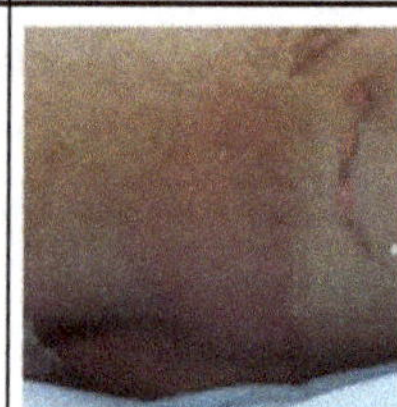
2: Partial-thickness skin loss with exposed dermis	The wound bed is viable, pink/red, and moist; may also present as an intact or ruptured serum-filled blister. Adipose and deeper tissue, granulation tissue, slough, and eschar are not seen.	This stage can be confused with incontinence-associated dermatitis* or traumatic wounds (e.g., skin tears, burns, abrasions).	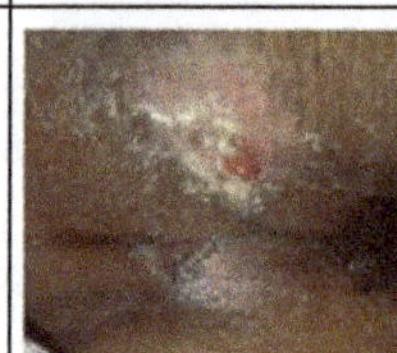
3: Full-thickness skin loss	***Adipose tissue, granulation, and epibole (rolled edges) are seen***. Slough and/or eschar may be seen but does not obscure the depth of tissue loss.	Depth of tissue damage differs by anatomical location, and areas of significant adiposity may portray as deep wounds. Undermining and tunneling may exist, but fascia, tendon, ligament, cartilage, and bone are not exposed.	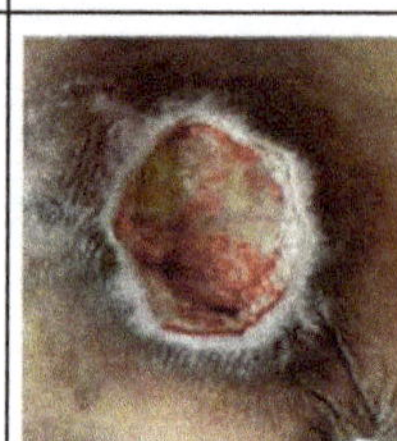

(*Continued*)

Stage	Appearance	Important to note	Illustrative examples
4: Full-thickness skin and tissue loss with extensive destruction	***Fascia, muscle, tendon, ligament, cartilage, or bone may be exposed or directly palpable.***	Depth of the wound varies by anatomical location. Rolled edges, undermining, and/or tunneling often occurs and slough and/or eschar may be seen.	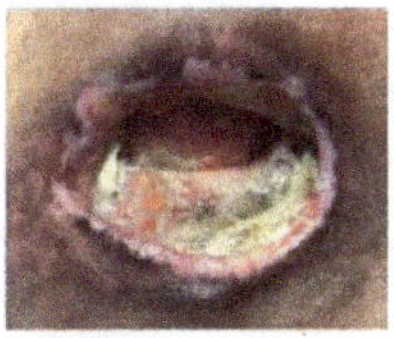
Unstageable: Obscured full-thickness skin and tissue loss	Extent of tissue damage or loss cannot be determined as the ***depth of the ulcer is obscured by slough and/or eschar***.	Debridement of the slough or eschar may reveal a Stage 3 or 4 pressure injury. NB. Stable eschar without erythema or presence of peripheral ischaemia over heel pressure injuries should not be softened or debrided. 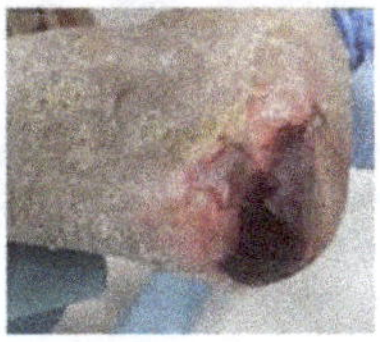	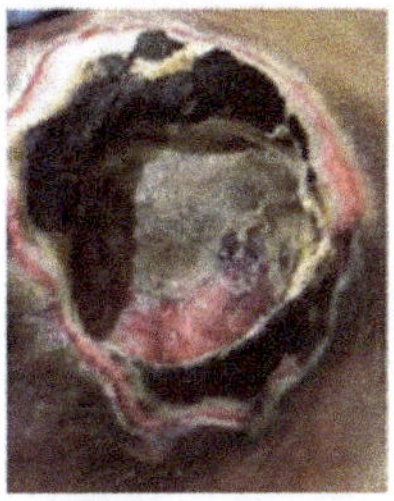 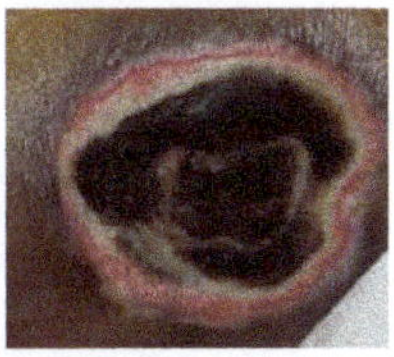
Deep tissue injury: Persistent non-blanchable deep red, maroon, or purplish discolouration	Can occur on intact or non-intact skin. Looks like Stage 1 but worse — colour is deeper. Epidermis may separate and appear as a dark wound bed or blood-filled blister.	Changes in pain and temperature change frequently precede skin colour changes. This injury is a consequence of intense and/or prolonged pressure and shear forces at the bone-muscle interface. NB. Deep tissue injury should not be used to describe vascular, traumatic, neuropathic, or dermatologic conditions.	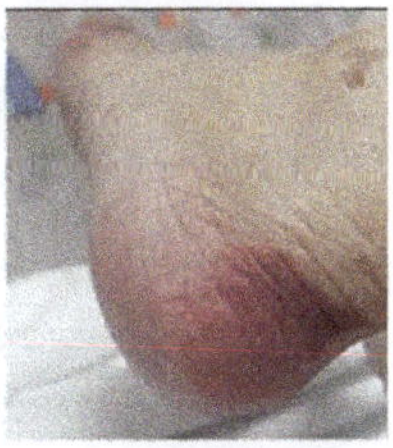 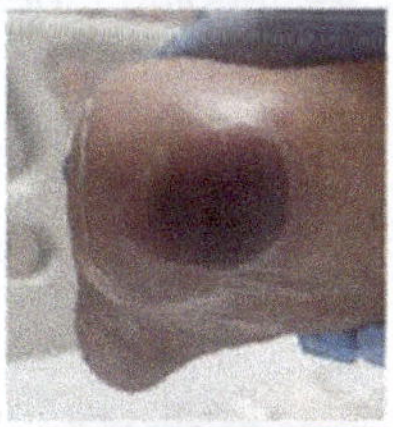 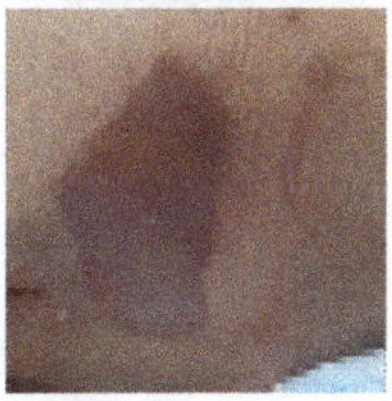

*Incontinence-associated dermatitis (Figs 33.2, 33.3) refers to skin erosions from urinary and/or faecal incontinence. Individuals on diaper care or with frequent loose bowel movements or urinary incontinence are at risk.

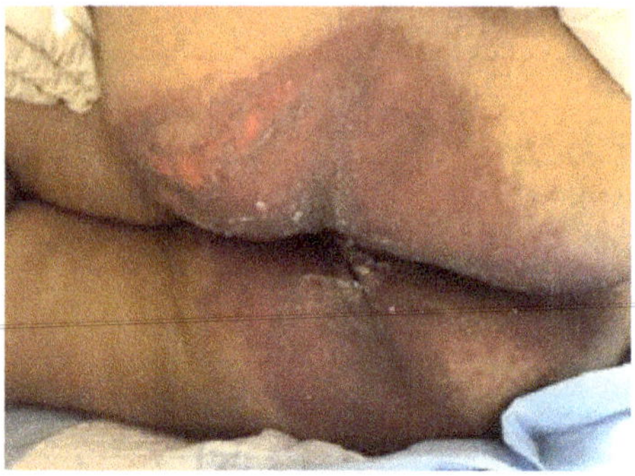

Fig. 33.2. Incontinence-associated dermatitis.

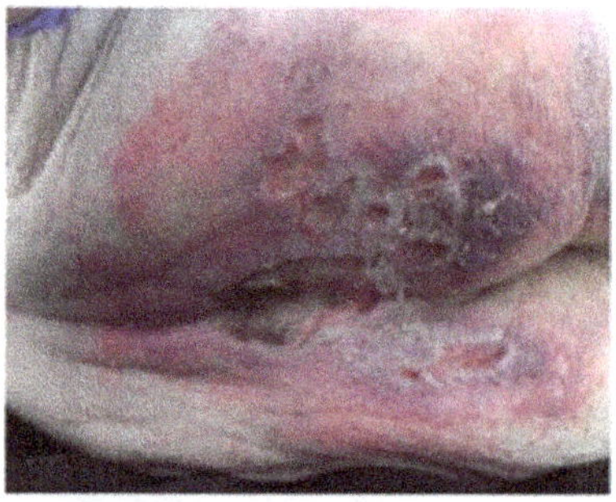

Fig. 33.3. Incontinence-associated dermatitis complicated with pressure injury.

Another form of pressure injury is classified under ***medical device-related pressure injury****. These injuries arise in connection with devices such as*

— *respiratory devices, e.g., nasal prongs, face masks, tracheostomy*
— *orthopaedic devices, e.g., braces, plaster casts*
— *urinary or faecal devices*
— *feeding tubes*
— *restraints*

Application of prophylactic dressings and proper anchoring of these devices can obviate pressure injury development in these individuals.

Pressure injuries are always staged at their worst associated tissue loss and cannot be reverse-staged when the wound improves. For example, a stage 3 pressure injury should not be re-classified as stage 2 when the wound granulates to the surface. Instead we will address it as a healing stage 3 pressure injury.

****

Pressure injuries pose significant health issues for susceptible individuals especially the frail, aged, immobile, cognitively or neurologically impaired. Evi-

Patient profile	Predisposing conditions	Triggering conditions
• Elderly • Long-term care home or community care residents	• Diabetes • Chronic neurological conditions	• Acutely and/critically ill • Hip fracture • Spinal cord injuries • Trauma and/ prolonged surgery

dence suggests that the following patients have multiple risk factors for increased probability of developing pressure injury:

All anatomical locations are at risk of pressure injury development from sustained or excessive pressure, shear, or friction. The areas most often affected are those over the bony prominences:

- In the sitting position: scapulae, ***sacrum***, ischium
- In the lateral position: ear cartilage, shoulder, trochanter, metatarsal, malleolus
- In the supine position: occiput, scapulae, spinous processes, elbows, iliac crests, ***heels***

The elderly, medically complex, and individuals in critical care are predominantly at risk of heel injuries. Peripheral vascular disease can delay healing and even potentiate the risk of amputation. Thus, checking for foot pulses in patients with heel pressure injury is a pivotal component in assessment as delayed referral to a vascular specialist can result in ongoing tissue death and subsequent risk of major amputation.

For a comprehensive evaluation to predict the development of a pressure injury, an assessment tool called the Braden scale is used. It encompasses the scoring of risk factors pertaining to activity, mobility, moisture, sensory perception, friction, and shear as well as general health status. The total score ranges from 6 to 23; the **lower** the score, the **higher** the risk.

Question 2: Mdm K has multiple risk factors that increase her likelihood of developing pressure injury as well as comorbidities that delay healing. Stratify her risk using the Braden score.

Link to Omni Braden Score Calculator

Question 3: Which of the following are appropriate primary dressings for Mdm K's pressure ulcer? Select one or more options.

a. **Alginate**
b. **Hydrocolloid**
c. **Hydrofibre**
d. **Hydrogel**
e. **Polymeric membrane dressing**

The ulcer should be gently cleansed and irrigated with normal saline via a syringe. Devitalised tissue (slough, eschar) should be debrided except in special situations such as a stable heel pressure ulcer or an ischaemic limb. If sharp debridement with scissors or scalpel is not available (due to the lack of an experienced clinician or wound nurse), you may consider enzymatic or autolytic debridement (interactive dressings as listed below).

The considerations for selecting appropriate wound dressings for pressure injuries are primarily based on a clinical assessment of the wound as well as the self-care abilities of the individual or caregiver.

Table 33.1. Common wound dressings used in pressure injury.

Pressure wound	Recommended dressing product	Frequency of change	Good clinical practice(s)
Stage 1	Polymeric membrane foam	3–5 days/PRN	• Daily skin checks are recommended
Stage 2	Hydrogels	2–3 days/PRN	• Monitor the edge and periwound for maceration
	Hydrocolloid (sheet)	3–5 days/PRN	• Carefully remove the dressing in patients with fragile skin as the adhesiveness of wafer dressings may cause skin injury • Protect periwound areas with barrier film products prior to hydrocolloid application
	Polymeric membrane foam	3–5 days/PRN	• Daily skin checks for improvement/ deterioration are recommended

Table 33.1. *(Continued)*

Pressure wound	Recommended dressing product	Frequency of change	Good clinical practice(s)
Stage 3 Stage 4	Primary^ dressing: Calcium alginates or hydrofibres Secondary^ dressing: Gauze or Gamgee pad (the latter is a thick layer of absorbent cotton wool between two layers of absorbent gauze)	2–3 days/PRN	• Undermining and tunneling should be packed to prevent premature superficial closure • Protect the periwound areas with barrier film products
Unstageable	Dressing product selection after wound assessment post-debridement		• In unstaged heel wounds with eschar/gangrene, assess for peripheral vascular disease
Deep tissue injury	Polymeric membrane foam	3–5 days/PRN	• Daily skin checks for improvement/ deterioration are recommended
Local wound infection	Antimicrobials: iodine, silver-based, honey-impregnated	PRN (use as per the manufacturer's recommendation)	• Choice and duration of antimicrobial dressing depends on the wound assessment and progress, respectively. Other factors to consider are affordability and caregiver ability to perform the dressing.

Note: ^"Primary" Refers to the Layer of Dressing that Directly Contacts the Wound while "Secondary" Refers to the Outer Layer of Dressing Used to Cover, Pad, or Attach the Primary Dressing. These dressings may be secured with film or adhesive tapes. Careful removal of adhesives to prevent skin injuries is advised particularly in elderly patients.

"Don't just treat the hole in the patient, but treat the patient as a whole!"

The management (and prevention) of pressure injuries is targeted with a bundle of strategies such as the following:

- **Support surfaces**

Support surfaces refer to specialised devices that redistribute pressures in managing tissue load and microcirculation. However, if the family is unable to access or afford these devices, the use of pillow or foam pads may be considered to reduce pressure over bony prominences. Heel pressure injuries can be prevented using polymeric membrane foam dressings and off-loading with pillows and heel cushions. Thirdly, for at-risk patients regardless of stage of pressure injuries if present, specialised devices that redistribute pressures to manage tissue load and the microcirculation may be employed. High-density foam or gel-foam mattresses as well as powered mattresses (either alternating pressure or low air-loss mattress systems) are suitable for patients prone to pressure injuries on their trunk or pelvis. Chair cushions (e.g., gel-foam seat cushions) are useful for sitting patients. With or without support surfaces, caregivers should be reinforced that repositioning and turning are still required. Recognising and minimising mucosal membrane and medical device-associated skin injury from tubes, catheters, and restraints is also fundamental for pressure injury prevention. Proper anchoring of tubes and catheters minimises risk of skin injuries.

- **Keep moving**

Immobility is the most significant risk factor for the development of pressure ulcers! Individuals at risk of developing pressure injuries are strongly recommended to be frequently repositioned. At the minimum, bedbound patients should be turned every two hours. When lying on one side, ensure that the patient is not positioned directly over the trochanter (hip) area. For sitting patients, encourage them to weight-shift every fifteen minutes, or reposition the patient every hour if he/she is not able to do so independently. Avoid prolonged sitting positions. Caregivers can plan an individualised schedule for extended periods of lying and sitting. You can consult the institution nursing team on turning and positioning techniques. Patients should be lifted off the bed or chair using transfer aids instead of being dragged so as to minimise friction and shear forces. For effective lifting and safe transfers, manual handling aids such as sliding sheets and transfer devices are recommended. Such medical assistive equipment can be obtained from medical supplies vendors as well. Passive bed exercises of the arms and legs prevent contracture and improve range of movement. The physiotherapist can be consulted for advice and training for these exercises.

- **Skin inspection**

Caregivers are encouraged to perform daily routine skin checks especially during bed-bath and diaper change or even during positioning to observe for early signs of pressure injury development such as redness. For patients with existing pressure ulcers, caregivers must learn how to look out for signs of infection.[γ] Application of barrier creams and sprays after each diaper change can protect the skin from continuous contact with urine or faeces. Moisturisers should be frequently and liberally applied on individuals with dry skin after bath and before sleep

- **Continence care**

The incontinence environment of prolonged excess moisture and chemical irritants (loose faecal matter is more damaging to the skin than urine, but the combination is more detrimental than either alone) on the skin can result in inflammation and maceration. This is further aggravated with the use of incontinence products that can alter the microclimate of the skin. A continence care plan can help to reduce the incidence of incontinent episodes. Instead of putting on diapers, suitable patients can be brought to the toilet at scheduled intervals for voiding. Prompt cleansing and use of high absorbency incontinence products such as diapers, underpads, or briefs together with skin protectants should be taught to family and caregivers.

- **Nutrition**

Inadequate nutritional intake is associated with pressure injury development, severity, and delayed healing. It is advisable to screen all patients at risk for inadequate nutrition. Malnourished individuals should be referred to a dietician for comprehensive assessment for implementation of a holistic nutrition care plan, focusing on energy and protein intake.

The Mini Nutritional Assessment — Short Form (MNA-SF) is a frequently used, validated, sensitive, specific, and simple to use tool for identifying malnourishment or risk of malnutrition in an elderly person.

Caregivers should be taught to look out for signs of infection in pressure injuries (Fig 33.4) such as

- pus
- increased redness, discharge, pain
- offensive smell

The pathogens are influenced by geographic and clinical settings, but commonly reported ones include *Staphylococcus aureus, Enterobacter, Proteus mirabilis,* and *Pseudomonas aeruginosa*. Antibiotics, surgical intervention (e.g., drainage of

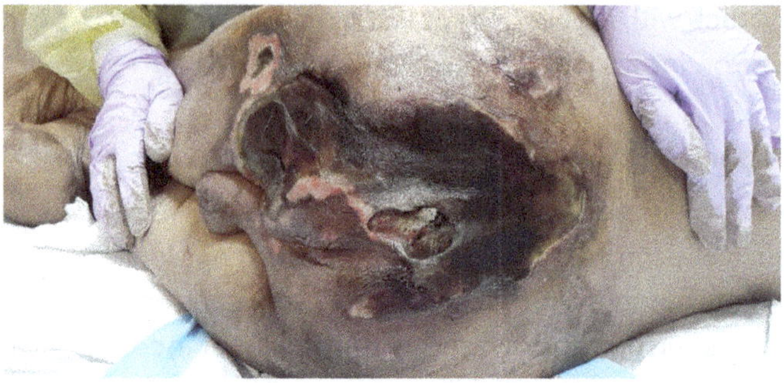

Fig. 33.4. Infected pressure wound.

local abscess), and topical antimicrobial dressings may be required. If exposed bone is present, osteomyelitis needs to be considered.

Key messages

1. The identification of risk factors is pivotal in predicting the development of a pressure injury and determining appropriate management strategies.
2. Be cognisant of pressure injuries in darkly pigmented individuals as it is under-detected.
3. Principles of pressure injury care are targeted at appropriate dressings; prevention and management strategies like support surfaces, turning and repositioning, regular skin inspections, attentive continence, and skin care as well as optimising nutrition.

Answer key

1. C. You may have mistaken the pressure injury as stage 3 or unstageable due to the presence of slough. However, the sloughy tissue is present only at the edges. Note that there is full-thickness skin and tissue loss, presence of undermining, necrotic slough tissue, and most importantly palpable bone.
2. Braden score is **7** [sensory perception: completely limited (1), moisture: constantly moist (1), activity: bedbound (1), mobility: completely immobile (1), nutrition: probably inadequate (2), friction and shearing (1)] which is considered as **HIGH** risk for pressure injury development.
3. A, C, E. Both alginates and hydrofibre dressings with an antimicrobial component would be ideal. As this is a chronic wound, bacterial burden is expected. It is

important to highlight to the caregiver that the undermining areas and tunnels should be packed with dressing to manage the exudate, prevent bacterial load accumulation, and prevent dead space formation. A polymeric membrane foam may be used as secondary dressing. If patients have faecal incontinence requiring frequent dressing changes or are financially challenged, a gauze/Gamgee pad can be considered as an alternative secondary dressing.

Reference

European Pressure Ulcer Advisory Panel, National Pressure Injury Advisory Panel and Pan Pacific Pressure Injury Alliance. Prevention and Treatment of Pressure Ulcers/Injuries: Clinical Practice Guideline. The International Guideline. Emily Haesler (Ed.). EPUAP/NPIAP/PPPIA: 2019.

34 Poor Oral Intake I (Advanced Dementia)

Lionel See Kee Yon, Victoria Wong Hwei May,
Lalmalani Roshan Mahesh

Mdm X is an 83-year old lady with moderately severe Alzheimer's disease, who has had multiple admissions in the past year for recurrent falls. She requires assistance in activities of daily living including showering, changing clothes, and feeding. She is only able to ambulate a few steps with a walking frame and one-person assistance. Her medical history includes hypertension, hyperlipidaemia, diabetes, and ischaemic heart disease. Her medications are enalapril 10 mg BD, simvastatin 20 mg ON, metformin 850 mg TDS, glipizide 5 mg BD, bisoprolol 2.5 mg OM, aspirin 100 mg OM, furosemide 20 mg OM, hydroxyzine 10 mg TDS, iron polymaltose 100 mg OM, and calcium/vitamin D 2 tabs OM. She is now admitted for poor oral intake. Her family is very concerned that she has been refusing food and drink and looking more dehydrated over the past week. In addition, Mdm X has been complaining of a burning sensation when passing urine. She is nursed on diapers and her helper has noted her urine to be more foul-smelling of late.

Question 1: What further history is important for a more comprehensive assessment of her present situation?

A decrease in oral intake is commonly seen in progression of dementia, but it may also be a result of other causes like infection, depression, pain, poor oral health, ill-fitting dentures, or polypharmacy. Hence, a comprehensive assessment is still required to exclude reversible or modifiable causes. Quantifying the amount of oral intake will also help us to understand the expectations of family or caregivers.

****

Mdm X normally takes about half a bowl of rice with finely minced vegetables and meat for her meals. This has since dropped to a few spoonfuls of food each meal over the past week. She says that she just does not have much appetite to eat.

She also drinks very little fluids, from her usual of 5–6 cups of fluids a day to barely 1–2 cups a day now. She denies feeling thirsty or hungry. Mdm X also denies any odynophagia or dysphagia, although her gums do hurt whenever she has to chew.

Mdm X has been complaining of a burning sensation whenever she passes urine for the past week. This was accompanied with low grade fever of 37.7–37.9°C, as well as increased foul-smelling urine reported by her helper. She denies any cough, increased sputum production, or shortness of breath. Her helper has not noticed any broken skin, pressure injuries, or increased redness or swelling in her limbs.

Her helper is still able to serve her medications regularly, which Mdm X takes very slowly each time. Mdm X denies early satiety, nausea, or vomiting. She opens her bowels regularly, approximately once every two days, and her stools are soft and brown.

Mdm X is widowed and lives only with her helper of two years. Her two sons usually visit her at least twice weekly, but have only managed to visit once over the past three months due to their work commitments. Her helper used to bring Mdm X out on the wheelchair to the park daily and she used to attend activities at the community centre weekly, but both activities have stopped owing to her increased difficulties with transfers. Furthermore, the children felt it was in her interest to remain indoors to minimise her exposure risk in view of the ongoing COVID-19 pandemic. Mdm X has been noted to be increasingly withdrawn lately, losing interest in her usual hobbies such as watching television or listening to the radio. She often spends her time in her bedroom taking naps.

On examination, Mdm X was alert though slightly lethargic looking. Her weight was 48.0 kg (it was 49.1 kg three months ago). Vital signs are temperature 38°C, heart rate 106/min, blood pressure 96/56 mmHg, respiratory rate 16/min, and SpO_2 *98% on room air. Her oral cavity and tongue were dry. When removing her dentures, her gums over the upper and lower molar regions were swollen, erythematous, and mildly tender. Heart and breath sounds were normal. Abdominal examination revealed suprapubic tenderness and a palpable bladder. Bowel sounds were normal. A bladder scan done after she had voided revealed a post-void residual urine of 500 mL. Her skin condition was dry with no broken skin or pressure injuries. Calves were normal and supple.*

Laboratory investigations showed:

Haemoglobin	*11.5 g/dL*	*(12–16)*
WBC count	*13.4 x* 10^9*/L*	*(4–10)*
Platelet count	*420 x* 10^9*/L*	*(140–440)*
Blood urea	*13.4 mmol/L*	*(2.7–6.9)*
Sodium	*152 mmol/L*	*(136–146)*

Potassium	*3.5 mmol/L*	*(3.6–5.0)*
Serum creatinine	*194 μmol/L*	*(54–101)*
Calcium	*2.40 mmol/L*	*(2.09–2.46)*
Phosphate	*0.89 mmol/L*	*(0.94–1.5)*
Magnesium	*0.77 mmol/L*	*(0.74–0.97)*
C-reactive protein	*83 mg/L*	*(0.2–9.1)*
Serum albumin	*27 g/L*	*(40–51)*
Thyroid-stimulating hormone	*2.05 mIU/L*	*(0.65–3.70)*
Free T4	*11.6 pmol/L*	*(8.8–14.4)*
HbA1c	*5.9%*	
UFEME	*3 RBCs/UL, 150 WBCs/UL, 0 epithelial cells/UL*	
Urine culture	*Pan-sensitive E coli, >100,000 cfu/mL*	
Blood cultures	*No bacterial growth*	

Question 2: List the medical issues to be addressed.

Poor feeding can be an atypical presentation of acute medical conditions in the elderly. The causes of poor feeding are often multifactorial and require a systematic and comprehensive assessment. Robbin's 9Ds of weight loss in the elderly can be used to assess for the causes of poor feeding.

Disease (acute and chronic):

Acute medical issues need to be assessed and treated as these can often lead to an abrupt loss of appetite. This involves screening for infections in the elderly, in particular pneumonia, urinary tract infections, pressure wounds, and cellulitis.

Poorly controlled pain from underlying illness can affect the patient's mood and oral intake. Pain assessment in patients with dementia is challenging as not all of them are able to self-report their pain. In patients who are unable to self-report pain, behavioural observation tools can be effective in quantifying the patient's pain. The tool used in our institution is the Pain Assessment in Advanced Dementia Scale. This and other tools such as the Pain Assessment Checklist for Seniors with Limited Ability to Communicate, Behavioural Pain Assessment Scale for the Elderly Presenting with Verbal Communication Disorders, and Abbey Pain Scale can be found online. (A free app — "Pain App" — which was developed by the University of Greenwich, adopts the Abbey Pain Scale, a commonly used tool in the UK, to help assess pain in older people with cognitive impairments.)

Metabolic and endocrinological abnormalities need to be assessed as well. Hyperthyroidism causes a hypermetabolic state that can cause loss of weight.

Hyperparathyroidism and hypercalcemia can lead to abdominal and bone pain, constipation, nausea, and dehydration, all of which can contribute to loss of appetite. Hypoadrenalism can cause increased lethargy, nausea, and anorexia. This may be caused by long-term usage of traditional medications containing steroids that sometimes can be seen in the elderly. Hyperglycemia from poorly controlled diabetes can result in drowsiness and reduced oral intake.

Chronic medical conditions can also lead to poor feeding. This may include chronic medical conditions of various organs, including congestive heart failure, chronic obstructive pulmonary disease, chronic kidney disease, and liver cirrhosis. Rheumatological conditions such as severe arthritis may also impact the patient's ability to eat independently. Treatment of the symptoms as well as the underlying medical condition in the first instance should be attempted as this may lead to an improvement in appetite.

The prevalence of cancer also increases with age, so screening for malignancy depending on other associated symptoms (early satiety, changes in bowel habits etc.) may need to be undertaken to exclude cancer as a cause.

Dementia/Delirium:

Patients with dementia and short-term memory loss may forget the task at hand or become easily distracted, resulting in poor oral intake. As dementia progresses, apraxia (the inability to perform skilled or purposeful movements) may result in difficulties with using eating utensils, while agnosia (impaired recognition or understanding of sensory stimuli) can impair the ability to recognise food. Furthermore, patients with behavioural and psychological symptoms in dementia (BPSD) may end up spitting their food or throwing tantrums at meal times — they are particularly challenging to feed!

In patients with more acute medical issues, delirium (hyperactive or hypoactive) can also impair feeding. Its management revolves around treatment of the underlying cause(s) of delirium.

Drugs:

It is essential to review medications because of polypharmacy, which is especially seen in the elderly with multiple chronic conditions. Certain medications may cause gastrointestinal-related side-effects including nausea, vomiting, or diarrhoea. Examples are antibiotics, digoxin, metformin, selective serotonin reuptake inhibitors (SSRIs), tricyclic antidepressants (TCAs), and dopamine agonists.

Acetylcholinesterase inhibitors (e.g., donepezil, rivastigmine, galantamine) used in the treatment of dementia have common side-effects of nausea, vomiting, and anorexia. Memantine, an NMDA receptor antagonist, can cause constipation which in turn can reduce appetite. In advanced dementia, consider discontinuing these drugs as they are deemed no longer efficacious.

Anticholinergic agents and many antihistamines (especially the H1-receptor antagonists which often have marked anticholinergic properties) may also cause xerostomia (dry mouth), which may affect appetite in the elderly. Furosemide is another medication that is often prescribed in the elderly which may contribute to dehydration and dry mouth.

Some medications may cause an altered sensation of taste or smell, including allopurinol, ACE-inhibitors, calcium channel blockers, propranolol, spironolactone, levodopa, and selegiline. Yet other medications may suppress appetite, including metformin, levodopa, bupropion, phentermine, methylphenidate, opioid analgesics, and theophylline.

Lastly, it is important to assess if certain medications may be causing pill oesophagitis or gastritis, including bisphosphonates often seen in osteoporosis treatment, or non-steroidal anti-inflammatory drugs (NSAIDs). Doxycycline, iron, and potassium supplementation may also contribute to dysphagia affecting swallowing and appetite.

Depression:

Depression in the elderly may contribute to reduced oral intake. Reduction in function, increased social isolation, neglect, and bereavement from the loss of lifelong partners or close friends can all contribute to depression in the elderly. Furthermore, medications prescribed in depression or for behavioural control in aggressive patients may result in somnolence and limit feeding.

Diarrhoea:

Medications are often the cause of diarrhoea in the elderly, with culprit drugs like metformin and omeprazole (chronic use causes small bowel intestinal overgrowth) as well as chronic laxative use. Diarrhoea in an elderly patient with recent use of antibiotics should prompt the exclusion of *Clostridium difficile* infection.

Other causes of diarrhoea may include an acute gastroenteritis, hyperthyroidism, inflammatory bowel disease, pancreatitis, or diverticulitis.

In the elderly, overflow diarrhoea may result from more proximal constipation. A digital rectal examination may need to be performed to exclude faecal impaction or a dilated rectum, which may indicate more proximal constipation. If present, manual evacuation of stools or a high fleet enema may have to be administered to clear the bowels adequately.

A detailed history has to be taken to exclude changes in bowel habits in the elderly, paying attention to red flags such as per rectal bleeding, melena, loss of weight, tenesmus, or narrowing calibre of stools which may suggest a colorectal malignancy.

Dysphagia and other swallowing issues:

The elderly may experience a range of swallowing issues that may limit their ability to consume food. Firstly, pain on swallowing (i.e., odynophagia) should be excluded. This is usually more acute and can be due to infections (e.g., Candidiasis, HSV, CMV, Streptococcal throat) or mucositis (chemotherapy or radiation therapy-related).

Patients with previous strokes, Parkinson disease, multiple sclerosis, scleroderma, or obstructive lesions may have difficulties with swallowing (i.e., dysphagia). This may be particularly problematic for patients with vascular dementia, who may have difficulties coordinating chewing and swallowing, resulting in gagging, coughing, or aspiration.

Yet other patients may have chronic reflux from gastro-oesophageal reflux disease or pill oesophagitis from bisphosphonates that may impact on their swallowing and desire for food. This may be particularly bothersome for the elderly as they may have decreased oesophageal sphincter tone, reduced gastric motility, and increased reflux.

Dental care:

Many elderly patients have poor dentition which may limit their ability to properly chew their food. Poorly fitting dentures may cause abrasions, gum swelling, stomatitis, and pain.

Xerostomia (dry mouth) often affects many elderly patients. This may be due to medications (especially drugs with anticholinergic properties), poor oral hydration, cancer therapy (e.g., previous head and neck radiation therapy) or poorly controlled diabetes.

Dysgeusia/Diets:

Patients with dementia may have increased impairment in olfaction and taste, resulting in poor appetite. In addition, certain chronic conditions including chronic kidney disease, liver cirrhosis, and hypothyroidism may contribute to an altered taste sensation. Xerostomia and poor oral hygiene can in turn lead to altered taste sensation, swallowing difficulties, and hence poor feeding. Patients with cancer also can have dysgeusia either from the malignancy itself or from underlying cancer treatments.

Common medications used in the elderly that can cause dysgeusia include the ACE-inhibitors, statins, anticholinergic agents, and proton-pump inhibitors.

Owing to their extensive comorbidities, many elderly patients are often placed on a range of therapeutic diets. Theses can range from low-salt diets in hypertensive patients, low-fat diets in those with metabolic syndrome, and low-carbohydrate diets in diabetics amongst others. Often, these diets are hugely unpalatable leading to reduced oral intake, and may be of limited therapeutic benefit for such patients in the longer term.

Patients with dysphagia are often placed on modified consistency diets including thickened fluids to reduce their risk of aspiration. The modification in the consistency in itself may lead to poor oral intake if the older person dislikes the proposed consistency.

Dysfunction (physical, psychosocial):

The reduced mobility of the elderly may inhibit their access to food. Some may have financial limitations that may affect their ability to acquire food. Socially isolated elderly may also have fewer social cues to have regular meals. Furthermore, studies have shown that older adults who eat in the presence of others consume more than those who eat alone. Homebound elderly may also opt to consume meals that are easier to prepare but which may not be as nutritious, including canned and preserved foods. Thus, a detailed diet history is important.

Chronic alcoholics may limit their oral intake and spend their money on the purchase of alcohol rather than food, resulting in malnutrition and weight loss. Elder abuse in the form of caregivers limiting their access to food and nutrition may also lead to weight loss.

Elderly patients with poor feeding are at risk of malnutrition, frailty, and sarcopenia (Fig 34.1).

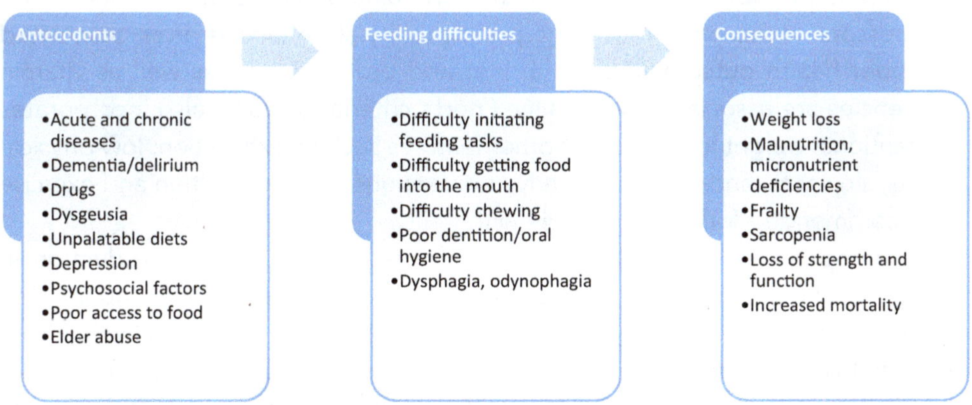

Fig. 34.1. Causes and consequences of poor feeding in older adults with dementia.

In 2018, the Global Leadership Initiative on Malnutrition developed a set of criteria to enable a global consensus on the identification and definition of malnutrition:

- ≥1 phenotypic criterion (involuntary weight loss, low BMI, reduced muscle mass) AND
- ≥1 aetiologic criterion (reduced foot intake/absorption, underlying inflammation due to acute or chronic disease)

Tools have also been developed to screen the elderly for malnutrition, and the Mini Nutritional Assessment-Short Form (MNA-SF) is a simple tool that can be used to screen for elderly patients who are at risk of developing malnutrition.

Malnutrition can result in poor physical function, poor recovery from an acute illness, increased health care utilisation, and lengthened hospital stay. Older adults are also less able to adapt to underfeeding following an acute illness. Thus, every attempt should be made to first treat acute medical causes that may contribute to poor feeding, such as infections or symptoms relating to chronic diseases. This lack of ability to compensate for periods of low food intake due to acute illness or other difficulties can result in long-term, persistent loss of weight and frailty.

Micronutrient deficiencies should also be evaluated in patients with poor feeding. This can include checking ***vitamin B12, vitamin D, and calcium levels***. Vitamin B12 deficiency can result in haematological, neurological, or psychological complications. Vitamin D deficiency can result in muscle weakness, functional impairment, increased risk of falls, and osteomalacia. Low calcium levels may result in cortical bone loss and predispose the patient to osteoporosis.

Frailty is a complex multi-system and multi-dimensional syndrome that is characterised by low reserves and increased vulnerability to internal and external stressors. It can often indicate a pre-disability state, and is often associated with poor health outcomes. Low nutrient and protein intake as well as vitamin deficiencies are associated with frailty. Fried's criteria for frailty also incorporates unintentional weight loss amongst other features such as exhaustion, low physical activity, slowness, and weakness. Early interventions such as nutrition and exercise are recommended for elderly people with frailty.

Sarcopenia describes a syndrome of muscle mass loss and reduction in strength and performance. It is associated with increased functional impairment, disabilities, falls, and mortality. The SARC-F screening tool comprises five components that can be easily assessed (strength, assistance in walking, rising from chair, climbing stairs, falls) to identify patients at risk of developing adverse outcomes from sarcopenia. A SARC-F score of ≥4 suggests the need for further, more comprehensive evaluation.

You may also conveniently screen for frailty and sarcopenia using the free app "RGA Clinic" which was developed by the National University Health System of Singapore.

Lastly, poor feeding and unintentional weight loss have been associated with increased mortality. This can be in the form of increased frailty and sarcopenia, reducing functional reserves and the ability to overcome acute medical issues such as infections, or predisposing them to falls and injuries. Thus, the involuntary loss of more than 5–10% of an elderly person's usual weight within one year should prompt a thorough evaluation as this is associated with increased mortality risk.

****

Question 3: Outline a management plan specifically to manage the poor feeding in this patient.

The approach should be to first address the reversible or modifiable causes followed by non-pharmacological and pharmacological interventions. Pay attention to acute infections that commonly occur in the elderly such as pneumonia, urinary tract infections, gastroenteritis, cellulitis, or infected pressure injuries. Other acute medical conditions to exclude include acute myocardial infarction, strokes, and electrolyte disturbances. In the elderly who are delirious, acute and reversible causes of delirium should be addressed (e.g., pain, constipation).

In elderly patients with chronic diseases, the associated symptoms need to be addressed and treated. For example, in an acute exacerbation of chronic obstructive pulmonary disease, symptom relief with inhalers along with treatment in the form of corticosteroids and antibiotics should be attempted first.

Dental referral should be made if there are poorly fitting dentures and/or for management of other oral pathologies. Xerostomia should be relieved with appropriate oral hygiene, including moisturising gels, mouthwashes (e.g., Oral7® or BioXtra®), or rinses with sodium bicarbonate powder mixed with water to remove coated tongue or oral debris. Medications that can cause xerostomia should be stopped if they are no longer needed.

Unnecessary therapeutic diets should be stopped if they are deemed to be of limited benefit. Finding the most palatable diet acceptable to the patient should be undertaken. A dietitian should be referred for dietary evaluation, appropriate dietary modifications, and oral nutritional supplementation if needed. A speech therapist may need to be referred to assess the swallowing in some patients as well as to determine if strategies to facilitate improved swallowing are required. This may include swallowing multiple times per bolus, limiting the bolus sizes per swallow, or altering the consistencies of food, amongst other strategies.

De-prescribing of medications should be attempted at every opportunity so as to prevent polypharmacy, especially those that can negatively impact feeding. The **SIRE acronym** (symptoms, indication, risks, end of life) can be used as a guide for de-prescribing. First, evaluate if the symptom that the medication is supposed to address has resolved, then review if there is still a valid indication for the medication, whether the risks of the medication outweigh the benefits, and lastly whether the patient has a short enough life expectancy that would limit the clinical benefit of the medication. The American Geriatrics Society (AGS) Beers Criteria as well as the Screening Tool of Older Persons' Prescriptions (STOPP) and Screening Tool to Alert to Right Treatment (START) are available tools that can be used to guide a clinician for specific medications that may be potentially inappropriate for older patients.

Concomitant low mood and depression should also be addressed. Psychotherapy and antidepressant medications may be necessary in patients with more severe depression. Improving social interactions may be useful, such as having fixed meal times with the rest of the family to improve the social cues for more regular meals, as well as reducing environmental distractions during dining. Increased physical activity can not only increase social interactions, physical function, and mood, but may also directly lead to an increase in appetite.

There is insufficient evidence to recommend the use of appetite stimulants (orexigenics). Dronabinol (cannabinoid agent not available in Singapore) has been shown to improve body weight and reduce negative affect in a small study, but its side-effects of risk of seizures, euphoria, somnolence, and tiredness limit its use. Megesterol acetate demonstrated benefit in patients with HIV or cancer. However, in older persons, there is limited evidence that it leads to significant weight gain or longer term health benefits. Furthermore, it may be associated with side-effects such as oedema, congestive heart failure, venous thromboembolism, impairment of the corticoadrenal axis, and insomnia. It has even been associated with increased mortality in nursing home patients. The AGS Beers criteria lists megesterol as potentially inappropriate for older adults aged >65 years.

Mirtazapine is a noradrenergic and specific serotonergic antidepressant that can be tried on patients with low mood or anxiety along with poor appetite. As its effects on weight gain in the elderly are modest at best, it should only be used when there is concomitant depressive or anxiety symptoms. Such patients should be monitored for side-effects such as increased somnolence, dry mouth, constipation, and hyponatremia. It is worth noting that to date no medications have been FDA approved for geriatric anorexia. Hence, if used, orexigenics should be used as a trial and regular review undertaken to monitor for their effectiveness while also evaluating for complications.

****

Question 4: Mdm X's family is extremely concerned about her starving in the ward and asks if tube feeding can be considered for her. What is the most appropriate advice?

a. Insert a nasogastric tube right away and start enteral feeding in gentle doses first.
b. Obtain collaborative evidence of dysphagia from speech therapy first before inserting a nasogastric tube for enteral feeding.
c. Arrange for percutaneous endoscopic gastrotomy insertion for feeding.
d. Start intravenous total parenteral nutrition to supplement her while waiting for her oral intake to improve.
e. Continue to encourage self or assisted feeding while treating the reversible causes of poor feeding.

It may seem intuitive to start tube feeding in a patient with advanced dementia and poor feeding to supplement nutrition and provide hydration and comfort. Despite these good intentions, there is actually limited evidence of clinical benefit for tube feeding in dementia. Furthermore, there are substantial risks associated with tube feeding. Thus, when a person with advanced dementia develops poor feeding, evaluating for reversible causes and addressing these should be the first step. Such interventions may also take time and patience is required to evaluate if poor feeding can be improved. Inserting a tube to commence feeding should never be the first or only treatment choice.

Tube feeding is most beneficial when used in the short term to correct deficits from the temporary inability to eat, such as recovery from surgery. It may also be useful in longer term scenarios such as to provide nutrition in patients who will never recover and be able to eat on their own (e.g., in a persistent vegetative state or irreversible neurological disorders). However, the decision for tube feeding has to be balanced with the complications associated with this potentially burdensome intervention (Table 34.1).

Tube feeding is associated with increased discomfort and agitation, particularly in dementia patients with BPSD who may attempt to pull out the tube. The associated increased use of physical and chemical restraints further adds to the agitation of such patients, limiting function and affecting mood. Indeed, the use of tube feeding also leads to increased hospital visits for tube-related complications such as tube dislodgement and agitation. The development of pressure ulcers has also been associated with tube feeding owing to the increased use of restraints and confinement to the bed.

Aspiration pneumonia involves the misdirection of contaminated pharyngeal contents (e.g., oral secretions) into the airway. The introduction of a large enough

Table 34.1. Burdens and Complications Associated with Tube Feeding. The most common complications are *italicised*.

	Nasogastric tube	Gastrostomy tube
Insertion	• *Discomfort* • *Tube coiling, misplacement*	• Sedation risks for procedure
Local/ mechanical	• Erosion/necrosis of the nasopharynx and oesophagus • Bleeding from trauma	• *Wound dehiscence* • *Skin excoriations* • Bleeding at the insertion site
Respiratory	• *Aspiration pneumonia* • Misplacement into the lung • Pneumothorax • Tracheobronchial perforation	• *Aspiration pneumonia*
Abdominal	• Reflux • Oesophageal perforation	• Gastric perforation • Peritonitis
Others	• *Deprives the patient of oral feeding and the pleasures of taste* • Tube blockages • Increased secretions • Fluid overload	
	• *Discomfort, agitation* • *Use of restraints may result in pressure injuries* • *Requirement for frequent repositioning and replacement* • *Tube migration*	• *Tube dislodgement*

inoculum of normally non-pathogenic organisms into the lung predisposes to pneumonia. Unfortunately, tube feeding does ***NOT*** reduce the risk of aspiration of oral contents or prevent the regurgitation of gastric contents. Furthermore, the insertion of a nasogastric tube may reduce the lower oesophageal sphincter pressure and contribute to an increased risk of reflux.

Tube feeding does not lead to clinically meaningful outcomes in patients with dementia. Tube feeding does not lead to a reduction in infections, improve nutritional status, or improve function. It is neither associated with the healing of pre-existing pressure ulcers nor prevention of new ones, and restraints placed on patients who are tube-fed and agitated may lead to new ulcer formation. Furthermore, data has also demonstrated consistently that mortality is not better in persons with advanced dementia who are tube fed compared to those who are not.

When difficulty with feeding arises in a patient with advanced dementia, careful hand feeding should be encouraged, while taking efforts to correct reversible causes.

This is because hand feeding, while challenging, has been shown to be as good as tube feeding for the outcomes of aspiration pneumonia, functional status, comfort, and mortality. Altering the environment and creating patient-centred approaches to encourage hand feeding should always be undertaken, and this includes the promotion of the enjoyment of food and empowering the caregiver to continue with hand feeding. Mealtime is one of the remaining pleasures in a patient with advanced dementia and should be regarded as an event of importance rather than a task that needs to be completed as quickly as possible. Other strategies would also involve making the food palatable, with adequate fluids to enhance hydration.

It should be emphasised that tube feeding should only be considered as a treatment modality of last resort in patients with advanced dementia who still have a reasonable prognosis. Often, the decision for tube feeding can be particularly challenging for family and surrogate decision-makers, given the complex interplay of cultural and religious beliefs, understanding of the natural progression of dementia, and the lack of awareness on the limitations and burdens of tube feeding.

Poor feeding is a part of the natural progression of the neurocognitive decline that occurs with dementia. Hence, the conversation regarding tube feeding in patients with dementia should begin early in the course of illness rather than when food refusal begins, or worse still, when the patient is no longer able to make decisions for himself.

In light of this, healthcare providers should not feel pressured into instituting tube feeding for a patient with advanced dementia who has lost mental capacity. Careful review of the patient's previously stated care plans and expressed wishes along with active and open discussions with the family and loved ones is crucial.

It is possible to consider a time-limited trial of tube insertion to assist with feeding and medication administration, but clear stipulations should be discussed beforehand regarding when not to consider re-insertion. For instance, if a patient with advanced dementia with BPSD pulls out the nasogastric tube more than two times, then he is clearly not tolerating it well and re-insertion should not be considered.

****

Mdm X was admitted and treated for urinary tract infection with a course of antibiotics. Her fever and urinary symptoms gradually subsided. Her hypernatraemia, hypercalcaemia, and acute kidney injury were corrected with appropriate hydration. She was reviewed by the speech therapist who recommended a blended diet. The dietitian gave appropriate dietary advice and recommended additional nutritional supplements for her.

Her medication list was reviewed and simplified. She had a good capillary blood glucose throughout her admission, and as her HbA1c over the previous checks were stably good, her metformin and glipizide were stopped. She had good lipid control, so her simvastatin was ceased. Furosemide was also stopped as it was deemed that the indication was not strong and she had no recent fluid overload symptoms. Hydroxyzine, prescribed for itch owing to dry skin, was stopped and replaced with topical moisturisers. She was also referred to psychiatry who diagnosed her with depression and started her on mirtazapine 7.5 mg ON, which was gradually uptitrated outpatient to 15 mg ON while monitoring for hyponatraemia and side-effects.

Advice was given for regular orientation and also to increase her social interactions and activities on discharge, including instituting regular meals, regular visits by family members, allowing the patient to be brought out into the community, resuming her activities in the community centre, and keeping her engaged in her hobbies.

She was reviewed by the dental specialist while admitted and she was assessed to have poorly fitting dentures. Appropriate advice was given for dental hygiene and following discharge, the family brought Mdm X to a dentist to make a new set of dentures.

With these efforts, Mdm X's appetite gradually improved during the admission and continued to do so over the next few months following her discharge.

Mdm X attended the clinic review three months later accompanied by her elder son, the main spokesperson. Mdm X had in fact gained about 1 kg over three months. Her son expressed that he felt that his mother's condition was worsening in that her moments of lucidity were getting shorter and her physical function was deteriorating. He asked, "how much time does she have left?"

Question 5: What would you like to address during the clinic consult?

Prognostication is a prediction of the possible outcome of a disease course based on medical knowledge and experience. It helps provide the patient and family with information on what to expect so that they can prioritise their goals and set expectations of care. This allows the patient to make an informed choice regarding ongoing care and plan for the future, including the goals of care.

A commonly used prognostication tool for dementia is the Functional Assessment Staging (FAST) score. A patient with dementia is likely to have a prognosis of 6 months or less if the FAST score is at least 7C and also exhibits one or more specific dementia-related comorbidities (aspiration, upper urinary tract infection, sepsis, multiple stage 3–4 pressure ulcers, persistent fever, weight loss >10% within 6 months). Another commonly used prognostic tool is the 12-item Advanced Dementia Prognostic Tool (ADEPT) to predict 6-month survival. The ADEPT tool was found to be 68% accurate while the FAST score was 55% accurate in predicting mortality over a 6-month period in patients living in a long-term care facility. Both tools should be used only as a guide — they should not replace consideration of patient's care preferences.

Advance care planning (ACP) is important in the management of patients with advanced dementia to avoid unwanted and unnecessary treatments. It is a process to discuss and document the patient's care preferences with loved ones. It is best to start the discussion early before the patient loses decision-making capacity. This will allow the patient to participate in deciding their goals and extent of care, and in the process ease the burden of decision-making for loved ones. The key things to consider addressing are:

— Identifying a nominated healthcare spokesperson (NHS)
— Discussing treatment plans and alternatives
— Understanding individual values, beliefs, and goals of care (e.g., tube feeding, desired functional outcomes, and acceptable versus unacceptable states)

There are three types of ACP that can be done:

(a) General ACP discussion: for relatively healthy individuals or patients with early chronic disease. Goals of treatment are considered in the event of a serious neurological injury.
(b) Disease-specific ACP: for patients with progressive, life-limiting illness (e.g., end organ failure) or frequent hospital admissions. The aim is to determine the goals of treatment as complications escalate.
(c) Preferred plan of care: for terminally ill patients (defined as prognosis <12 months) and/or patients requiring long-term institutional care. A specific plan of care is established in the event of patient deterioration including care options on CPR, care goals for medical intervention if the patient deteriorates, preferred place of care, and death.

The completion of ACP can be done in a single visit or over multiple visits. After completing an ACP, a copy will be uploaded to the *Living Matters* website so that it can be accessed via the National Electronic Health Record. ACP requires regular revisiting especially when there is a change of NHS or major life events (e.g., hospital admissions) to check if there are any changes in the values or goals of care. More information on ACP and how to initiate an ACP discussion can be found at this link:

****

Mdm X was assessed to have adequate mental capacity and she completed her ACP over two clinic visits. She decided that her elder son will be her NHS. From Mdm X's point of view, she is agreeable for a limited trial of treatment if the healthcare team thinks she will benefit from it. However, she feels that there is no longer much quality of life when she becomes uncommunicative and bedbound. Hence, she would not want to insert a nasogastric tube in the event that she is unable to swallow. She has no preferred place of death; all she asks for is to preserve her dignity.

Over the course of a year, Mdm X subsequently declined. She gradually started speaking less and by one year later was barely communicative. Her dementia was assessed to have progressed to FAST 7 dementia.

Mdm X was eventually admitted for a severe pneumonia and started on intravenous antibiotics. Despite this, her oxygen requirements continued to remain high and her pneumonia was not improving. She became increasingly drowsy and refused all food, drink, and medications. She became increasingly hypotensive. Her healthcare team assessed that Mdm X was actively dying.

Her doctors arranged to speak to Mdm X's family members to prepare them for her impending demise. The topic of tube feeding was brought up, but remembering her ACP discussion, her elder son was able to communicate with the rest of the family that this would not be what Mdm X would have wanted. Her family agreed that Mdm X would not have wanted to be burdened with tubes that would not offer much in the way of comfort and symptom relief. The family members instead learned how to participate in oral hygiene for Mdm X which they found meaningful as they were able to contribute to her care in her dying phase. Mdm X passed away a few days later peacefully with her family members at her bedside.

Key messages

1. Poor feeding is common in advanced dementia and is a natural part of the disease process.
2. Poor feeding in the elderly is often multifactorial and reversible causes should be addressed in the first instance.
3. When persistent, poor feeding may characterise end-stage dementia. In such situations, every attempt to encourage continued hand feeding (i.e., self or assisted feeding by hand or using cutlery) should be performed.
4. Enteral feeding (nasogastric tube or percutaneous endoscopic gastronomy) in advanced dementia does not prevent aspiration pneumonia.
5. Tube feeding has not shown much clinically meaningful benefits in advanced dementia.

6. Proper goals of care discussions in advance of poor feeding is important to educate on the limitations of artificial nutrition and hydration in advanced dementia.

Answer key

1. You can think about assessing poor feeding in the elderly in these four domains:

FEEDING SYSTEM	COMORBIDITY INFLUENCES
• Oral intake — quantify oral intake prior to and during current food refusal, consistencies of food the patient has been taking, and the patient's own cited reasons for food refusal. • Issues relating to the oral cavity such as loose teeth, poorly fitting dentures, pain on chewing, painful conditions like aphthous stomatitis, or autoimmune blistering conditions such as bullous pemphigoid or mucous membrane pemphigoid. • Swallowing issues causing odynophagia or dysphagia (throat infections, Parkinson's disease).	• Infection screen — most common infections in the elderly include pneumonia, urinary tract infection, infected pressure sores, cellulitis. • Red flags — early satiety (gastric cancer), changes in bowel habits (colorectal cancer). • Psychiatric — depression, delirium, progression of dementia.
MEDICATION ISSUES	**ENVIRONMENTAL FACTORS**
• Those causing gastrointestinal side-effects like nausea and vomiting (metformin, antibiotics, SSRIs, TCAs). • Those that can alter sense of taste or smell (ACE-inhibitors, calcium channel blockers, allopurinol). • Those that can cause xerostomia (anticholinergics, antihistamines). • Those that can suppress appetite (anticonvulsants, metformin, theophylline). • Those that can cause dysphagia (bisphosphonates, doxycycline, NSAIDs, potassium supplements).	• Therapeutic diets that may be unpalatable — e.g., diabetic diet, low salt diet, modified diet (blended food), hospital food.

2. Mdm X has poor feeding and dehydration that is multifactorial:
   a. *E. coli* urinary tract infection, contributed by her reduced mobility.
   b. Poor oral dentition with poorly fitting dentures resulting in gum abrasions.
   c. Polypharmacy, with culprit medications that can directly contribute to her poor oral intake including metformin, simvastatin, enalapril, furosemide, hydroxyzine, and iron polymaltose.
   d. Low mood likely from reduced visits from her family, reduced social interactions, and isolation at home.
   e. Underlying moderately severe Alzheimer's disease with functional dependence.

   Her poor oral intake has been complicated with hypernatraemia, hypercalcaemia, and acute kidney injury.
3. Antibiotics to treat urinary tract infection;

   Referral to dietitian;

   Dental referral for evaluation, fixing of dentures, and advice on dental hygiene;

   De-prescribing of unnecessary medications;

   Start mirtazapine 7.5 mg ON;

   Increase social interactions
4. E.
5. Known tools for prognostication in dementia can be used to estimate prognosis in advanced dementia, including the FAST score (based on function) and the ADEPT tool. ACP should also be proactively done to understand the patient's values and preferences, as well as to allow the identification of a NHS who can assist in advocating the patient's care preferences when he/she is no longer able to communicate.

References

American Geriatrics Society Ethics Committee and Clinical Practice and Models of Care Committee (2014) American Geriatrics Society feeding tubes in advanced dementia position statement. *J Am Geriatr Soc* **62**(8): 1590–1593.

Hanson LC, Ersek M, Gilliam R, Carey TS (2011) Oral feeding options for people with dementia: a systematic review. *J Am Geriatr Soc* **59**(3): 463–472.

Mitchell SL, Miller SC, Teno JM, Kiely DK, Davis RB, Shaffer ML (2010) Prediction of 6-month survival of nursing home residents with advanced dementia using ADEPT vs hospice eligibility guidelines. *JAMA* **304**(17): 1929–1935.

Navia RO, Constantine LA (2022) Palliative care for patients with advanced dementia. *Nursing* **52**(3): 19–26.

Robbins LJ (1989) Evaluation of weight loss in the elderly. *Geriatrics* **44**(4): 31–34, 37.

35 Poor Oral Intake II (Poor Oral Health)

Dorcas Lim Shao Jiao, Lalmalani Roshan Mahesh

Mr L is an 84-year-old gentleman who was admitted to the general medicine ward for worsening oral intake over two weeks. He currently takes only a few spoonfuls of porridge per meal and one to two cups of water per day. This is on the background of progressive poor oral intake and weight loss of 10 kg over the past year. His past medical history is significant for Parkinson's disease and he is taking L-dopa/benserazide 125 mg QDS. He also recently started to take loratadine 10 mg BD and hydroxyzine 10 mg ON from his general practitioner for itch due to xerotic eczema. He does not smoke or drink.

Clinical examination showed a thin alert man. Vital signs were normal. His oral mucosa was dry and he was edentulous (his daughter clarified that despite having dentures fitted one year ago, he rarely used them due to gum pain). His skin was dry with scattered excoriations. His cardiorespiratory and abdominal systems were normal. No peripheral lymphadenopathy was detected. He exhibited a stable Parkinsonian gait but otherwise was functionally independent. Depression screen was unremarkable.

Laboratory investigations on full blood count, renal and liver panels, thyroid function, and urinalysis were normal. CT neck, thorax, abdomen, and pelvis were unremarkable. Upper and lower gastrointestinal endoscopy was unremarkable except for one benign colonic polyp.

Question 1: What is the most likely cause(s) of Mr L's unintentional weight loss?

Unintended weight loss and poor oral intake is a common phenomenon amongst elderly patients. Please refer to the chapter on "poor oral intake in advanced dementia" for a general approach to poor oral intake.

Poorly fitted dentures cause gum irritation including inflammation, erosions, blisters, and bleeding. The oral cavity is innervated by the superior and inferior dental plexus, both of which are branches of the mandibular nerve. The mandibular nerve transmits sensory information from the lower third of the face as well as the mandible, preauricular, temple, meninges, anterior, and middle cranial fossa. Hence, nerve root irritation due to poorly fitted dentures may result in earaches and headaches.

Due to significant local and transmitted pain, chewing becomes a challenge and this may result in reduced oral intake. Furthermore, the dentures may "become loose" as the gum and jawbone shrink due to lack of stimulation of the tooth root.

The American Dental Association recommends regular dental visits at six-monthly intervals to ensure proper denture fit and to evaluate for signs of oral disease. Dentures may need to be re-aligned or remade due to normal wear and tear or age-related changes to gums and jawbones.

To acclimatise to a new set of dentures, one should ideally start with soft foods cut into small pieces and chewed slowly. Normal diet can be resumed when one gets used to the dentures. Hot foods or hard foods with bones or shells should be avoided to minimise further discomfort.

Oral health is a prevalent problem in the elderly:

- Nearly all adults aged 65 years and older have had a cavity; 1 in 5 have untreated tooth decay;
- 2 out of 3 older adults have gum disease;
- About 1/3 of older Singaporeans (according to a 2016 survey) have lost all their teeth.

In Singapore, MediSave is a national medical savings scheme that helps individuals set aside a proportion of their income to pay for healthcare expenses including hospitalisation, day surgery, and certain outpatient expenses. However, the majority of dental services is *not* included in the list of claimable expenditure:

- Tooth extraction
- Scaling and polishing
- Braces
- Dentures
- Crowns
- Non-surgical root canal treatment

Whilst the local healthcare economics setup proves to be a challenge to improving oral health, the government has implemented further subsidy programmes (Fig 35.1) such as the Community Health Assist Scheme (CHAS), Merdeka

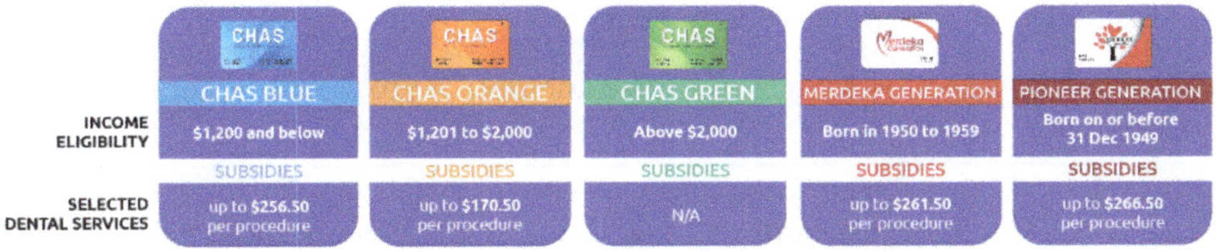

Fig. 35.1. Community Health Assist Schemes in Singapore (2022).

Generation, and Pioneer Generation to help residents with the costs of health and dental services.

Poor oral hygiene can be caused by problems with the gums, teeth, tongue, or salivation. Chronic smoking, low socio-economic status, and elderly who are homebound or institutionalised greatly increase the risk of having poor oral health.

A. Periodontal disease

Gingivitis is the inflammation of the gums, characterised by gingival erythema, swelling, and bleeding. Healthy gingival tissue appears pink and firm and should not bleed while brushing or flossing.

Gingivitis may progress to periodontitis, which is gingival inflammation with the loss of supportive connecting tissues including the periodontal ligament and alveolar bone. Gingival recession reduces the stability of the tooth and may lead to subsequent loss of the tooth.

Chronic diseases, such as diabetes, increase the risk of periodontal disease. These patients are also less likely to seek dental care.

To reduce the risk of gingivitis, encourage good oral hygiene with regular brushing (at least twice a day) and flossing (at least once a day) to remove dental plaque between teeth where a toothbrush cannot reach. In an elderly person with impaired finger dexterity due to osteoarthritis, a floss pick or a water flosser may be considered.

B. Tooth disorder — Dental caries

Dental caries ("tooth decay") is the erosion of the tooth enamel. Plaque is constantly being formed by bacteria within the oral cavity. It converts sugar and carbohydrates into acids which erode the tooth enamel and lead to the formation of cavities over time. The resultant exposure of the nerves of the underlying dentin and pulp causes increased pain and sensitivity especially when consuming hot or cold food and drinks.

Early caries can be reversed with good oral hygiene and regular brushing with a fluoride toothpaste. However, the damage is irreversible once the enamel is completely destroyed.

C. Disorders of the tongue (Table 35.1)

Table 35.1. Common tongue disorders contributing to poor oral hygiene in the elderly.

Features	Geographic tongue (benign migratory glossitis)	Atrophic glossitis	Median rhomboid glossitis (oral thrush)
Clinical presentation	Smooth areas of papillary atrophy surrounded by whitish serpiginous borders, with spontaneous shape-shifting and expansion, resolution, and migration	Smooth and glossy dorsal tongue with a red or pink background	Smooth shiny erythematous plaque along the dorsal midline of the tongue
Causes	Unknown, but associations have been drawn with ***nutritional deficiencies***, coeliac disease, and dermatologic diseases (e.g., psoriasis, atopic dermatitis)	Nutritional — protein-calorie malnutrition, deficiencies in ***iron, vitamin B12***, ***folate*** etc; Systemic disease (e.g., diabetes mellitus, coeliac disease); Dermatologic disease (e.g., lichen planus)	*Candida albicans*, a known coloniser in the oral cavity, may flourish rapidly in the elderly or immunocompromised person
Symptoms	Mostly asymptomatic; some have increased sensitivity, soreness, burning pain, or taste dysfunction; may be exacerbated by spicy or acid foods	Xerostomia; Sore, tender, or swollen tongue impairing ability to speak or eat properly	Dysphagia
Management	Reassurance of benign nature; Avoidance of irritants such as tobacco or spicy/acidic foods; Mouthwashes with local anaesthetic properties; Topical tacrolimus 0.1% ointment BD may be considered	Treat underlying condition; Mouthwashes with local anaesthetic properties	Mild oropharyngeal candidiasis is treated with miconazole oral gel QDS or nystatin 100,000 IU/mL suspension 5 mL QDS "swish (as long as possible) and swallow" for 7–14 days. Note that nystatin contains sucrose, so prolonged use may cause dental caries! Moderate to severe cases can be treated with oral fluconazole 50 mg OM for 7–14 days

D. Xerostomia

In the maintenance of good oral hygiene, saliva does the following:

- lubricates the oral cavity
- protects against microbial and fungal growth
- neutralises acids that break down tooth enamel
- aids in remineralisation of damaged enamel

Xerostomia, or dry mouth, is a subjective perception of dryness of the mouth. It may occur when there is hyposalivation due to salivary gland hypofunction. Reduced saliva flow increases the risk of cavities and can significantly impact quality of life by affecting eating and swallowing. It affects every one in five individuals, with a rising prevalence amongst the elderly population.

The xerostomia inventory is a multi-item inventory that can be used to assess the presence and magnitude of xerostomia. It is found in the Appendix at the end of this chapter.

As our population ages and develops more chronic medical conditions, the incidence of polypharmacy rises.

Table 35.2. Common medications used in the elderly that may contribute to xerostomia (non-exhaustive list)

Drugs with Anticholinergic Activity	
Classes	Examples
Atropine and analogues Antidepressants (tricyclics) Antipsychotic agents Antihistamines Anti-emetics Anti-Parkinson's Bronchodilators	Atropine, Benztropine Amitriptyline, Nortriptyline Quetiapine, Risperidone, Lithium Loratadine, Promethazine, Hydroxyzine Scopolamine Levodopa, Amantadine Ipratropium, Tiotropium
Drugs with Sympathomimetic Activity	
Classes	Examples
Antidepressants (SSRI, SNRI, NaSSA) Antihypertensives (α/β-blockers) Anti-migraine Bronchodilators	Venlafaxine, Duloxetine, Mirtazapine Bisoprolol, Prazosin, Terazosin Zolmitriptan Salbutamol
Drugs with Synergistic Action (Anticholinergic + Sympathomimetic)	
Classes	Examples
Opioids Benzodiazepines	Fentanyl, Morphine, Tramadol Alprazolam, Lorazepam

(*Continued*)

Table 35.2. *(Continued)*

Others	
Classes	Examples
H2-antagonists/proton-pump inhibitors Antibiotics Antivirals	Famotidine, omeprazole Amoxicillin, tetracycline, metronidazole Lamivudine, ritonavir

Note: Adapted from Han P, Suarez-Durall P, Mulligan R (2015) Dry-mouth: a critical topic for older patients. *J Prosthodont Res* **59**(1): 6–19.

****

Question 2: What is your plan of management for Mr L?

As with most things, prevention is better than cure. These constitute a multi-pronged approach to maintain good oral health:

Patient	Caregiver	Doctor
• drink fluoridated water and brush with fluoride toothpaste (Singapore is the first country in Asia to institute community water fluoridation to cover 100% of the population) • practice good oral hygiene; brush teeth twice daily and floss between teeth to remove dental plaque • visit the dentist once a year, even if one has no natural teeth or has dentures • avoid tobacco products and limit alcoholic drinks • see the doctor or dentist if one notices a change of taste or smell	• help older individuals brush and floss their teeth • remind and bring them for dental follow-ups	• control chronic health diseases, especially diabetes, as good diabetic control reduces risk of gum diseases; conversely, treating gum disease will also improve blood sugar level • watch for anticholinergic drugs which cause dry mouth and increase risk of dental caries; if unavoidable, ensure that patient drinks plenty of water

Key messages

1. Oral pathology is an important and often treatable cause of poor feeding. Don't forget to look into the mouth of the older person with poor feeding as it may provide the answer to the cause!
2. With increasing prevalence of cognitive impairment and dementia, the older person may not be able to complain of pain or discomfort; hence it is important to examine the oral cavity thoroughly even in the absence of a suggestive history.
3. Due to a lifetime of low awareness on the importance of good oral hygiene, many older people have significant issues with their dentition. It is never too late to try to arrest oral pathology — make a prompt referral for dental consultation and provide encouragement to see a dentist. Improvement in oral health and dentition will in turn help with improving nutrition and quality of life.
4. A detailed review of medications is useful in identifying the culprits of xerostomia. It is useful to review the indications of culprit medications and consider ceasing them should they no longer be needed.

Answer key

1. Poor oral intake secondary to poorly fitted dentures, exacerbated by iatrogenic xerostomia (sedating H1-antihistamine ± L-dopa).
2. Dental review to evaluate denture fit as well as oral hygiene;

   Ensure regular dental follow-up;

   Stop the oral antihistamines as they are unlikely to help with the itch and instead moisturise liberally and frequently;

   Dietician review for optimisation of oral intake.

References

Chiu CT, Malhotra R, Tan SM, *et al.* (2016) Dental health status of community-dwelling older Singaporeans: findings from a nationally representative survey. *Gerodontology* **34**(1): 57–67.

Han P, Suarez-Durall P, Mulligan R (2015) Dry-mouth: a critical topic for older patients. *J Prosthodont Res* **59**(1): 6–19.

Appendix

The Xerostomia Inventory *is an 11-item summated rating scale where each item is scored for never (1), hardly ever (2), occasionally (3), fairly often (4), and very often (5). A minimum score of 11 indicates mild xerostomia whilst a maximum score of 55 indicates severe xerostomia.*

1. *I sip liquids to help swallow food.*
2. *My mouth feels dry when eating a meal.*
3. *I get up at night to drink.*
4. *My mouth feels dry.*
5. *I have difficulty in eating dry foods.*
6. *I suck sweets or cough lollies to relieve dry mouth.*
7. *I have difficulties in swallowing certain foods.*
8. *The skin of my face feels dry.*
9. *My eyes feel dry.*
10. *My lips feel dry.*
11. *The inside of my nose feels dry.*

36 Dying from Advanced Malignancy

Kayleigh Ho Huimin, Victoria Wong Hwei May,
Anupama Roy Chowdhury

Mr O is an 82-year-old Chinese gentleman with a past medical history of diabetes mellitus, hypertension, and hyperlipidaemia. He was diagnosed with prostate cancer 5 years ago with metastasis to the bones and small volume metastasis in the lung and liver. His cancer was initially controlled with hormonal therapy, but unfortunately it progressed and was not responsive to subsequent lines of chemotherapy.

Mr O was referred to the Advance Care Planning (ACP) team for a discussion regarding his care preferences.

Question 1: Which of the following statement(s) regarding ACP is true?

a. **It is a legally binding document which cannot be changed or reversed once signed.**
b. **It is meant only for people who are terminally ill.**
c. **It takes into account a patient's values and personhood.**
d. **Its main purpose is to establish resuscitation status and extent of care.**

ACP is not a legally binding document. It is the process in which we communicate and document our values and wishes regarding future medical care. The aim of ACP is to promote care that is consistent with one's values and preferences, empowering patients to choose how they want to be cared for and helping them communicate with their loved ones and healthcare team these preferences in the event that they are unable to make decisions or speak for themselves.

While ACP does guide loved ones in decision-making when the patient loses mental capacity, we need to remember that preferences and priorities can change over time. It requires regular revisiting, especially when there is a change of nominated healthcare spokespersons (NHS) or major life events (e.g., hospital admissions), to check if there are any changes in values or goals of care.

Advance medical directive (AMD) is a legal document signed in advance by the patient to inform the treating doctor (in the event they become terminally ill and unconscious) not to use any extraordinary life-sustaining treatment to prolong their life. The AMD will come into force once it is determined that the patient has a terminal illness. Three doctors (of which at least 2 out of 3 must be specialists empaneled for the purpose of such assessments) must unanimously agree that the patient is terminally ill. After an AMD is signed, it will be registered with the Registrar to AMD at the Ministry of Health. It is an offence to enquire whether an AMD had been made.

An AMD can be revoked in the presence of at least one witness in writing, orally, or in any other way in which the patient can communicate. Submit the notice of revocation to the Registrar containing: (A) the name and NRIC of both the person and the witness along with addresses and phone numbers, and (B) the time, date, and place where the revocation was made.

Lasting power of attorney (LPA) is a legal instrument which allows a person who is at least 21 years of age ("donor") to voluntarily appoint one or more persons ("donees") to make decisions and act on their behalf should they lose mental capacity one day. A donee can be appointed to act in the two broad areas of (1) personal welfare and (2) property and affairs matters. The donees must act in the best interest of the donor. After an LPA has been lodged, the Office of Public Guardian will verify your documents and accept your application for registration. If no valid objections are received in the following three weeks, the LPA will be registered at the end of that period. There are some restricted/excluded decisions that the donees cannot make:

(a) Personal welfare
  - Life-sustaining decisions, AMD, medical treatment, organ donation
  - Consent to marriage, divorce, adoption
  - Decisions related to religion, abortion

(b) Property and affairs
  - Execute a will
  - Make or revoke insurance/CPF nominations
  - Make gifts from the donor's property

****

Mr O nominated his son as his NHS, and his ACP was done with his son as witness. During the process of discussion, Mr O shared that he is someone who values his independence and does not like to trouble other people. He is a retired teacher. In his free time, he enjoys taking long walks with his wife and spending time at home with his family or cycling around his neighbourhood. It is important to him that he remains as independent as possible as he does not want to be a burden to his family. While he still hopes for life prolongation, he is also clear that quality of life is more important than number of days left. He hopes to remain as symptom-free as possible. If possible, he would prefer to pass away at home in the presence of his family.

One month later, he is admitted to hospital following a fall with right hip pain. Scans show a pathological fracture of his right hip.

Question 2: What would affect your treatment decision for the hip fracture?

I. Prognosis

II. Functional status

III. ACP

IV. Comorbidities

V. Whether or not he is still on active chemotherapy

Options

a. I and II only

b. I, II, III, and IV

c. I, II, and V

d. All of the above

The patient's prognosis, functional status, and goals of care should be taken into account when deciding whether or not the patient is a surgical candidate. The general rule of thumb is that the patient should have a prognosis and functional status that are good enough for them to recover from and reap the benefits of the various interventions. We should also take into consideration the patient's preferences for their care. A patient on best supportive care does not preclude them from being offered surgery and/or other invasive therapies to manage symptoms.

Skeletal-related events (SREs) are morbidity events that result from bony metastasis. These include pain, hypercalcaemia, pathological fractures, and spinal cord/nerve root compression. The management of SRE can be categorised into surgical intervention, non-pharmacological and pharmacological.

Surgical management is reserved for lesions with complete or impending pathological fracture, or for spinal metastasis causing mechanical instability or spinal cord compression. There are a few scoring systems available to aid us in assessing the need for surgical intervention.

(1) Mirel's score is used to assess the risk of fracture for long bones and the role of prophylactic nailing.
(2) The Spinal Instability Neoplastic Score is used to assess spinal stability and need for surgical consultation.
(3) The Tokuhashi Score is used to predict the survival period for patients with metastatic spine tumour.

Post-operative radiation therapy is generally given after an intervention to stabilise the spine, promote re-mineralisation and bone healing, alleviate pain, improve functional status, and reduce the risk of subsequent fracture/loss of fixation by treating the residual disease. Radiation therapy should be started only after the wound is fully healed to prevent any wound breakdown. The mean time to response is about 3 weeks, and the mean duration of remission (of pain) is about 4–5 months.

Osteoclast inhibitors: Once cancer cells are established in the bone, the interaction between tumour cells, osteoblasts, and osteoclasts creates a vicious cycle that increases bone turnover. In prostate cancer, the bone metastasis is predominantly osteoblastic but bone resorption is also increased. Hence, agents that block bone resorption can also help to decrease pain from the bone metastasis and also reduce the risk of SREs.

Osteoclast inhibitors are used as an adjuvant in the management of non-fracture bone pain as well as to reduce SREs.

Examples of osteoclast inhibitors are bisphosphonates (e.g., pamidronate, zoledronic acid) and denosumab.

Bisphosphonates absorb calcium to provide physicochemical protection, suppress normal functioning osteoclasts, and prevent osteoclast precursors from maturing. It helps to prevent SREs and is used in the treatment of bone loss in patients at high risk of fracture who are receiving hormone deprivation for early prostate or breast cancer as well as in the treatment for tumour-induced hypercalcaemia. Patients with renal impairment will require dose adjustments. It is important to be cognizant of the risks and precautions with the use of bisphosphonates

Adverse Event	**Preventive measures**
Osteonecrosis of the jaw	Dental clearance prior to treatment; Regular oropharyngeal examination before administration
Hypocalcaemia	Routine monitoring of calcium and albumin
Renal dysfunction	Routine creatinine clearance monitoring and dose adjustment accordingly
Fever	Prophylactic/adjuvant use of antipyretics
Nausea	Anti-emetics prior to administration

Note: Risks and precautions for use of bisphophonates.

Denosumab ($403.53 per 60 mg SC injection every 6-monthly) is a receptor activator of nuclear factor kappa-B ligand (RANKL) inhibitor. It does not undergo hepatic or renal metabolism, hence it can be used in patients with advanced renal impairment. In patients with hypercalcaemia of malignancy, the dose interval of denosumab is 4-weekly compared to when used in osteoporosis which is 6-monthly.

****

In view of Mr O's good functional status and prognosis as well as his wish to remain as independent as possible, he was offered nailing of the right hip as well as post-operation radiation therapy. He recovered well from these treatments and was discharged with PO tramadol 25 mg as needed, up to 4 times daily, for pain management.

Nine months later, Mr O returned to the Emergency Department with severe back pain. He described it as a severe deep aching pain with a pain score of 8. It was constantly present with exacerbations upon movement. There was no radiation of pain, allodynia, or any neurological deficits. He denied any issues with passing urine or passing motion. Physical examination did not reveal any signs of cord compression. After he was admitted to the ward, he continued to complain of poorly controlled pain which was affecting his mood and appetite despite taking regular PO tramadol 50 mg TDS.

Question 3: What would you do next? Select the two most appropriate options.

a. Give IM Pethidine 50 mg stat

b. Increase tramadol to 100 mg QDS and use oral morphine 15 mg Q1H PRN as breakthrough

c. Keep tramadol 50 mg TDS but add oxycodone immediate release capsule (OxyNorm) 5 mg TDS

d. Start fentanyl patch 12 mcg/hr and add a breakthrough dose of 25 mcg Q1H PRN

e. Start on morphine infusion 0.6 mg/hr and add a breakthrough dose of 1.2 mg Q1H PRN

f. Stop tramadol, start on oral morphine syrup 5 mg Q4H, and add a breakthrough dose of 5 mg Q1H PRN

The patient is having poorly controlled pain. A quick clinical assessment should be made to elicit the nature and aetiology of pain and determine what medications have been given so far, with the aim of providing pain relief as soon as possible. A full and detailed history and physical examination can be done when pain is better controlled.

The use of strong opioids is considered in patients with severe pain and who are no longer getting pain relief from mild opioids (as in Mr O's case!). Ideally, parenteral strong opioids should be used as the onset of action is much quicker than oral options. ***A referral to inpatient pain service or palliative medicine should be made if rapid bedside titration of parenteral opioids is required***. In the meantime, a dose of opioids should be given to the patient. If the patient is opioid-naive, give a stat dose of IV or subcutaneous morphine 1 mg (normal renal function) or fentanyl 10–25 mcg (impaired renal function).

The strong opioids that are typically used in Singapore are morphine, fentanyl, and oxycodone. The choice of opioid depends on renal and hepatic function as well as the effective route of administration. Pethidine is generally avoided as it incurs a significant risk of developing dependence and drug-seeking behaviour. Furthermore, repeated doses lead to accumulation of the toxic metabolite norpethidine, which lowers the seizure threshold.

<u>Morphine</u> is the drug of choice for patients with good renal and hepatic function as this is readily available and most physicians are familiar with it. There are two formulations of oral morphine available in Singapore: morphine sulfate tablets (MST) and morphine mixture.

Morphine mixture is short-acting and lasts about 4 hours. Start at 2.5 mg every 4 hours. In patients with impaired renal or liver function, reduce the dose of morphine and/or increase the dosing interval. The doses are then titrated according to the patient's response and symptoms. When the required dose of morphine is stable, it can be converted to MST which is long-acting (the duration of action is 8–12 hours).

In patients who are unable to take orally, a good starting dose of subcutaneous/IV morphine is 1 mg Q1H PRN. However, if the patient is already on oral opioids, convert to the equivalent parenteral dose and administer 1/10th of the total daily dose (i.e., if patient is on a total of 90 mg of oral morphine, the parenteral equivalent dose is 90 mg/3 = 30 mg per day; to give 3 mg as a stat dose).

<u>Fentanyl</u> comes in two different formulations: transdermal patches and parenteral. The transdermal fentanyl patches available in Singapore are at fixed doses of 12 mcg/hr, 25 mcg/hr, and 50 mcg/hr. Fentanyl patches can be changed every 72 hours and are ideal for patients with renal or liver impairment or those who are unable to take orally. In patients with severe pain and who require frequent adjustment of opioids, fentanyl patches will not be suitable because it takes 8–12 hours for the analgesic effect to be optimum.

In patients who require parenteral fentanyl, we can start with 10–25 mcg Q1H PRN and titrate according to symptoms and response. Once the analgesic dose reaches a steady value, we can consider switching to a fentanyl patch to ensure better compliance.

Oxycodone has two oral formulations: short-acting ones are oxycodone immediate release capsules (OxyNorm) 5 mg, 10 mg, and oxycodone liquid (OxyNorm liquid) 1 mg/ml; long-acting ones are oxycodone extended release tablets (OxyContin) 10 mg, 20 mg.

Scanning this code brings you to the opioid conversion table from the Lien Centre for Palliative Care SG Pall eBook which you can refer to when you need to opioid-rotate to an equivalent dose.

After converting, we usually attenuate the starting dose by ~30% to avoid unintentional overdose due to incomplete cross-tolerance (there may be individual variations in opioid pharmacokinetics).

Illustrative example 1: a patient is currently on oral morphine 100 mg/day and a decision is made to convert to long-acting oxycodone for ease of dosing. After conversion, the daily equivalent dose of oxycodone is 50 mg. Attenuating the dose by 25% gives 40 mg. A reasonable starting dosing of Oxycontin-CR would be 20 mg ($3.36) OM and 20 mg ($3.36) ON.

Illustrative example 2: Mr O's pain is controlled on morphine infusion 0.6 mg/hr with additional four breakthroughs of 1.2 mg per day. He is going to be discharged with oral MST. What dose do you think is needed? (read on to find out)

For geriatric patients it is important to be careful with dose titration of opioids. We should give the lowest effective dose and monitor closely for signs of opioid toxicity such as myosis, respiratory depression (manifested by respiratory rate <8/min), and myoclonic jerks. If there are signs of opioid toxicity, we should assess the patient and decide if the opioid should be stopped or reduced. Please consult the palliative care physician or pain specialist if there are any concerns.

Also, be mindful that constipation is an exceedingly common side-effect of strong opioids especially in the elderly. Concomitant regular laxatives are highly recommended. Stimulant laxatives such as senna and bisacodyl are appropriate choices. Avoid bulk laxatives (e.g., Fybogel) as these require the intake of adequate amounts of fluid to be effective and the older person with terminal illness or severe pain may not be able to drink enough. Less frequent side-effects are nausea or vomiting and sedation, but patients normally develop tolerance within a week or so. If the nausea or vomiting is distressing, PO haloperidol 0.5–1.5 mg at bedtime is helpful.

****

The palliative team comes to see Mr O and rapid bedside titration is done. His pain is better controlled and he is maintained on morphine infusion of 0.6 mg/hr with breakthrough of 1.2 mg Q1H as needed.

Further history is taken from Mr O. He says that apart from pain, he has been having exertional dyspnoea over the past few months. His family has also noted that he is pale looking. He is easily fatigued and tires on minimal exertion.

His blood tests are reviewed and it is noted that his haemoglobin level is 7.2 g/dL (baseline 10 g/dL). He has no signs of bleeding. Further investigation is done and it is determined that the anaemia is likely due to marrow involvement from the extensive bone metastasis. Mr O was given blood transfusion with good symptomatic relief with an improvement in his energy level and breathlessness. He was later counselled on the pros and cons of blood transfusion. He understands that the anaemia will recur as the aetiology is due to marrow involvement from the cancer. He is still keen for transfusion if it helps him feel better. However, should the interval of blood transfusions required grow shorter and burden of care increases, he is not keen for multiple repeated transfusions and the goal of care is to be kept comfortable. Mr O's ACP was updated to reflect this decision regarding his extent of care preferences. Mr O's morphine infusion was converted to PO MST 20 mg Q12H prior to his discharge home.

In the following half a year, Mr O had multiple admissions for anaemia. Initially the intervals between each blood transfusion was about 6 weeks; of late, it has become shorter with intervals of less than 2 weeks. Mr O is beginning to find that he no longer benefits from the transfusion. He remained lethargic and fatigued despite the transfusions.

A few days later, Mr O developed severe chest pain and was diagnosed with a myocardial infarction. He declined any further intervention and requested for comfort care and symptom control only. He refused all further blood investigations. It was noted that Mr O was getting weaker and had problems swallowing. His PO MST 20 mg Q12H was converted to a fentanyl patch of 18 mcg/hr with breakthrough of oral morphine 7.5 mg Q1H PRN in preparation for home.

While preparations were made for him to be discharged, Mr O continued to decline and his healthcare team assessed him to be actively dying. He grew more lethargic and was unable to eat or drink. Mr O's family is now asking for him to be placed on IV fluids or have a nasogastric tube (NGT) inserted for feeding since he is unable to take orally as they did not want him to starve to death.

Question 4: What would you do or say in response to this request?

a. **Explain that inserting a NGT (or IV cannula) is distressing to the patient, discourage it, and offer subcutaneous fluids instead.**
b. **Insert a NGT for feeding but hold off on IV fluids as it is cruel to subject the patient to multiple IV insertions.**
c. **Speak to the family to understand their concerns and expectations, then explain the utility of artificial nutrition and hydration at the end of life.**
d. **Start IV fluids and insert a NGT for feeding as per their request so that the patient does not starve to death.**

Hydration and nutrition are essential for the maintenance of life. However, at the end of life, artificial nutrition and hydration offer very limited utility. There is actually no strong evidence supporting their use for the majority of terminally ill patients. In spite of this, artificial nutrition and hydration pose serious clinical and ethical dilemmas that clinicians often have to face, especially when coupled with mounting pressure from the families of patients to initiate such treatment. Indeed, there are also wide variations in practice depending on the culture, field of expertise, and even location of practice in caring for patients at the end of life.

In the last days to weeks of life, anorexia often occurs. Families may express a desire to initiate artificial feeding, often as a grieving response in wanting to do something for the dying patient. Such requests often occur in the form of wanting to insert a NGT for nutrition. However, the psychological benefit associated with tube feeding has to be closely balanced with the burden of having an artificial tube inserted, which can be associated with distress during and after the insertion process. Tube feeding may deny patients of the simple pleasures of oral feeding, limit meaningful interactions with loved ones in the remaining time that the patient has owing to discomfort, and worse still precipitate agitation.

Artificial nutrition is most beneficial when it is used for a short period of time to allow the patient to recover from surgery or sudden illness. However, at the end of life, the caloric requirements of a dying patient are naturally reduced, so the clinical benefit is not apparent. In fact, the current evidence is that ***artificial feeding does not meaningfully prolong survival in a dying patient***. Artificial nutrition can also increase the risk of aspiration pneumonia, cause unnecessary secretions, and lead to fluid overload. In an anorexic patient who has not been fed for some time, complications such as re-feeding syndrome may occur and lead to discomfort from arrhythmias and in the worst case hasten death. Regular blood investigations to monitor for and correct electrolyte abnormalities also result in greater distress at the end of life.

Another less common form of artificial nutrition that families may request would be parenteral nutrition. This involves administering nutrition parenterally, either via a central line (total parenteral nutrition) or via a peripheral cannula (peripheral parenteral nutrition). Again, this can result in unnecessary needle pricks for IV access, and in the case of total parenteral nutrition may result in complications of the pneumothorax, catheter infections, and pain. Indeed, such traumatic methods to ensure artificial nutrition that may not produce any clear benefits hardly seem warranted when comfort should be of utmost importance at the end of life.

Infusion of fluids is one of the most common medical treatments. It is not difficult to see why such treatment would continue even when the patient is at the end of life. Fluids can be administered intravenously, subcutaneously (hypodermoclysis), or via a NGT.

Often, thirst is cited as a reason for administering artificial hydration in a dying patient who can no longer have easy access to fluids. However, studies have shown that there is only a modest correlation between the sensation of thirst and hydration status at the end of life. Furthermore, thirst can be symptomatically managed with small amounts of oral fluids by mouth, wetting the lips, as well as vigilant oral care. Products that moisten the oral cavity, including mouth gels and mouthwashes as well as the use of sodium bicarbonate powder dissolved in water to clean debris in the mouth, are simple techniques that can be taught to the loved ones of dying patients to involve them in the precious act of caring for such patients in their final stages of life.

A plausible use for artificial fluids administration that may be cited would be for delirium and myoclonus in terminal patients. Such symptoms may occur due to the accumulation of toxic metabolites from certain medications being administered such as opioids. Hydration may be able to prevent or reverse such symptoms, but the available evidence is weak and inconsistent. Furthermore, there are other ways to manage these symptoms at the end of life, including pharmacological and non-pharmacological approaches.

Indeed, a large body of evidence suggests that there are minimal clinical benefits for hydration in the management of other symptoms at the end of life, such as fatigue and hallucinations. It also does not confer any quality of life and survival benefits in terminally ill patients. Often times, the dying patient who is comatose does not experience symptoms distress. Furthermore, there would be less respiratory secretions and pulmonary oedema with less artificial hydration at the end of life.

When the families of dying patients strongly insist for artificial fluids to be administered, isotonic fluids may be provided subcutaneously as an alternative

to intravenous hydration. This is an underutilised method of administration which avoids the need to locate a vein and may be less painful for the patient given the small needle size. Family members can be informed that small volumes of fluids can be administered (500–1,000 mls) subcutaneously, with the caveat to stop should the patient develop complications (secretions or fluid overload).

Families should be ***educated that the withdrawal or withholding of artificial nutrition and hydration does not hasten death or constitute euthanasia.*** Oftentimes, a request for artificial nutrition and hydration reflects a lack of clear understanding and acceptance about the true prognosis and nature of the illness among the loved ones of the dying patient. In fact, such requests may reflect a need to do something for the patient simply because it can be done, rather than because of any measurable benefit or relief of suffering. More importantly, such requests present an opportunity to explore the family's fears, anxieties, and goals of care for the patient, and to reassure them that the patient will not be abandoned as he or she approaches death.

****

Mr O continued to deteriorate over the next few days and became increasingly drowsy and was unable to communicate. His family was in agreement that he would not have wanted to be burdened with injections and tubes that would not offer much in the way of comfort and symptom relief. A subcutaneous drip was similarly declined.

It was noted that Mr O started to make some rattling noises when breathing which distressed his family greatly as they thought that he was drowning in saliva.

Question 5: How do you manage this problem of respiratory secretions? Select all that apply.

a. **Deep suctioning as needed**
b. **No need to do anything as patients are not distressed by it**
c. **Re-position the patient**
d. **Subcutaneous hyoscine (Buscopan) to dry up the secretions**
e. **Stop feeding the patient**

Terminal secretions have been described in up to 23–95% of patients in various palliative units. It is a good predictor of "impending demise" and prognosis of short days. Terminal secretions occur because patients get weaker at the end of life and are unable to swallow and/or clear their oral secretions which then pool in the airways. The sound can be distressing for family members to hear as they often perceive it as their loved ones drowning in their secretions.

It is important to differentiate between terminal secretions and increased sputum production from a chest infection as the treatment for each is different.

Non-pharmacological methods to handle terminal rattling include repositioning the patient and allowing them to lie on the side or in a semi-prone position as this allows for postural drainage of the oral secretions. Gentle suctioning can be done if the patient is not distressed by it. Otherwise, suctioning is generally discouraged as it can cause discomfort to the patient, and most secretions tend to be inaccessible to suctioning as it occurs below the level of the larynx. Any ongoing feeding or parenteral fluids should be reduced or stopped if needed.

Pharmacological agents to manage terminal rattling can be administered by the following routes:

A. Parenterally (intravenously or subcutaneously)
   i. Hyoscine butylbromide (Buscopan) 20 mg up to every 4 hours as needed. This does not cross the blood-brain barrier. (Oral bioavailability is poor, hence the oral formulation may not be effective for secretion management.)
   ii. Glycopyrrolate 100–400 mcg up to every 6 hours as needed.
B. Sublingual
   i. Atropine 1% ophthalmic 1–2 drops every 4–6 hours. More often used in the homecare setting for ease of administration by family members.

****

In accordance with his preference to be cared for at home, preparations were made for Mr O to be terminally discharged. He eventually passed away a few days later at home with his immediate family members at his bedside.

Question 6: Which of the following statements concerning terminal discharge are correct? Select all that apply.

a. All parenteral medications should be switched to oral or transdermal formulations as IV and subcutaneous medications cannot be given at home.

b. If the patient's family is unable to cope with care of the patient at home, then it is not wrong to keep the patient in the hospital for terminal care even though the patient's wish is to die at home.

c. If the patient is actively dying, then we should not terminally discharge the patient as there is a possibility that the patient will die in the ambulance en route home.

d. The goal of terminal discharge is for the patient to reach home to pass away, hence time is of essence and the main priority is to book an ambulance to send the patient home as soon as possible.

e. We should refer the patient to a home hospice as soon as possible.

While going home as soon as possible is important in planning for a terminal discharge, it is important that we ensure that the patient receives good care at home as well. Caregiver training should be carried out prior to sending the patient home, and this includes general care of the patient (e.g., changing of clothes and/or diapers, cleaning the patient, oral care), basic nursing care (e.g., wound care if applicable, prevention of pressure injuries), and subcutaneous medicine administration. If care at home is going to be suboptimal or if there is no identified caregiver, then it is not wrong to keep the patient in the hospital for terminal care.

Before the patient is discharged, a referral should be made to the home hospice team to help support the patient and the family at home. In addition, contacts for private home medical support for emergency should be provided.

It is important to note that home hospice care does not help with the basic and nursing care of the patient. Their role is to provide support with symptom management as well as psychosocial support. If the family needs help with nursing care, private nursing services can be engaged.

As the patient is deteriorating and at the terminal phase, increasing drowsiness is expected and they will be unable to take medications orally. Hence most, if not all, medications will have to be given via non-oral routes such as transdermal, subcutaneous, or suppository. If infusions are needed, home hospices can also support with drug infusions via infusion pumps.

All patients who are terminally discharged have a chance that they will pass on en route home. This is not a contraindication to allowing a terminal discharge. As part of the preparation for home, the primary team should provide three memos:

1. Memo to the ambulance service to continue the journey to the patient's home even if they should demise en route.
2. Memo to a general practitioner stating the cause of death so that the doctor can help to write the death certificate.
3. Memo to the home hospice service with a handover of the patient's condition.

Key messages

1. ACP is important as it helps the patient's family and medical team understand how they would like to be cared for in a way that is consistent with their values and preferences.
2. The management of bone metastasis and impending fractures includes both optimal pain control as well as consideration of surgery and/or other interventions. Doses of medications should be reviewed with caution in the elderly population.

3. In an acute pain crisis, it is important to quickly serve parenteral opioids to control the pain after a rapid clinical assessment of the nature and aetiology of the pain. A referral to palliative medicine should be made as rapid bedside titration of opioids may be required.
4. Artificial hydration and nutrition at the end of life do not add to survival or mortality benefit. Proper goals of care and the family's concerns and expectations should be addressed. It is also important to balance the family's request for feeding and nutrition against the problems it may cause to the patient.
5. The management of terminal secretions includes non-pharmacological methods and medications like hyoscine butylbromide which can help to dry up secretions. Avoid suctioning and invite the family to participate in care of the patient (e.g., oral toileting).
6. Terminal discharge can be considered if the patient had stated that their preferred place of death is at home. Preparation is needed including caregiver training and a referral to home hospice services.

Answer key

1. C.
2. B.
3. E, F.
4. C.
5. C, D, E.
6. B, E.

References

Chai HZ, Krishna LK, Wong VH (2014) Feeding: what it means to patients and caregivers and how these views influence Singaporean Chinese caregivers' decisions to continue feeding at the end of life. *Am J Hosp Palliat Care* **31**(2): 166–171.

Clark K, Butler M (2009) Noisy respiratory secretions at the end of life. *Curr Opin Support Palliat Care* **3**(2): 120–124.

Dev R, Dalal S, Bruera E (2012) Is there a role for parenteral nutrition or hydration at the end of life? *Curr Opin Support Palliat Care* **6**(3): 365–370.

https://www.aic.sg/care-services/advance-care-planning.

Swarm RA, Paice JA, Anghelescu DL, *et al.* (2019) Adult Cancer Pain, Version 3.2019, NCCN Clinical Practice Guidelines in Oncology. *J Natl Compr Canc Netw* **17**(8): 977–1007.

Index

Contents (Back)

www.ingramcontent.com/pod-product-compliance
Lightning Source LLC
Chambersburg PA
CBHW081416220926
51613CB00011B/258